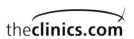

CRITICAL CARE NURSING CLINICS OF NORTH AMERICA

Pediatric Critical Care

GUEST EDITOR
Patricia A. Moloney-Harmon, RN, MS,
CCNS, CCRN, FAAN

CONSULTING EDITOR
Suzanne S. Prevost, PhD, RN

December 2005 • Volume 17 • Number 4

SAUNDERS

An Imprint of Elsevier, Inc.
PHILADELPHIA   LONDON   TORONTO   MONTREAL   SYDNEY   TOKYO

W.B. SAUNDERS COMPANY
A Division of Elsevier Inc.

Elsevier Inc., 1600 John F. Kennedy Blvd., Suite 1800, Philadelphia, PA 19103-2899.

http://www.theclinics.com

CRITICAL CARE NURSING CLINICS OF NORTH AMERICA   Volume 17, Number 4
December 2005   ISSN 0899-5885
Editor: Maria Lorusso   ISBN 1-4160-2653-3

Reprints. For copies of 100 or more, of articles in this publication, please contact the Commercial Reprints Department, Elsevier Inc., 360 Park Avenue South, New York, New York 10010-1710. Tel. (212) 633-3813 Fax: (212) 462-1935 e-mail: reprints@elsevier.com

The ideas and opinions expressed in *Critical Care Nursing Clinics of North America* do not necessarily reflect those of the Publisher. The Publisher does not assume any responsibility for any injury and/or damage to persons or property arising out of or related to any use of the material contained in this periodical. The reader is advised to check the appropriate medical literature and the product information currently provided by the manufacturer of each drug to be administered to verify the dosage, the method and duration of administration, or contraindications. It is the responsibility of the treating physician or other health care professional, relying on independent experience and knowledge of the patient, to determine drug dosages and the best treatment for the patient. Mention of any product in this issue should not be construed as endorsement by the contributors, editors, or the Publisher of the product or manufacturers' claims.

Critical Care Nursing Clinics of North America (ISSN 0899-5885) is published quarterly by W.B. Saunders Company. Corporate and editorial offices: Elsevier Inc., 1600 John F. Kennedy Blvd., Suite 1800, Philadelphia, PA 19103-2899. Accounting and circulation offices: 6277 Sea Harbor Drive, Orlando, FL 32887-4800. Periodicals postage paid at Orlando, FL 32862, and additional mailing offices. Subscription prices are $105.00 per year for US individuals, $175.00 per year for US institutions, $55.00 per year for US students and residents, $135.00 per year for Canadian individuals, $215.00 per year for Canadian institutions, $145.00 per year for international individuals, $215.00 per year for international institutions and $75.00 per year for Canadian and foreign students/residents. To receive student/resident rate, orders must be accompanied by name of affiliated institution, date of term, and the *signature* of program/residency coordinator on institution letterhead. Orders will be billed at individual rate until proof of status is received. Foreign air speed delivery is included in all *Clinics* subscription prices. All prices are subject to change without notice. POSTMASTER: Send address changes to *Critical Care Nursing Clinics of North America,* W.B. Saunders Company, Periodicals Fulfillment, Orlando, FL 32887-4800. **Customer Service: 1-800-654-2452 (US). From outside of the US, call 1-407-345-4000.**

Critical Care Nursing Clinics of North America is covered in *International Nursing Index, Nursing Citation Index, Cumulative Index to Nursing and Allied Health Literature, and RNdex Top 100.*

Printed in the United States of America.

GOAL STATEMENT

The goal of *Critical Care Nursing Clinics of North America* is to keep practicing critical care nurses up to date with current critical care clinical practice by providing timely articles reviewing the state of the art in critical care.

ACCREDITATION
The *Critical Care Nursing Clinics of North America* is planned and implemented in accordance with the Essential Areas and Policies of the Accreditation Council for Continuing Medical Education (ACCME) through the joint sponsorship of the University of Virginia School of Medicine and Elsevier. The University of Virginia School of Medicine is accredited by the ACCME to provide continuing medical education for physicians.

The University of Virginia School of Medicine designates this educational activity for a maximum of 60 category 1 credits per year, 15 category 1 credits per issue, toward the AMA Physician's Recognition Award. Each practitioner should claim only those credits that he/she actually spent in the activity.
NOTE: The American Nurses Credentialing Center (ANCC), and many State Boards accept AMA category 1 credit issued by an ACCME provider to maintain ANA certifications or licensure. 15 AMA category 1 credits are equivalent to 18 ANA contact hours.

The American Medical Association has determined that physicians not licensed in the US who participate in this CME activity are eligible for AMA PRA category 1 credit.

Category 1 credit can be earned by reading the text material, taking the CME examination online at http://www.theclinics.com/home/cme, and completing the evaluation. After taking the test, you will be required to review any and all incorrect answers. Following completion of the test and evaluation, your credit will be awarded and you may print your certificate.

FACULTY DISCLOSURE/CONFLICT OF INTEREST

The University of Virginia School of Medicine, as an ACCME accredited provider, endorses and strives to comply with the Accreditation Council for Continuing Medical Education (ACCME) Standards of Commercial Support, Commonwealth of Virginia statutes, University of Virginia policies and procedures, and associated federal and private regulations and guidelines on the need for disclosure and monitoring of proprietary and financial interests that may affect the scientific integrity and balance of content delivered in continuing medical education activities under our auspices.

The University of Virginia School of Medicine requires that all CME activities accredited through this institution be developed independently and be scientifically rigorous, balanced and objective in the presentation/discussion of its content, theories and practices.

All authors/editors participating in an accredited CME activity are expected to disclose to the readers relevant financial relationships with commercial entities occurring within the past 12 months (such as grants or research support, employee, consultant, stock holder, member of speakers bureau, etc.). The University of Virginia School of Medicine will employ appropriate mechanisms to resolve potential conflicts of interest to maintain the standards of fair and balanced education to the reader. Questions about specific strategies can be directed to the Office of Continuing Medical Education, University of Virginia School of Medicine, Charlottesville, Virginia.

The authors/editors listed below have identified no professional or financial affiliations for themselves or their spouse/partner:
Marie Antonacci, BScN; Dorothy M. Beke, RN, MS, CPNP; Jennifer E. Bevacqua, RN, BSN, CCRN; Nancy J. Braudis, RN, MS, CPNP; Beverley Copnell, RN, RSCN, BappSc, PhD; Jill Renee Hecker Fernandes, MSN, RNC, APRN-FNP; Frances Fothergill-Bourbonnais, RN, PhD; Allen D. Frye, RN, C, BS, CCRN; Patricia Lincoln, RN, MS; Maria Lorusso, Acquisitions Editor; Linda Masse, MScA, LLM; Carla Nelson, MPH, CPHQ; Bonnie A. Rice, ARNP, MSN, CCNS; Janlyn R. Rozdilsky, RN, MN, CNCCP; Lauren R. Sorce, RN, MSN, CCRN, CPNP; and Margot Thomas, RN, MScN, CNCC.

The authors listed below have not provided disclosure for themselves or their spouse/partner:
Dirk R. G. Danschutter, RN, CCRN, CP; Erwin Ista, RN; Koen Josten, MD, PhD; Maureen A. Madden, MSN; Kelly Keefe Marcoux, MSN, CPNP-AC, APRN_BC, CCRN; Patricia A. Moloney-Harmon, RN, MSN, CCNS, CCRN, FAAN; and Kathryn E. Roberts, MSN, CRNP, CCRN.

Disclosure of Discussion of non-FDA approved uses for pharmaceutical products and/or medical devices:
The University of Virginia School of Medicine, as an ACCME provider, requires that all faculty presenters identify and disclose any "off label" uses for pharmaceutical and medical device products. The University of Virginia School of Medicine recommends that each physician fully review all the available data on new products or procedures prior to instituting them with patients.

TO ENROLL

To enroll in the Critical Care Nursing Clinics of North America Continuing Medical Education program, call customer service at 1-800-654-2452 or visit us online at **www.theclinics.com/home/cme**. The CME program is available to subscribers for an additional fee of $99.00

CONSULTING EDITOR

SUZANNE S. PREVOST, PhD, RN, Nursing Professor and National HealthCare Chair of Excellence, Middle Tennessee State University, School for Nursing, Murfreesboro, Tennessee

EDITORIAL BOARD

RUTH KLEINPELL, PhD, RN, ACNP, FAAN, Associate Professor, Department of Adult Health Nursing, Rush University, Chicago, Illinois

STEPHEN D. KRAU, PhD, RN, Associate Professor, School of Nursing, Middle Tennessee State University, Murfreesboro; and Staff Nurse, Coronary Care Unit, Vanderbilt University Medical Center, Nashville, Tennessee

JANE LESKE, PhD, RN, Associate Professor, School of Nursing, University of Wisconsin-Milwaukee, Milwaukee, Wisconsin

CAROL A. RAUEN, MS, RN, CCRN, Instructor, School of Nursing and Health Studies, Georgetown University, Washington, DC

PAMELA RUDISILL, MSN, RN, CCRN, Associate Executive Director of Nursing, Lake Norman Regional Medical Center, Mooresville, North Carolina

MARILYN SAWYER SOMMERS, PhD, RN, FAAN, Professor, College of Nursing, University of Cincinnati, Cincinnati, Ohio

CATHY J. THOMPSON, PhD, RN, CCRN, Assistant Professor, School of Nursing, University of Colorado Health Sciences Center, Denver, Colorado

MARITA TITLER, PhD, RN, FAAN, Director of Nursing Research, Quality and Outcomes Management, Department of Nursing Services, University of Iowa Hospitals and Clinics, Iowa City, Iowa

MICHAEL WILLIAMS, MSN, RN, Assistant Professor, Department of Nursing, Eastern Michigan University, Ypsilanti, Michigan

GUEST EDITOR

PATRICIA A. MOLONEY-HARMON, RN, MS, CCNS, CCRN, FAAN, Advanced Practice Nurse/Clinical Nurse Specialist, Children's Services, Sinai Hospital of Baltimore, Baltimore, Maryland

CONTRIBUTORS

MARIE ANTONACCI, BScN, Assistant Head Nurse, Pediatric Intensive Care Unit, Montreal Children's Hospital, McGill University Centre, Montreal, Quebec, Canada

DOROTHY M. BEKE, RN, MS, CPNP, Clinical Nurse Specialist, Cardiac Intensive Care Unit, Children's Hospital, Boston, Massachusetts

JENNIFER E. BEVACQUA, RN, BSN, CCRN, Staff Nurse, Pediatric Intensive Care Unit, Emanuel Children's Hospital; Staff Nurse, Pediatric Post-Anesthesia Care Unit, Doernbecher Children's Hospital; Pediatric Nurse Practitioner Student, Oregon Health & Science University, Portland, Oregon

NANCY J. BRAUDIS, RN, MS, CPNP, Clinical Nurse Specialist, Cardiac Intensive Care Unit, Children's Hospital, Boston, Massachusetts

BEVERLEY COPNELL, RN, RSCN, BAppSC, PhD, Postdoctoral Research Fellow, The Royal Children's Hospital; Murdoch Children's Research Institute, Melbourne, Australia

DIRK R.G. DANSCHUTTER, RN, CCRN, CP, Chief Nurse, Pediatric Intensive Care Unit, Free University Hospital, Brussels, Belgium

JILL RENEE HECKER FERNANDES, MSN, RNC, APRN-FNP, Clinical Instructor, Department of Family Health Nursing, University of Wisconsin Eau Claire, College of Nursing and Health Sciences, Eau Claire, Wisconsin

FRANCES FOTHERGILL-BOURBONNAIS, RN, PhD, Full Professor of Nursing, School of Nursing, Faculty of Health Sciences, University of Ottawa, Ottawa, Canada

ALLEN D. FRYE, RN C, BS, CCRN, Clinical Leader, Division of Pediatric Critical Care, Children's Hospital, Columbus, Ohio

ERWIN ISTA, RN, Department of Pediatrics, Pediatric Intensive Care Unit, Erasmus MC - Sophia Children's Hospital, Rotterdam, The Netherlands

KOEN JOOSTEN, MD, PhD, Department of Pediatrics, Pediatric Intensive Care Unit, Erasmus MC - Sophia Children's Hospital, Rotterdam, The Netherlands

PATRICIA LINCOLN, RN, MS, Clinical Nurse Specialist, Cardiac Intensive Care Unit, Children's Hospital, Boston, Massachusetts

MAUREEN A. MADDEN, MSN, PNP-AC, FCCM, Assistant Professor of Pediatrics, Division of Critical Care Medicine, UMDNJ-Robert Wood Johnson Medical School; Pediatric Critical Care Nurse Practitioner, Bristol-Myers Squibb Children's Hospital at Robert Wood Johnson University Hospital, New Brunswick, New Jersey

KELLY KEEFE MARCOUX, MSN, CPNP-AC, APRN-BC, CCRN, Clinical Assistant Professor of Pediatrics, UMDNJ/Robert Wood Johnson Medical School; Pediatric Critical Care Nurse Practitioner, Bristol-Myer's Squibb Children's Hospital, New Brunswick, New Jersey

LINDA MASSÉ, MScA, LLM, Advanced Practice Nurse/Clinical Nurse Specialist, Pediatric Intensive Care Unit, Montreal Children's Hospital, McGill University Centre, Montreal, Quebec, Canada

PATRICIA A. MOLONEY-HARMON, RN, MS, CCNS, CCRN, FAAN, Advanced Practice Nurse/Clinical Nurse Specialist, Children's Services, Sinai Hospital of Baltimore, Baltimore, Maryland

CARLA NELSON, MPH, CPHQ, Outcomes Coordinator, Quality and Outcomes Department, All Children's Hospital, Saint Petersburg, Florida

BONNIE A. RICE, ARNP, MSN, CCNS, RN, Systems Administrator, Quality and Outcome Department, All Children's Hospital, Saint Petersburg, Florida

KATHRYN E. ROBERTS, MSN, RN, CRNP, CCRN, Clinical Nurse Specialist, Pediatric Intensive Care Unit, The Children's Hospital of Philadelphia, Philadelphia, Pennsylvania

JANLYN R. ROZDILSKY, RN, MN, CNCCP(C), Clinical Nurse Educator, Pediatric Intensive Care Unit, Royal University Hospital, Saskatoon, Saskatchewan, Canada

LAUREN R. SORCE, RN, MSN, CCRN, CPNP-AC/PC, Pediatric Nurse Practitioner, Pediatric Critical Care, Children's Memorial Hospital, Chicago, Illinois

MARGOT THOMAS, RN, MScN, CNCCP(C), Advanced Practice Nurse, Pediatric Intensive Care Unit, Children's Hospital of Eastern Ontario, Ottawa, Canada

CONTENTS

unscathed from the use of the medications, some suffer adverse responses. This article elucidates adverse responses to these medications for the APN, including withdrawal syndrome, muscle weakness, decreased gastric motility, corneal abrasions, and costs associated with these morbidities.

FORTHCOMING ISSUES

RECENT ISSUES

THE CLINICS ARE NOW AVAILABLE ONLINE!

Access your subscription at:
www.theclinics.com

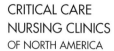

CRITICAL CARE
NURSING CLINICS
OF NORTH AMERICA

ELSEVIER
SAUNDERS

Crit Care Nurs Clin N Am 17 (2005) xv – xvi

Preface

Pediatric Critical Care

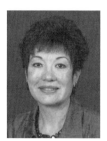

Patricia A. Moloney-Harmon, RN, MS, CCNS, CCRN, FAAN
Guest Editor

Pediatric critical care nursing as a specialty has evolved tremendously since the 1950s when the first pediatric ICU (PICU) programs were developed. The knowledge explosion brought about by the increasingly complex technology, the ongoing development of new treatments, and the pressure of regulatory agencies provide pediatric critical care nurses with new challenges and opportunities. Practicing as a nurse in this complex environment requires a strong foundation in the fundamentals, skilled evidence-based clinical practice, a thirst for ongoing learning, and a desire to provide a reassuring presence to child and family. Pediatric critical care nurses establish an environment in which critically ill infants and children and their families are the recipients of the coordinated efforts and observant care of a extremely well-skilled group of pediatric health care professionals [1]. In addition, pediatric critical care nurses ensure that patients and families are not only recipients of care, but that they become partners with the health care team in assuring the best possible outcome. As a distinguished nursing leader from the United States noted, nursing is the intensity in ICU care [2]; the constant within the intensity of the pediatric critical care environment is the pediatric critical care nurse [1]. The components of pediatric critical care nursing practice include the nurse at the bedside, professional development which assures that lifelong learning can occur, and nursing leadership

who facilitates a healthy work environment so that nurses can make their optimal contribution [1]. Indeed, the art and science of pediatric critical care have matured over the past 5 decades.

As the art and science of pediatric critical care nursing practice has evolved, it has become more global. There have been four World Congresses of Pediatric Intensive Care; establishment of the International Pediatric Intensive Care Nurses Association in 2003 (which meets regularly by way of a list serve); publishing of *Pediatric Intensive Care Nursing*, the official journal of the International Pediatric Intensive Care Nurses Association; and development of the World Federation of Pediatric Intensive and Critical Care Societies. All of these provide a forum for pediatric critical care nurses from around the world to come together electronically or in person to exchange ideas and focus on the care of critically ill infants and children and their families. Because of this ability to interface, barriers have come down and our specialty has benefited greatly.

This issue of *Critical Care Nursing Clinics of North America* is dedicated to nurses from around the world who have chosen to care for critically ill infants and children and their families. This is an outstanding compendium of contributions that deals with issues in pediatric critical care nursing, not only from the United States, but also from Canada, Europe, and Australia. These authors exemplify a commitment to

0899-5885/05/$ – see front matter
doi:10.1016/j.ccell.2005.08.003

establishing that environment in which critically ill infants and children and their families benefit from the expertise of the nurses who are caring for them. Frye discusses the care of the child who has acute lung injury and acute respiratory distress syndrome, a devastating final common pathway that is seen in the PICU. Fernandes advances the science of pediatric critical care nursing by discussing the results of a study that examined parents' experiences with a child who has a congenital heart defect. Thomas also advances the science by discussing the results of her study, which examined the cues that expert pediatric critical care nurses use in making clinical judgments about suctioning intubated and ventilated, critically ill children. Bevacqua describes the expert nursing management of the child in diabetic ketoacidosis, a frequently encountered endocrine emergency in the PICU. Copnell reviews current research concerning end-of-life care in the PICU, thus increasing knowledge for pediatric critical care nurses to act as advocates for patients and families. Roberts stimulates critical thinking by presenting case studies in fluid and electrolyte balance. Masse and Antonacci discuss the challenges of caring for the child who has low cardiac output syndrome, increasing knowledge in this area. Appropriate nutritional support is key to assuring a good outcome; Ista and Joosten provide information about nutritional assessment and enteral support in the critically ill child. Madden provides an in-depth examination of caring for the pediatric victim of toxic ingestion, a preventable cause of morbidity and mortality. Moloney-Harmon discusses pediatric sepsis, which remains a major cause of mortality in the pediatric critical care setting. Beke, Braudis, and Lincoln present a comprehensive discussion of caring for the child after cardiac surgery and describe the subtleties that the nurse must look for in managing this challenging patient population. Rice and Nelson address the issue of patient safety in the PICU, which is critically important to all of us in our roles as patient advocates. Sorce presents an update on the adverse response to sedation, analgesia, and neuromuscular blocking agents in critically ill children, which is another challenge for pediatric critical care nurses. Rozdilsky educates pediatric critical care nurses about the needs and reactions of well siblings which enables the nurse to optimize support. Marcoux reviews the care of the child who has status asthmaticus, one of the most common reasons for admission to the PICU, and thus, provides current information to facilitate optimal care. Finally, Danschutter describes in vivid detail his experience as a member of a disaster response team from Belgium that cared for the pediatric victims of the tsunami of 2004. His story is a tribute to all of the victims as well as his colleagues and the profession of nursing.

This issue celebrates the global commitment that pediatric critical care nurses make to their patients and families every day. It also acknowledges the incredible contributions that are made by nurses to caring for children and families. I am proud to be a colleague of these dedicated professionals and I thank them for their contributions and their commitment.

Patricia A. Moloney-Harmon, RN, MS,
CCNS, CCRN, FAAN
Children's Services, Sinai Hospital of Baltimore
125 West Lafayette Avenue
Baltimore, MD 21217, USA

References

[1] Curley MAQ. The essence of pediatric critical care nursing. In: Curley MAQ, Moloney-Harmon PA, editors. Critical care nursing of infants and children. 2nd edition. Philadelphia: WB Saunders; 2001. p. 3–16.
[2] Diers D. Nursing: implementing the agenda for social change. Presented at the 50th Anniversary Symposium: Nursing as a force in social change. University of Pennsylvania School of Nursing, Philadelphia, September 20, 1985.

CRITICAL CARE
NURSING CLINICS
OF NORTH AMERICA

Crit Care Nurs Clin N Am 17 (2005) 311–318

Acute Lung Injury and Acute Respiratory Distress Syndrome in The Pediatric Patient

Allen D. Frye, RN C, BS, CCRN

Division of Pediatric Critical Care, Children's Hospital, 700 Children's Drive, Columbus, OH 43205, USA

The ultimate goal of pediatric critical care is to meet the challenge of balancing oxygen delivery with oxygen demand. This challenge is clearly evident in patients who are admitted to the pediatric ICU with an acute lung injury (ALI). ALI encompasses a spectrum of inflammatory responses to the inciting event. ALI can result from a direct insult to the lung from aspiration of gastric content, pneumonia, inhalation of toxic vapors, or pulmonary contusion. Secondary or indirect lung injury can occur as the result of systemic inflammatory mediators being activated by acute pancreatitis, cardiopulmonary bypass, multisystem trauma, reaction to transfusion therapy, drug overdose, and sepsis. The final common pathway of ALI is an inflammatory-mediated response at the level of the alveolar capillary membrane which results in membrane destruction [1]. The spectrum of ALI ranges from mild to the most severe injury known as Acute Respiratory Distress Syndrome (ARDS). Over the past decade, research efforts have been aimed at understanding, modulating, and decreasing the inflammatory response experienced at the alveolar capillary membrane level, improving gas exchange, and preventing further injury induced by mechanical ventilation. Despite our advances in understanding the cellular mechanisms at work and providing targeted interventions, the mortality for ARDS continues to be significant and ranges from 5 to 30% [2]. The care of these critically ill children requires a fundamental understanding of the physiologic mechanisms at work, and implementation of evidenced-based practices that decrease morbidity and mortality.

Common ground: a working definition

In 1994, the North American–European Consensus Conference (NAECC) on ARDS proposed a definition for ALI and ARDS [3]. The NAECC recommendations acknowledged that pediatric patients experienced a similar physiologic response to ALI as did adult patients. The committee recommended that the name be changed from adult respiratory distress syndrome to acute respiratory distress syndrome. The current criteria for the diagnosis of ALI and ARDS include: an acute and persistent pulmonary process that demonstrates radiographic evidence of bilateral opacities in the absence of left-sided heart failure or clinical evidence of left atrial hypertension. The severity of lung injury is determined by evaluating the relationship of the patient's PaO_2 and the fraction of inspired oxygen (FIO_2) given to the patient. This relationship known as the P:F ratio is used to determine where in the spectrum of ALI the patient falls. The NAECC oxygenation criteria identifies a $PaO_2:FIO_2$ ratio of less than 300, regardless of positive end-expiratory pressure (PEEP), for patients who have ALI, and a $PaO_2:FIO_2$ ratio of less than 200, regardless of PEEP, for patients who have ARDS [3].

Pathophysiology

The functional unit of gas exchange in the pulmonary system is the alveolar–capillary membrane, across which the exchange of oxygen and carbon dioxide takes place by diffusion of gases. A thin layer of alveolar fluid—which is a complex mixture of

E-mail address: fryea@chi.osu.edu

doi:10.1016/j.ccell.2005.07.008

phospholipids and lipoproteins, called surfactant—lines the alveolus and reduces surface tension. By reducing the surface tension of the alveolus, surfactant diminishes the tendency for complete collapse. As gas diffuses across the alveolar–capillary membrane, oxygenated blood enters the capillary where oxygen attaches to the hemoglobin molecule, and carbon dioxide diffuses into the alveolus to be exhaled. This diffusion relationship—referred to as ventilation (V) and perfusion (Q) matching—requires adequate perfusion of the alveolus and effective ventilation to remove carbon dioxide.

When the alveolar–capillary membrane is subjected to toxic substances, such as gastric content, infection, or toxic vapors, an inflammatory-mediated response occurs. Proinflammatory cytokines, such as tumor necrosis factor, interleukin (IL)-1, and IL-8, are released in response to invasion of a foreign substance at the level of the alveolar–capillary endothelium [4]. As part of the inflammatory cascade, neutrophils are recruited to the lungs and release toxic mediators which further damage the alveolar endothelium and capillary endothelium. As a result, the normal protective barriers of the alveolar capillary membrane are lost, and protein is allowed to escape from the vascular space. During the acute derangement of the alveolar capillary environment, the ability to up-regulate alveolar fluid clearance may be lost [5]. The end result of the initial inflammatory cascade is that the alveolar spaces fill with bloody, proteinaceous edema and cellular debris. Functional surfactant is lost which results in alveolar collapse.

Clinical features

Early clinical features of ALI or progressive ARDS result from the effects of acute alveolar damage. Because the alveolar capillary membrane is injured, the V/Q mismatch results in hypoxemia. This is manifested clinically by an increasing oxygen requirement without noticeable increase in the PaO_2. Increased physiologic dead space by collapsed alveoli initially may not result in hypercarbia; however, the increased minute ventilation that is required to maintain a normal $PaCO_2$ results in tachypnea. A decreased pulmonary compliance is one of the hallmarks of ARDS. The low compliance or small physical lung volume, termed "baby lung," results in retractions to overcome the increased resistance to inspiration. On expiration, grunting may be noticeable in the nonintubated patient in an attempt to increase functional residual capacity (FRC) and improve oxygenation. As the diseases progresses, hyp-

oxemia and respiratory failure ensue which require endotracheal intubation and mechanical ventilation.

Mechanical ventilation strategies

Modern advances in the understanding and definition of ARDS have led to a change in the treatment modalities. As recently as a decade ago, ARDS was viewed as a homogeneous illness with poorly compliant lungs that required high pressures to ventilate [1,2,6]. The treatment aim in that philosophy was to ventilate the patient with the goal of maintaining control of $PaCO_2$. This treatment strategy often required high ventilating pressures that were counterintuitive. High ventilating pressures resulted in overdistention of the lung and tissue injury due to stretching of the air spaces. A second cause of tissue injury in this ventilation strategy was the repetitive collapse of edematous and surfactant-deficient alveoli at end-expiration, followed by forced reopening and distention during inspiration that produced a shearing-type injury to the tissue. In the early 1990s, understanding of the clinical illness of ARDS as a homogeneous process was challenged by Pelosi and colleagues. Through the use of CT, they were able to show that ARDS is a heterogeneous process with areas of dependent atelectasis, hyperinflation, and edema interspersed with normal regions [7–9]. Pelosi and colleagues asserted that what previously were believed to be stiff, noncompliant lungs actually were "small" lungs. This paradigm shift, coupled with the concepts of permissive hypercapnia and relative permissive hypoxemia, set the stage for the current strategic management of ARDS [10]. The strategic goals of ventilatory management in a patient who has ARDS include maintaining adequate gas exchange while avoiding ventilator-induced lung injury. In an attempt to provide direction in achieving these goals, investigators used the assertions of Pelosi and colleagues, as well as the concepts of ventilator-induced lung injury to reshape ventilatory management in this complex disease process.

Lung protective strategies

In 1998, Amato and colleagues published a study in the *New England Journal of Medicine* that outlined a "protective ventilation strategy" [11]. In this study, patients were randomized to a conventional treatment group or the "lung protective group." Patients who were randomized to the conventional group had volume-controlled ventilation titrated so that the

$PaCO_2$ was 35 to 38 mm Hg. Patients randomized to the "lung protective group" were ventilated with a lower tidal volume (<6 mL/kg) and a plateau pressure was kept at less than 20 cm H_2O greater than the PEEP. The 28-day mortality was significantly better in the low tidal volume group (38% versus 71%). This study set the stage for a change in practice in the treatment of patients who have ARDS. The largest study to date was published by the ARDS Network in the *New England Journal of Medicine* in 2000 [12]. This study randomized patients in a two-arm study that included a conventional treatment group and a lung protective group. Patients who were randomized to the conventional group received mechanical ventilation with tidal volumes of 12 mL/kg and a peak pressure of less than 50 cm H_2O. Patients who were randomized to the lung protective group received mechanical ventilation with the goal of a tidal volume of less than 6 mL/kg and a plateau pressure of less than 30 cm H_2O. In this study, the primary end point was mortality. After randomizing 861 patients, the study was stopped because there was a significant reduction in mortality among the low tidal volume strategy. These two studies provide evidence-based practice for using low tidal volumes and lower plateau pressures.

High-frequency oscillatory ventilation

The use of high-frequency oscillatory ventilation (HFOV) for ARDS is a topic of high-spirited debate among pediatric ICU clinicians. The advantages of using high-frequency ventilation therapies include: (1) the use of low tidal volume with improved lung recruitment and avoidance of alveolar shearing injury, and (2) the maintenance of near normal $PaCO_2$ with improved minute ventilation. Clinical evidence for the use of HFOV is lacking. Arnold and colleagues [13] published a report that was made up of data obtained from five tertiary pediatric ICUs. In this study, patients were randomized into HFOV with an "ideal lung recruitment" strategy or to a conventional ventilation group in which the main ventilation goals were limiting the FIO_2 and peak airway pressure while maintaining adequate oxygenation. Patients who failed the conventional ventilation arm were allowed to cross over to the HFOV group. The results of this study were interesting in that those who were randomized into the HFOV group had better outcomes than those who crossed over to HFOV [14]. This would seem to indicate that early intervention with HFOV provides a better outcome.

Adjunctive therapies

The patient who experiences ALI or ARDS requires a multifaceted approach to their care. Although effective mechanical ventilation strategies are essential in supporting the patient, the use of adjunctive therapies may contribute to decreased mortality, improved gas exchange, and decreased ventilator days.

Inhaled vasodilator therapy

Patients who experience ALI and ARDS develop some degree of pulmonary hypertension and increased pulmonary vascular resistance. Increased pulmonary pressures can have a negative effect on right ventricular function and result in dysfunction. In an attempt to minimize this effect, investigators have proposed the use of inhaled nitric oxide (iNO). Nitric oxide is a free radical gas produced in the lung that causes pulmonary vasodilatation and reduction in pulmonary vascular resistance. Improving pulmonary blood flow by selective pulmonary vasodilatation may improve oxygenation. Approximately 60% of patients who had ARDS or ALI of all causes responded to iNO, which increased their PaO_2 by more than 20% [15]. In theory, the use of iNO may yield improved oxygenation and pulmonary blood flow; however, in practice it did not demonstrate improved outcomes in clinical trials [15–18].

Corticosteroids

The use of corticosteroids remains controversial in the treatment of ALI and ARDS. As an adjunctive therapy, corticosteroids reduce the production of inflammatory and profibrotic mediators. Clinical trials in the 1980s demonstrated that the use of steroids early in the course of ARDS did not change outcomes or mortality. Some trials demonstrated an increased risk of infection, lower rates of reversal of ARDS, and increased mortality associated with the use of high-dose steroids. [19–22]. Although the use of corticosteroids in the early phases of ARDS has not shown to be beneficial, their use in the late phases (7–14 days from diagnosis) has not been abandoned. In one randomized trial, 24 patients who had "unresolving" ARDS of more than 7 days' duration received methylprednisolone in divided doses with an incremental taper. The patients in the steroid group all survived and were extubated. In the nonsteroid group, 5 of the 8 patients who were randomized to the placebo group died [22]. A larger National Institutes of Health ARDS Network Late Steroid Rescue Study may provide more sound evidence for prescribing low-dose steroids in late ARDS.

Prone positioning

Prone positioning, first proposed by Bryan in 1974 [23], has been shown to be beneficial in improving oxygenation in multiple clinical trials over the past 2 decades [24,25]. Understanding of the physiologic influences that prone positioning provides has been enhanced greatly through technologic advances and multiple clinical investigations. The mechanisms of improved oxygenation with prone positioning seem to be multifactorial. The primary beneficial effects include changes in perfusion and ventilation distributions. Secondary effects include mobilization and redistribution of secretions and pulmonary fluids.

The effects of prone positioning on ventilation can be theorized by first understanding the role of transpulmonary pressure (Ptp) [26]. Ptp is the difference between airway pressure and pleural pressure. This relationship estimates the alveolar distending pressure. Pleural pressures change in relation to gravitation influences. In the prone position, pleural pressure is minimized. Pleural pressures also may be influenced by the compressive effects of the heart on the lung parenchyma as well as the effects of transmitted pressure to the pleural space across the diaphragm. In the supine position, FRC is decreased secondary to upward displacement of the diaphragm due to intra-abdominal pressure. Loss of diaphragm tone or function secondary to sedation or chemical relaxation may increase this effect and further decrease FRC. Placing patients in the prone position with the abdomen unsupported allows abdominal weight to become less restrictive and the diaphragm can move downward, thereby increasing FRC. This concept is essential to understand, as it often is the practice to place the patient in the prone position with the abdomen supported. Positioning so that the patient's chest and pelvis are supported while the abdomen hangs free often can present a challenge, depending on the size of the patient's abdomen.

The second factor in influencing Ptp is manipulating the airway pressure. Airway pressures can be manipulated by changing PEEP in an effort to recruit nonventilated regions of the lung. Prone positioning may allow for redistribution of lung water, improved secretion clearance, and redistribution of lung density. The addition of PEEP assists in recruiting nonventilated regions of the lungs by preventing complete collapse of the alveoli. Recruitment of alveoli improves the ventilation component of V/Q matching at the level of the alveolar capillary membrane.

Responders versus nonresponders

Clinical trials that focus on prone positioning classify patients primarily into two categories: responders and nonresponders. A responder is defined as a patient who demonstrates an appreciable change in oxygenation, as evidenced by a 20 mm Hg or greater improvement in their $PaO_2:FIO_2$ ratio, when changed from the supine to prone position. Nonresponders lack a favorable change in oxygenation when placed in the prone position. Patients who are nonresponders during one episode of prone positioning may convert to being a responder in another episode of prone positioning. Although methods of predicting who will have a positive response to prone positioning are not well-studied, patients with certain pathophysiology are more likely to respond to prone positioning than others. Patients who present with early diffuse injury that is characterized by edematous lungs and dependent (posterior) collapse are expected to have the best positive response to prone positioning. Patients who have fibrosis or predominately anterior infiltrates are less likely to respond to prone positioning. Patients who have high intra-abdominal pressures may benefit from prone positioning, provided that the abdomen is allowed to hang unsupported.

Timing of prone positioning

The use of prone positioning is a widely accepted adjunctive therapy in the management of patients who have ALI and ARDS. The concept that is not as widely accepted among clinicians is the duration of prone positioning that yields the most benefits. Curley and colleagues [27] were among the first investigators to describe the benefit of prolonged periods of prone positioning in the pediatric patient. In this study, they implemented prone positioning early in the patients' clinical course and maintained the prone position for greater than 20 hours daily. In a study published in *Chest*, Relvas and colleagues [28] attempted to determine if pediatric patients who were placed in the prone position continued to receive the benefit of prone positioning past 12 hours. In this study, they divided pediatric patients into two groups, those who were prone from 6 to 10 hours and those who were prone for a prolonged period of time (18–24 hours). They found that patients who were prone for prolonged periods (18–24 hours) had a more pronounced and stable reduction in their oxygen index values in comparison with those who were prone for short periods of time.

Nutrition

Among the adjunctive therapies for ALI and ARDS, probably the most important intervention that will have a sustained measurable impact is nutritional supplementation. Patients who are critically ill often experience barriers to receiving optimal nutrition, such as fluid restriction, gastrointestinal hypoperfusion, paralytic ileus, and pancreatitis. To recover from serious illness, nutritional stores must be repleted and caloric requirements must be met to avoid metabolic acidosis. The overall goals of nutritional support for pediatric patients who have ALI and ARDS are to modulate the immune response to disease, prevent bacterial translocation from the gut, and support the patient during his hypermetabolic state to reduce the risk of protein energy malnutrition [29].

Nutritional support is available for critically ill children primarily in two forms. Parenteral nutrition can be used to meet the macronutrients and micronutrients of the patient who may not be able to absorb nutrients from the gut, or has some abdominal pathology that prohibits using the gastrointestinal tract. When initiating parenteral nutrition, the primary goal is to increase the glucose concentration incrementally to avoid hyperglycemia while attempting to maximize caloric intake. Protein in parenteral nutrition is provided in the form of amino acids which are necessary for tissue growth, enzymatic reactions, and nitrogen balance. The amino acid compound in parenteral nutrition for infants less than 6 months of age is provided as TrophAmine, which is based on the protein makeup of breast milk. Children older than 6 months of age are given amino acids in the form of Aminosyn, which is similar to the protein required for adult metabolism [29]. In addition to carbohydrates and amino acids, patients on parenteral nutrition also receive lipid emulsion supplementation.

Enteral nutrition, if tolerated, is the preferred route of nutrition for all patients. Enteral nutrition has several advantages over parenteral nutrition, including maintenance of a protective barrier in the intestine which prevents bacterial translocation, maintenance of gut function, and possible enhancement of immune modulation. When selecting an enteral formula the clinician must consider the patient's age, gastrointestinal function, and the caloric density of the formula. The American Academy of Pediatrics recommends the use of breast milk when possible for infants. Commercially available infant formulas are designed to mimic the contents of breast milk when breast milk is not available [30]. Patients who are 1 to 10 years of age may be started on a commercially prepared enteral formula which typically provides a higher caloric value with higher amounts of calcium, phosphorus, and vitamins than infant formulas. Patients who are older than 10 years of age can tolerate formulas that are prepared for adult enteral nutrition.

Immune modulation using enteral formulas is an up and coming area of research that has shown promise in the adult population. Patients who have ARDS may benefit from a diet that is low in carbohydrates and high in linolenic acid and antioxidants. Formulas that have antioxidant properties may enhance immune function, which ultimately improves patient outcomes and shortens the hospital length of stay. Further research is necessary to evaluate the efficacy of these formulas in the pediatric population.

Rescue therapy

Despite the combination of mainstay and adjunctive therapies for pediatric ARDS, the mortality remains significant. In an effort to gain recovery time for the lungs, extracorporeal membrane oxygenation (ECMO) may be used as a rescue therapy. ECMO is not curative, but is palliative in an attempt to support oxygenation requirements until the lungs are healed enough to resume physiologic function. Depending on the support needed, EMCO may be used as pulmonary support by using veno-venous ECMO, or cardiopulmonary support by using veno-arterial ECMO. Patients who are placed on ECMO for ALI and ARDS typically require a prolonged period of support.

Nursing care

Care of the pediatric patient who is experiencing ALI or ARDS requires input from all members of the critical care team. A plan of care that incorporates input from critical care physicians, highly skilled bedside nurses, respiratory therapists, and ancillary staff is essential to coordinating care that meets the patient's needs. Pediatric patients who experience respiratory distress often are irritable and tire easily. Stimulation should be kept to a minimum, whereas comfort measures should be maximized. Early discussion with the parents of the pediatric patient who is experiencing respiratory distress from an ALI should include the potential for necessary mechanical support. The primary goal of nursing care is to maximize oxygen delivery and minimize oxygen consumption through the use of collaborative, coordinated care.

Assessment

The nurse who is providing care for the patient who has an ALI must be able to detect subtle changes so that early intervention can be provided. Pediatric patients who experience altered pulmonary function often have a prolonged period of compensation that is followed by an acute decompensation when reserves are exhausted. Prevention of a clinical crisis for the patient can be achieved by frequent assessment of the patient's vital signs, careful attention to changes in lung compliance and oxygen requirements, observation of changes in level of consciousness, and changes in peripheral perfusion. Hemodynamics and ventilator parameters should be assessed frequently to note subtle changes.

Sedation

The use of judicious sedation is essential in the management of patients who are mechanically ventilated. A certain amount of discomfort is inherent to being intubated and mechanically ventilated; it is incumbent on the nurse to ensure adequate sedation. Agitation and anxiety may increase oxygen consumption by as much as 18%, whereas sleep, relaxation, and pain relief may decrease oxygen consumption by 25% to 50% [30].

Benzodiazepines and opioids are the mainstay in the sedation arsenal of the pediatric ICU. Continuous opioid infusions, such as fentanyl or morphine, may be necessary to achieve adequate sedation. Some clinicians may prefer to provide synergy with the sedative and anxiolytic properties of benzodiazepines in addition to continuous opioids [31]. Patients who are on continuous infusions of benzodiazepines, such as lorazepam and midazolam, should be monitored for development of an anion gap metabolic acidosis which may develop secondary to the alcohol-based preservative.

Chemical relaxants

The routine use of chemical relaxants to achieve paralysis has fallen out of favor over the past few years. The use of chemical relaxants should be limited to patients who experience patient-ventilator asynchrony, despite deep sedation. Prolonged muscle weakness has been attributed to the long-term use of chemical relaxants, especially when used in combination with steroids or some antimicrobial agents [32]. If chemical relaxation is used, it is imperative that adequate sedation is provided.

Pulmonary hygiene

Pulmonary hygiene maneuvers, such as chest physiotherapy and suctioning, are used often as a method of clearing bronchial secretions and recruiting atelectatic lung. These maneuvers often are considered standard care practices, despite limited evidence of their effectiveness [33]. These maneuvers may have a profound effect on the patient's oxygen consumption and result in a 30% to 35% increase in consumption [34]. Care must be taken by the bedside nurse to coordinate pulmonary hygiene maneuvers with the respiratory therapist so that the sedation level may be adjusted to account for the potential agitation and anxiety that occur during chest physiotherapy and suctioning. During suctioning, patients may require preoxygenation and manual ventilation with low tidal volumes and prolonged inspiratory times with PEEP that matches that of the ventilator settings. Patients who are on high-frequency oscillation should have limited disruption in the maintenance of mean airway pressure by using a closed-suction system for suctioning.

The nurse's role in positioning

Placing a critically ill patient in the prone position requires planning, team collaboration, and frequent assessment. The bedside nurse needs to develop a carefully thought out plan that addresses patient safety, security of invasive lines and tubes, appropriate amount of staff necessary to complete the procedure safely, anticipation of how care will be delivered in the prone position, and an emergency supine procedure if it should be necessary. Before the team is assembled to turn the patient in the prone position, the bedside nurse systematically performs an assessment of baseline hemodynamics and respiratory parameters and takes inventory of all appliances and invasive lines that need to be secured. All invasive lines that are inserted from the waist up are positioned toward the head of the bed. All invasive lines that are inserted from the waist down are positioned toward the foot of the bed. Chest tubes are positioned so that the tubing and collection chamber is toward the foot of the bed. The endotracheal tube is assessed to ensure that it is taped securely to avoid unplanned extubation. All extremity and abdominal dressing changes and oral care, including suctioning of the naso-oropharynx, are completed before the proning procedure. Eye care is performed to decrease the incidence of corneal abrasions. Enteral feeds are stopped 1 hour before the turn to decrease the risk of aspiration of gastric content. Several prone positioning methods have been published to accomplish safe patient management [35,36]. Once in the prone position, the patient is reassessed paying careful attention to the placement of the endotracheal tube, invasive lines, and appliances. An evaluation of the patient's hemodynamic status and respiratory parameters are noted for baseline data. Patients in the prone position for long periods of time will develop dependent facial edema. Care is taken to monitor the placement of the endotracheal tube in relation to the teeth or gums, rather than in relation to the lip as a reference mark. Extremities are in neutral positions and the head, neck, chest, and pelvis are supported. Pressure ulcers are the most common complication that is experienced by patients in the prone position. This complication may be minimized by frequently rotating the patient slightly so that weight is redistributed. Care of the patient in the prone position can present a logistical challenge. Careful planning and collaboration with team members is the key to providing safe care with minimal complications.

Summary

Despite the tremendous advances in our understanding of the pathophysiology at work in patients who have ALI, few interventions actually demonstrate decreased mortality and morbidity in patients who have ALI or ARDS. Data extrapolated from adult studies have shown some promise in the treatment of pediatric patients; however, clinical trials that address the unique features of the pediatric population are necessary for further advancement in the management of this devastating disorder. Care of these complex patients requires the efforts of the entire health care team.

References

[1] Anderson MR. Update on pediatric acute respiratory distress syndrome. Resp Care 2003;48(3):261–78.

[2] Dahlem P, van Aalderen WM, de Neef M, et al. Incidence and short-term outcome of acute lung injury in mechanically ventilated children. Eur Respir J 2003; 22(6):980–5.

[3] Bernard G, Artogas A, Carlet J, et al. The American-European Consensus Conference on ARDS: definitions, mechanisms, relevant outcomes, and clinical trial coordination. Am J Respir Crit Care Med 1994;149:818–24.

[4] Martin TR. Lung cytokines and ARDS. Chest 1999; 116:2S–8S.

[5] Ware LB, Matthay MA. Alveolar fluid clearance is impaired in the majority of patients with acute lung injury and the acute respiratory distress syndrome. Am J Respir Crit Care Med 2001;163(6):1376–83.

[6] Carpenter T. Novel approaches in conventional mechanical ventilation for paediatric acute lung injury. Ped Respir Rev 2004;5(3):231–7.

[7] Pelosi P, D'Andrea L, Vitale G, et al. Vertical gradient of regional lung inflation in adult respiratory distress syndrome. Am J Respir Crit Care Med 1994;149: 8–13.

[8] Pelosi P, Crotti S, Brazzi L, et al. Computed tomography in adult respiratory distress syndrome: what has it taught us? Eur Respir J 1996;9:1055–62.

[9] Gattinoni L, D'Andrea L, Pelosi P, et al. Regional effects and mechanisms of positive end-expiratory pressure in early adult respiratory distress syndrome. JAMA 1993;269:2122–7.

[10] Pierson DJ. The future of respiratory care. Respir Care 2001;46:705–18.

[11] Amato MB, Barbas CS, Medeiros DM, et al. Effect of a protective-ventilation strategy on mortality in the acute distress syndrome. N Engl J Med 1998;338(6): 347–54.

[12] The Acute Respiratory Distress Syndrome Network. Ventilation with lower tidal volumes as compared with traditional tidal volumes for acute lung injury and the acute respiratory distress syndrome. N Engl J Med 2000;342(18):1301–8.

[13] Arnold JH, Truog RD, Thompson JE, et al. High-frequency oscillatory ventilation in pediatric respiratory failure. Crit Care Med 1993;21(2):272–8.

[14] Arnold JH, Hanson JH, Toro-Figuero LO, et al. Prospective, randomized comparison of high-frequency oscillatory ventilation and conventional mechanical ventilation in pediatric respiratory failure. Crit Care Med 1994;22(10):1530–9.

[15] Dellinger RP, Zimmerman JL, Taylor RW, et al. Effects of inhaled nitric oxide in patients with acute respiratory distress syndrome: results of a randomized phase II trial. Inhaled Nitric Oxide in ARDS Study Group. Crit Care Med 1998;26:15–23.

[16] Michael JR, Barton RG, Saffle JR, et al. Inhaled nitric oxide versus conventional therapy: effect on oxygenation in ARDS. Am J Respir Crit Care Med 1998; 157(5 Pt1):1372–80.

[17] Troncy E, Collet JP, Shapiro S, et al. Inhaled nitric oxygen in acute respiratory distress syndrome: a pilot randomized controlled study. Am J Respir Crit Care Med 1998;157(5 Pt 1):1483–8.

[18] Lundin S, Mang H, Smithies M, et al. Inhalation of nitric oxide in acute lung injury: results of a European multicentre study. The European Study Group of Inhaled Nitric Oxide. Intensive Care Med 1999;25: 911–9.

[19] Weigelt JA, Norcross JR, Borman KR, et al. Early steroid therapy for respiratory failure. Arch Surg 1985; 120:536–40.

[20] Bernard GR, Luce JM, Sprung CL, et al. High-dose

corticosteroids in patients with the adult respiratory distress syndrome. N Engl J Med 1987;317:1565–70.

[21] Bone RC, Fisher Jr CJ, Clemmer TP, et al. A controlled clinical trial of high-dose methylprednisolone in the treatment of severe sepsis and septic shock. N Engl J Med 1987;317:653–8.

[22] Meduri GU, Headley AS, Golden E, et al. Effect of prolonged methylprednisolone therapy in resolving acute respiratory distress syndrome: a randomized controlled trial. JAMA 1998;280:159–65.

[23] Bryan AC. Comments of a devil's advocate. Am Rev Disease 1974;110(6, pt2):143–4.

[24] Stocker R, Stein S, Ecknauer E, et al. Prone positioning and low-volume pressure limited ventilation improves survival in patients with severe ARDS. Chest 1997;111:1008–17.

[25] Gattinoni L, Pesenti A, Taccone P, et al. Effects of prone positioning on the survival of patients with acute respiratory failure. N Engl J Med 2001;345:568–73.

[26] Culver B. Respiratory mechanics. In: Albert RK, editor. Clinical respiratory medicine. 2nd edition. Philadelphia: Mosby; 2004. p. 65–9.

[27] Curley MAQ, Thompson JE, Arnold JH. The effects of early and repeated prone positioning in pediatric patients with acute lung injury. Chest 2000;118: 156–63.

[28] Relvas MS, Silver PC, Sagy M. Prone positioning of pediatric patients with ARDS in improvement in oxygenation if maintained >12 h daily. Chest 2003; 124(1):269–74.

[29] Heird W. Amino acids in pediatric and neonate nutrition. Curr Opin Clin Nutr Metab Care 1988;1: 73–8.

[30] American Academy of Pediatrics. Breastfeeding and the use of human milk. Pediatrics 1997;100:1035–9.

[31] Brinker D.. Sedation and comfort issues in the ventilated infant and child. Crit Care Nurs Clin North Am 2004;16:365–77.

[32] Vender JS, Szolo JW, Murphy GS, et al. Sedation, analgesia, and neuromuscular blockade in sepsis: an evidence-based review. Crit Care Med 2004;32(11): S554–61.

[33] Main E, Castle R, Newham D, et al. Respiratory physiotherapy vs. suction: the effects on respiratory function in ventilated infants and children. Intensive Care Med 2004;30:1144–51.

[34] White KM, Winslow EH, Clark AP, et al. The physiologic basis for continuous mixed venous oxygen saturation monitoring. Heart Lung 1990;19:548–51.

[35] Balas MC. Prone positioning of patients with acute respiratory distress syndrome: applying research to practice. Crit Care Nurs 2000;20:24–36.

[36] Vollman KM. Manual pronation therapy. In: Lynn-McHale DL, Carlson KK, editors. AACN procedure manual for critical care. 4th edition. Philadelphia: WB Saunders; 2001. p. 83–94.

ELSEVIER
SAUNDERS

Crit Care Nurs Clin N Am 17 (2005) 319 – 327

CRITICAL CARE
NURSING CLINICS
OF NORTH AMERICA

The Experience of a Broken Heart

Jill Renee Hecker Fernandes, MSN, RNC, APRN-FNP

Department of Family Health Nursing, University of Wisconsin Eau Claire, College of Nursing and Health Sciences,
3624 Glen Way, Eau Claire, WI 54701, USA

Giving birth is usually a joyous occasion; however, the diagnosis of congenital heart disease (CHD) is difficult for families to understand. Many times these infants appear normal on the outside while their life-giving organ, "the heart," attempts to sustain life in its state of abnormality. Throughout history, the heart has been viewed by humanity not only as a life-sustaining organ, but also as a home for the soul, personality, and the very essence of the person's being [1].

The phenomenon of interest for this study was to discover what it is like, as the parent of a newborn infant, to be faced with the diagnosis of CHD. An inquiry into this area was done to help nurses and physicians better understand the emotional, physical, and psychologic needs of parents when they are faced with the diagnosis of CHD. Such knowledge is necessary because these infants present a physical challenge to the health care team and a psychologic challenge to the parents. Nurses who participate in the care of these infants and families need to realize what is necessary from the family's point of view, not to fix the "broken heart," but to assist in the "process of living, not just life itself" [1]. Further exploration of parental conceptions and feelings about CHD may be important in understanding how this diagnosis affects the family [2]. The results of this study present a useful addition to the care of families with infants who are diagnosed with CHD.

Studies that attempt to explain the emotional and spiritual needs in relation to patient care are common.

The studies attempt to quantify patient needs. In the world of family-centered care, quantification may not be enough to allow the nurses to connect with families at their level in that moment. The mother's experiences after learning her child's diagnosis include grief, loss of her imagined healthy child, lack of knowledge of the disease, anger, and difficulty in caregiving, among other issues [3]. A qualitative study that uses phenomenology can allow nurses to become as close as possible to the lived experience of the parents of these infants. Nurses interact with mothers on a more consistent basis than any other member of the health care team, and, thus, must seize these moments to provide adequate support and information [3]. A phenomenologic study of this experience will assist in narrowing the gaps that nurses may experience in relating to the parents of infants and responding to their emotional and physical needs.

Background

As far back as 1964, studies have attempted to understand what parents needed, experienced, and felt in relation to their child being diagnosed with CHD. In 1967, a study that examined the impact of CHD on the family concluded that this diagnosis often produces a harmful material and emotional impact on the family. The effects of the impact are determined largely by the parental characteristics, and certain families are "at risk." Other influences are the severity of the cardiac disorder and the quality of medical management and communication [4]. A study that examined the reactions of parents to the diagnosis of CHD was done by giving the parents a

---

E-mail address: rfernan9@aol.com

doi:10.1016/j.ccell.2005.08.001

list of words. The parents were asked to indicate the degree to which the words described a feeling that they may have felt. The data from this study demonstrate that all parents experience sadness, anger, and fear [5]. The results indicate a need to obtain more empiric data in relation to the reaction to the diagnosis of CHD. This study was a quantification of the degree of emotion; however, it is necessary to take this study one step further and understand the underlying real emotional reaction that exists for all parents. In 2002, a retrospective study was performed to clarify whether differences exist in parental stress when a child has complex versus minor CHD. The findings demonstrated that the severity of the child's CHD is of no distinct importance to the degree of parental stress. All families with the experience of CHD need the same amount of support and understanding, irrespective of the severity of diagnosis [6].

Several studies that are related to this topic described themes that were uncovered in the present study. An examination of the emotional implications of CHD in children noted a description of vague apprehension by parents. In this study, more than half of the mothers interviewed recalled that they had suspicions well before the diagnosis was made. Sometimes this feeling was based on nothing more than intuition [7]. Patients and families consistently describe the "feeling that something is not quite right." The mothers in this study had this feeling in relation to the pregnancy and birth of their infant.

The goal of an inquiry into the effects on the family with a child who is diagnosed with tetralogy of Fallot was to discover the practical problems with which these mothers are faced, and to document how the family as a whole, and the mother in particular, is affected and overcomes the disaster that has occurred [8]. The expressions that were used repeatedly by most parents to describe their feelings when they were told that the child had a heart defect were "absolutely shattered" and "shocked." They felt as if there was no hope for the baby [8]. These results coincide with the third theme that was uncovered in the present study.

The issues of communication, honesty, and information are constants in nurses' relationship with patients and families. Family members need a clear and concise explanation of the diagnosis. Health professionals' medical jargon fosters a superior–subordinate relationship between the team and the family and can confuse family members. Family members prefer an honest, friendly, and professional manner, rather than a businesslike or authoritative one [9]. Understanding the diagnosis is based on four major sources of information: what health care

professionals tell them, what they read, what they hear from others, and their past experiences [10]. Caregivers can provide the best care when there is understanding of the need for information; allowing the parents to describe their experience provides a picture of their needs. It is important for those who work with these parents to remember that the parent's ability to absorb information is reduced; information must be given in small amounts and wording so that parents can understand [11].

The current study was necessary to examine the issues that were discussed above and to take analysis of the experience of CHD to a more human experience level. Two parents explained, "Remember we don't have your experience. We don't see children everyday with congenital heart disease" [12]. Most nurses will not have the personal experience of giving birth to an infant who has CHD. The parents in this study attempted to provide a glimpse into their reality so that the experience can be understood and parents can be assisted to cope at whatever stage necessary.

Method of inquiry

The approach to inquiry for this study was phenomenology. Phenomenology is a philosophy. As a philosophy, its main interest is in the phenomenal question, what is the meaning of being human? [13]. Phenomenologic research is based on the belief that no single reality exists and that individuals have unique and separate realities [14]. The interview process of phenomenology allows the uniqueness of reality to be expressed by the participants. This study used the method of phenomenology to identify the separate reality that parents experience when their infant is diagnosed with CHD. The point of this research method is to borrow other people's experiences and their reflections to come to an understanding of the deeper meaning or significance of an aspect of human experience [15]. This method allowed the participants to reflect and share the meaning of a difficult time in their lives so that nurses and physicians who were involved in the care of these infants and families could understand this experience at a deeper, more emotional level.

Relevance to nursing

Nursing is thought of as a caring profession. The "caring" is of the whole person—the body, mind, heart, and soul of each patient. The care of the heart in this case was examined from two perspectives. The care of the physiologic condition of the infant's heart and the care of the emotional heart of the parents of the infant.

Methodology

Phenomenology is a systematic attempt to uncover and describe the internal meaning of a lived experience [15]. Through reflection, discussion, and analysis, the goal of this study was to provide such a description. The specific approach used in this study was based on van Manen. The steps according to van Manen [15] are:

- Turning to the nature of the lived experience
- Investigation of the experience as it is lived
- Reflection on the essential themes that characterize the phenomenon
- Description of the phenomenon through the art of writing and rewriting

The data were collected by obtaining experiential descriptions from the parents of the children. The descriptions were obtained during an interview and the process of reflection on the human experience.

Sample

The participants in the study were 10 parents (five couples) who had given birth to an infant who had CHD within 3 years from the date of the study (May 1997). The infants were living with CHD or had the defect repaired by surgery. Both parents were interviewed together when possible after giving informed consent for inclusion in the study. Gaining access was achieved by an initial phone call to the participants. The study, the process involved in the interview, and how the results would be used were discussed. Verbal consent was obtained followed by written consent at the time of the interview.

Setting

The setting for the interviews was the home of the participants, except for one interview, which was done over the phone because of distance issues. The home setting allowed for comfort and security for the participants which was important because of the personal nature of the interview.

Process

The interviews began with an open-ended question, "Will you tell me about the birth of your infant?". The interviews continued with leading questions and conversations based on specific participant responses. Participants were encouraged to share photographs, music, and poetry as it related to their experience. The interviews were tape recorded and the data were transcribed to allow for examination of themes and concepts. Thematic analysis was used in the reading of each interview through a detailed or line by line approach. These were compared with the themes that were noted in the interviews of other participants and reflected upon to discover meaning. No thematic formulation can completely unlock the enigmatic aspects of the meaning [15]; however, through analysis and extraction of themes, an attempt was made to provide a complete description of the parents' lived experience when a child is born with CHD.

Consideration of human subjects

Consideration of human subjects was provided for by a consent letter explaining the reason, goal of the study, the provision of privacy of the participants, and the fact that the participant had the ability to withdraw from the study at anytime without repercussion. No names were used. The study was approved by the hospital and university institutional board review. Upon completion, all participants received a copy of the study for review.

Results

The experience of a "broken heart" is significant in many ways. The interviews related to the study are significant in that parents were able to share a vivid description of what the diagnosis of CHD was like for them. These descriptions can assist nurses to see the reality of the experience through the eyes of the parents. Many themes were brought out during the interviews. The themes are described in the most vivid manner possible so that all who read them may be witness to the parent's "experience of a broken heart."

- Several themes were unique to each parent's experience; however, one theme that was consistent was that of an unconditional love expressed by all of the parents for their infants. The eyes of the parents truly see differently than any doctor or nurse when looking at a patient.

A mother's intuition: "something's just not right"

The parents who participated in the interviews, as well as most parents who have this experience, are not health care professionals. It is said that mothers have a special instinct. They know when something is not right with their child whether the child is next to them, far away, or in this case, new to the world as an infant. The infant is new to the world but not to the mother who has spent 9 months with the child growing and thriving. The parents described their "instinct" about the birth of their child.

> "There was a different sense when she was born, I was happy but it was like I had a feeling. I cannot explain it."
>
> "When they brought him to me, I was going to breastfeed. He seemed very tired, and we started joking around, 'He's just like his daddy. He likes to sleep too much, little sleepyhead.' So we just joked around, but my gut gave me a bad feeling. I just didn't tell anybody, didn't discuss it, and put it aside."

The parents know how sick their infant is, maybe before a nurse or doctor knows. It is important to listen to, and not doubt, the parents' intuition. They know their baby, at all levels and stages of life. They have a bond that the health care team will never achieve, no matter how much time passes.

Is it a dream?

Is it possible to imagine the feeling of being awakened out of a sound sleep, following the joyous occasion of the birth, waiting for the new baby to arrive for the first feeding, and instead, the doctor walks in. The parents described trying to imagine that it was all a bad dream, and if they could open their eyes again, it would all be right. One parent described the feeling of being in a dream when she was told the diagnosis of her infant. She did not have a sense of disbelief, but felt that it was a dream that the physician came into the room at such an odd hour to tell her that the child had a life-threatening defect and may even die.

> "He (the doctor) came at two o'clock in the morning. He brings a model of a heart and says 'your baby's got a problem.' He had another guy

with him and I remember thinking, 'This is a dream. Why are you here'?." She continued, "I just sat there by myself, I was just like, in shock." She stayed by herself and then in a "dream state" although she had just had a C-section, walked by herself to see her baby. She "just sat there looking at him."

These mothers had hope that it was just a dream, but the reality of CHD was true to fact.

The need for support and encouragement begins at the time of diagnosis. Mothers and families should be given the opportunity to choose how they would like to be told of their child's diagnosis. Nurses can facilitate and support families by allowing for a safe and comfortable environment, scheduling a meeting time where all support persons can be present, and being truthful [3]. An awareness of the effects of the diagnosis can assist nurses to be better prepared to walk the parents through the beginning stages of the diagnosis of CHD.

Shock, disbelief, lives shattered

The dreams and nightmares brought the parents to the actual reality that their baby was sick. During the interviews the parents voiced vivid descriptions of the life-shattering experience of CHD. For one family, the emotions and tears were as real as 3 years earlier when the infant was born.

> "When the doctor first came to see us, we were still in the emergency room and he goes, 'This is not good news. Your baby can't go home with you tonight.' And my just...my total disbelief. I mean we had him home. Five days of nursing him and loving him and having him and it was like this disbelief that he couldn't go home. That was shattering in itself."
>
> "They said, 'Your son has a very severe heart condition. We're very sorry.' Well, I screamed, my husband cried. I hit the wall, and stomped my feet, my husband did the same. My sister and my mom just hugged us. We all screamed and were hysterical for that moment." She remembered saying, "No, you've got the wrong child. You know, you guys got your tests mixed up. You guys screwed up. That's not my child you're talking about, my child is healthy, I saw him."

How can a child have such a serious condition? It is a difficult question to answer; listening to the responses of the parents can help the health care team to examine the words and techniques that are used when communicating with families during critical illness. Children who are born with significant health impairments also may elicit unique parental responses. How parents respond over time can influence the children's short- and long-term developmental outcomes [16]. It is necessary to examine the questions to provide gentle guidance and understanding.

Time stops

This theme was brought out in many ways by all of the parents. The parents make many trips in and out of the ICU. The nurses and doctors come and go, talk to the families, sympathize, attempt to empathize, but life for the health care team continues on as normal. For the parents, the life they had no longer exists. The happy moment of giving birth has changed to days and nights in the ICU with fluorescent lights, no windows, no privacy, public bathrooms, soda and snack machines, and public telephones.

"You know it's just absolutely shocking. I mean if your whole world never, ever, ever stops, your work schedule, your life, your phone, your voice mail, your beeper, your mobile phone, you know? Suddenly you will just stop. You're just, all you want to know is...that your baby will be okay."

"You lose track of time. You don't know what time it is, what day it is. You really don't care because nothing else matters. You're just focusing on day to day; getting through the day. You're living for the moment. You're not thinking about tomorrow or yesterday. You're living for the moment. And you don't want to go far, so you end up sleeping on a sofa in a waiting room, you know fully dressed."

Time stopped for the parents when the diagnosis was made. Waiting for time to start again coincides with the diagnosis not being real or with the child's heart being "fixed." The possibility of this not happening creates actual timeless moments between the child and their parents. Timeless moments that will go on forever if the child dies, but will take the parents from one moment to another as the child survives.

The last kiss

The parents described leaving as one of the hardest things to do. They felt better if they were just a rocking chair away. They wanted to be there in case something happened. They did not want to miss

their baby's eyes opening, even if it were just for a moment.

"It was hard, any time I left the room, you always think could this be the last kiss? And even now, could this be the last Christmas? Could this be? You know? You can't help to think it, but it's a reality."

There are many moments of discomfort for health care professionals when parents and families are present at the bedside. Encouraging family presence is key to assisting parents to comfort and love their infants. Their baby's life is of primary focus. The health care team can embrace families by welcoming their presence at the bedside.

Words, words, beeps and buzzers, nothing makes sense

The ICU staff speak in a language foreign to anyone who is unfamiliar with the environment. This is important to remember in providing care to an infant or child of parents who do not understand. Translator services can be used for patients who actually speak another language. Nurses are the translators of ICU language.

"Don't assume because we've been around for some time and picked up the jargon, that we really know everything. Things that may seem little and routine to you, like faulty equipment, this can scare terribly. We don't know what is life saving or life threatening. Don't assume that because we don't ask, that we know. We're probably afraid to ask or think we know, but we really don't. Don't ever stop explaining to us. We need to hear it. No matter how much we seem to know, we're not experts [12]."

The caregiver has the ability to increase comfort and simplify what can be complex and overwhelming. It is necessary to reach their level, wherever that may be. Just a little attention to details may help to make some sense of it all.

Lack of information versus too much information

Watching procedures and seeing the baby in pain is a well-documented stressor for parents [17].

"What would have helped is if before, there was a minute or two before all the stuff took place that they would say, 'you know what, this is what we got to do. The reason we got to do it is...What your baby is going to feel is...' and just a little bit of information. But many times there is little or no information. That leaves it open for your mind to go wild about what your baby is going through."

Providing education to parents is a key component in empowering them to make decisions about their child's health care [3]. It is important to encourage questions by the parents so that they can feel knowledgeable and less anxious. Talking the parents through procedures and having them hold their child's hand may stop the torment of the unknowns.

Trust

The parents of hospitalized children place a great deal of trust in the health care team that is providing life support to their newborn child.

"Anxious, wanting to know where is my baby? Who is touching him? Who's doing what? It's motherly instinct to protect your child, and it's hard to give up your child into the care of someone else and totally trust them and their capabilities."

"The experience of being totally out of place and totally in an arena I know nothing about, where you have to turn your child over to somebody that you don't really know. I just got to trust you, there is nothing you can do to change things. You have to let go. You have to trust."

Although the staff of the ICU are familiar and known to each other, to the parents they are strangers. Parents are asked to entrust the life of the newborn child to someone they do not know. Returning to the basics may be the only intervention to ease this transition. Health care team members need to introduce themselves, provide explanations, and obtain contact information. Ask them about their baby, what to do when he/she cries, and encourage personalization of the child's bedside.

Loss of control

Trust coincides with loss of control in many ways. Hugs, kisses, and time spent with the baby are lost in the ICU environment for a variety of reasons. The control of who, what, where, and when in reference to the family's life are surrendered to the staff and the rules of the ICU. A second part of the loss of control is not being able to make the child better or change the potential outcome for the child.

"I felt helpless, because there was nothing I could do about it. I like to be in control over my environment and situations, I had no control over this."

"I mean I felt a lot like I was overstepping my welcome because I wanted to touch my baby."

Encourage the parents to be a part of the care for their child. Parents need to be parents, even in the ICU. Discussions with the parents about the plan of care and the part that they play in that plan will assist in regaining some of the control and help them to feel a part of the health care team.

The baby's experience

The baby as the patient is part of this experience.

"What did I do? Who are these people? This doesn't feel good. That baby has a sense of feeling, the baby senses it all. And I think any baby as soon as it's here, it has a whole sense of everything going on, and they know when they're separate, and they know when it's not their mom or dad who's holding them."

Infants need to be sung to, talked to, held, and cuddled. Touch is healing. Encouraging parents to help their child heal is a part of nursing the family as well as the patient. Often, in the ICU environment the emotional aspects of care become secondary because the technical component is the focus. Refocusing to the emotional aspects is necessary. Although all of the parents did not bring out the theme of sensing, the idea was described in many ways. Parents felt that it was necessary to be there and let the baby know that they were present. Parents wanted to appeal to the sense of hearing and touch and help their baby get through the experience of hospitalization.

Parental perception

This theme was brought out by the parents in a discussion of how the baby looked to them. The parents come into the ICU and look, trying to find a little bit of normalcy in their infants' appearance. It is important to take time to discuss parental perceptions of the child and the child's health. It is essential to emphasize ways in which infants and children who have heart disease are behaviorally normal [18]. There were differences in the parents' perception seen in their descriptions.

"It was intense, because obviously, physically what your baby looks like, because you know their body has been almost completely shut off to have the procedure, and he's just coming back alive and being turned back on. It's really intense to know that your little baby went through that, that your little baby was almost shut off, and cut, and his breastbone broken. That's serious, I mean you're afraid to even cut your baby's nails, and now somebody else is going to cut him open and break his breastbone, and get to their heart and start messing with it."

"He seemed so lifeless, when he was sedated. They flopped him this way and that, and most people were gentle but sometimes, he seemed like a piece of meat. It was hard to see him treated...I don't know...It was like he wasn't a child. It was like he wasn't a baby. It was like he was something else. He was a thing rather than a person. Laying there with all these enormous tubes and everything."

"He was doing well and I went to see him on Sunday. His chest was still open, and you could see a mound of red, I didn't know what that was. I asked, and they said it was his heart. I just about fell out of my chair, you know, seeing this thing move up and down, knowing that it was his heart and it was keeping him alive. He looked good after surgery. He wasn't as blue as before. He looked good. He looked healthy. He still had all the tubes and oxygen in him, and a lot of medicine in him. But I knew he was doing good."

The thoughts of the parents help to remind nurses that many times parents have difficulty processing what is actually happening to their child. Being positive and describing some of the positive features re-humanizes the baby to the parents.

The closing of the curtain

What exactly goes on behind the curtain? Curtains are closed in the ICU for several reasons: for procedures, to bathe a patient, change the bed, when a patient is decompensating or dying, or when the patient is dead. The parents described their perception of closing the curtain in the ICU. One mother described everybody scurrying around doing things, then

"quiet. The curtain. You can't see this. You can't watch this. It's like 'Why?'".

A second mother described a critical moment during her baby's hospitalization:

"And then they told me to leave. And they go 'now you have to wait outside.' That's when I lost it. That's when I screamed and I threw myself on the floor. You feel like, at least if you are there and seeing that he's being worked on, there's a chance. When you're asked to leave, you feel like that's it. He's gone. You have a feeling of not being part of the team, not knowing what's going on, so you have more anxiety."

The parents should always have a feeling of being part of the team. If the curtain needs to be closed for whatever reason, parents should have the option of staying. This may actually change their anxiety into trust.

The emotional roller coaster

This ride described by parents was not one of excitement, but of exhaustion, shock, and emotional and physical stress.

"The thrill of giving birth naturally and then to be separate. It was thrilling, and then it came crashing down. You know, it's like the most incredible experience you can ever go through in a lifetime. You feel it. And then a short time later, you're faced with the most traumatic, heart wrenching feeling that you can ever be faced with. You know it was thrilling, then devastating, all in a little short period. Kind of like a roller coaster, an emotional roller coaster."

One mom explained:

"...and then another pump will come on, but the next day, two will come off. It's like an emotional roller coaster ride."

CHD became an up and down process for many of the parents. It was the excitement of the birth and then the agony and sadness of having a child diagnosed with a life-threatening defect. Many of the infants, children, and families who deal with this diagnosis accept a life-long commitment of doctors' appointments, medications, procedures, surgeries, and hospitalizations along with the financial burden of it all. The roller coaster ride may end at some point, but for other parents it is a ride that they may continue for life.

Just wait until this time tomorrow

Each day in the ICU brings new challenges to the family and the child. Each tomorrow hopefully brings the baby closer to leaving the ICU and going home. One family used a poem to describe this experience (Appendix 1).

The memory doesn't fade

The infants, now children, have visible scars which have faded with time, and the stretching of the skin over the chest. Many times, the memory for parents seemed like it all just happened yesterday and for others, like it never happened.

> "I like to believe everything is going to be okay. One time I visited the pediatrician and he asked me if they had told me his life span. I told him that I didn't want to know. I don't know my life span, and I don't want to know his. You know, if they were to tell me that when he is 5 years old, he will die, then when he gets to be 5, I'm going to wake up everyday thinking, 'Is this the day?'."

> "You don't even think about it. I see him everyday in the swimming pool and he's getting bigger and taller, that scar is just shrinking down a little bit more, and it's toned up exactly the same as his body. But you don't think about it much."

> "I think about it everyday, I swear. Everyday when I look at him, or give him a bath, or change a diaper, you'd see the scar, and you'd think about it. It was an ordeal, but we got through it, and I guess the only reason we got through it is everyone's telling us that he's doing really good and being so positive."

Summary and reflections

The results of this study can assist nurses and physicians to see the emotional impact for parents of children who have CHD. Parents can be helped during this experience to continue parenting—and even during a difficult time—to experience the joy of life in their new infant. The health care team as a whole has the ability to help them be parents, even in the ICU, and to let them see the beauty of their child, no matter how sick. Calling the child by his/ her first name, remembering the sex of the child, telling the parents about the child's long eyelashes, tiny toes, cute nose, and beautiful hair may seem like small, insignificant details in comparison with the child's diagnosis, but it can make a big impact on the parents. This will let them see the child behind the defect, and let them know that their child is seen by the nurses and doctors as a baby, not just another patient who has CHD.

Nursing is a caring profession. With each intervention, nurses show the patients and families that they care about them, their illness, and how they are feeling at that moment in time. Nurses provide comfort, alleviate pain, and improve quality of life. The parents who participated in this study provided an opportunity for all health care professionals to see what it is like for a parent and infant who is diagnosed with CHD. They have provided a description so vivid, that it is hoped that all members of the health care team will understand this experience more clearly.

Appendix 1. Just Wait 'Til This Time Tomorrow

It was 6:26 on the eve of March 3rd that I finally decided to come out
After nine months inside my mom
I'm finally able to shout
I'm here, I'm here is what I felt first
When I looked into my mom's eyes, and that English voice
and not one but three midwives.
I'm sorry to take so long to come,
But there's something you don't know
I have a heart that needs to be fixed, and I'm kind of afraid to say so.
All I need is my mom and dad in the day and in the night
And we will be separate soon
The transport team and I will take a flight
I know my eyes weren't open yet, but I heard my mom and dad cry
When each of the doctors explained the truth
It was possible I could die
Though I could not speak any words just yet, I wanted to yell and yell
I'll be okay, really I will
This is something I've got to live and tell.
But at the time, only I knew the truth, I was going to live
I'm still very close to God you know,
I'm a gift he wants to give
The next morning, at 9 am I felt kisses on my cheek
It's surgery time, mom and dad are afraid
How I wish that I could speak.
I'll be back in just a few hours
Dr. P. will fix me right, and Dr. H. will keep you posted
In the day and in the night
It's hard for a new mom and dad to hide this kind of pain
and I heard them cry as they rolled me away, so unsure about this game
Just four hours later, my heart was all fixed, and I remained asleep
My little body needs to start up again from my head down to my feet.
The staff explained what could happen in the recovery period to follow
And what kept my mom and dad sane was saying
"JUST WAIT 'TIL THIS TIME TOMORROW"

When that time tomorrow came I was back in newborn ICU

With Annette and Helmut, doctors galore

with Vicki and Mary Lou

I can't forget about Donna, she called me mister Shaun

and Jill with her wild hair ties the colors kept me up 'til dawn.

I'll toot here and there for Nora, cuz I like to hear her laugh,

and Debbie I know you appreciated me tooting in the bath.

I'll never forget the compassion Kim showed me through her eyes,

or Mary, as they flew me here in the midnight skies.

As a result of all your sincere love, I recovered so heckin' fast

And I'm alive to write this poem

I'm all fixed up at last.

I'll be eternally grateful for what you helped me through.

I thank you with my whole heart and soul,

I'll never again be "blue"

Reprinted with permission from the author on March 24, 1998.

References

[1] Norris MK. A parent's perspective. Crit Care Nurs Clin North Am 1994;6(1):111–9.

[2] Goldberg S, Simmons R, Newman J, et al. Congenital heart disease, parental stress, and infant mother relationships. J Pediatr 1991;119(4):367–79.

[3] Upham M, Medhoff-Cooper B. What are the responses & needs of mothers of infants diagnosed with congenital heart disease. MCN Am J Matern Child Nurs 2005;30(1):24–9.

[4] Apley J, Barbour R, Wesmacott I. Impact of congenital heart disease on the family: a preliminary report. BMJ 1967;1:103–5.

[5] Cohn J. An empirical study of parent's reaction to the diagnosis of congenital heart disease in infants. Soc Work Health Care 1996;23(2):67–79.

[6] Mörelius E, Lundh U, Nelson N. Parental stress in relation to the severity of congenital heart disease in the offspring. Pediatr Nurs 2002;28(1):28–32.

[7] Glaser H, Harrison G, Lynn D. Emotional implications of heart disease in children. Pediatrics 1964;33:367–79.

[8] Boon A. Tetralogy of Fallot—effect on the family. Br J Prev Soc Med 1972;26:263–8.

[9] Kashani I, Higgins S. Counseling strategies for families of children with congenital heart disease. Pediatr Nurs 1986;12(1):38–40.

[10] Gottesfield I. The family of the child with congenital heart disease. Am J Matern Child Nurs 1979;4:101–4.

[11] Bowen J. Helping children and their families cope with congenital heart disease. Crit Care Nurs Q 1985;8(3):65–74.

[12] Schrey C, Schrey M. A parent's perspective. Our needs and our message. Crit Care Nurs Clin North Am 1994;6(1):113–9.

[13] Munhall P. Revisioning phenomenology: nursing and health science research. New York: National league for Nursing Press; 1994.

[14] Massey V. A study and learning tool for nursing research. Springhouse (PA): Springhouse Corporation; 1995.

[15] van Manen M. Researching lived experience. human science for an action sensitive pedagogy. London: State University of New York Press; 1990.

[16] Carey L, Nicholson B, Fox R. Maternal factors related to parenting young children with congenital heart disease. J Pediatr Nurs 2002;17(3):174–83.

[17] Curley MAQ, Meyer EC. Caring practices: the impact of the critical care experience on the family. In: Curley MAQ, Moloney-Harmon PA, editors. Critical Care Nursing of Infants and Children. 2nd edition. Philadelphia: WB Saunders; 2001. p. 47–64.

[18] Uzark K, Jones K. Parenting stress and children with congenital heart disease. J Pediatr Health Care 2003;17(4):163–8.

ELSEVIER
SAUNDERS

Crit Care Nurs Clin N Am 17 (2005) 329–340

CRITICAL CARE
NURSING CLINICS
OF NORTH AMERICA

Clinical Judgments About Endotracheal Suctioning: What Cues Do Expert Pediatric Critical Care Nurses Consider?

Margot Thomas, RN, MScN, CNCCP(C)[a],*,
Frances Fothergill-Bourbonnais, RN, PhD[b]

[a]*Pediatric Intensive Care Unit, Children's Hospital of Eastern Ontario, 401 Smyth Road, Ottawa, Ontario K1H 8L1, Canada*
[b]*School of Nursing, Faculty of Health Sciences, University of Ottawa, 451 Smyth Road, Ottawa, Ontario K1H 8M5, Canada*

Making accurate and appropriate judgments based on multiple ways of knowing is an essential skill in critical care nursing practice. Studies have proposed that positive patient outcomes are linked to expert judgments in a variety of critical care situations [1–6]; however, little is known about clinical judgments related to specific critical care nursing interventions. The skills inherent in the thinking that precede and accompany the action are as critical as the action itself. Endotracheal suctioning (ETS) is one intervention that requires acute assessment and judgment skills, in addition to specific psychomotor skills, to ensure positive patient outcomes. Yet how nurses make judgments as to when and how to suction is not well understood. The purpose of this article is to describe a study that examined the cues that expert pediatric critical care nurses used in making clinical judgments about suctioning intubated and ventilated, critically ill children. By examining cues that participants identified as meaningful, the study was able to describe an aspect of nurses' practice that has not been explored completely.

This work was supported by funding from the Research Institute of the Children's Hospital of Eastern Ontario, Ottawa, Canada.

* Corresponding author.
E-mail address: thomas@cheo.on.ca (M. Thomas).

Background

Multiple terms, including decision making [7], critical thinking [8–12], diagnostic reasoning [13–15], and clinical judgment [16,17], have been used in nursing research to examine a concept that some investigators propose roughly describes a single phenomenon with overlapping competencies [9,11, 18–20]. This study used the definition of clinical judgment, "the ways in which nurses come to understand the problems or concerns of clients/patients, to pay attention to specific information and to respond in concerned and involved ways in providing nursing care" [16]. Although a significant body of knowledge about the importance of clinical judgment in nursing has been developed, there is not one theoretic perspective that has been accepted widely as an explanatory framework. Initial nursing studies [21,22] concluded that the nurses' cognitive tasks were complex with respect to the number of cues involved, the number of responses to tasks, and the relation between cues and actions. Studies using the analytic linear framework for decision making, as proposed in the medical literature, have concluded that nurses make judgments in rational ways that are influenced by situational, personal, and contextual variables [23–38]; however, some researchers have suggested that this linear approach does not predict the ways in which expert nurses make judgments [1,26,34, 39–43]. Alternative frameworks, such as nursing scripts, and heuristics, drawn from other disciplines and from an intuitive perspective, have been suggested to explain the effects of expertise on nurses' judgments [44–49]. Although research examining judgment in clinical practice [50], simulation exercises [37], and narrative inquiry [45] has suggested that nurses attend to specific cues to make clinical judgments, there is a lack of knowledge as to the specific cues that nurses consider for specific nursing interventions.

Endotracheal intubation and mechanical ventilation are fundamental interventions in caring for critically ill children. Numerous studies suggest that the complications that are associated with intubation and ETS may contribute to potentially negative patient outcomes [51–64]. As well, failure to perform ETS appropriately has been proposed to lead to the accumulation of pulmonary secretions and tube obstruction [56,60]. Studies have identified that nurses may suction according to a prescribed frequency (eg, every 4 hours), as part of the unit routine and according to patient criteria [52,65]; however, it is unknown how expert nurses determine patients' needs for suctioning, and whether that need consistently directs the clinical judgments about the timing of ETS. Published protocols for artificial airway suctioning are variable, and in general, are not based on rigorous evidence [66–70]. A Canadian survey [68] identified practice variations related to frequency, use of saline instillations, and discipline of the practitioner who is performing the skill. Recent clinical practice guidelines do not give specific direction as to the indications for, or the frequency for, suctioning [71].

The recognition of cues has been proposed as an initial step in the clinical judgment process [50]. To understand the nature of clinical judgments, it is necessary to examine the cues that nurses consider. Because experience and expertise have been proposed as factors that influence the nature of clinical judgment, this study was undertaken to describe how expert nurses use cues to make judgments about the timing for ETS and asked the following research question: What are the cues that expert pediatric critical care nurses recognize in determining the need for ETS when caring for mechanically ventilated children?

Method

A descriptive, qualitative study as described by Sandelowski [72], was conducted in the critical care unit (CCU) of a Canadian pediatric care institution after receipt of ethical approval. Three data collection methods were used: (1) participant observation (field notes), (2) think aloud (concurrent verbalization), and (3) semi-structured interviews (retrospective verbalization), to enable nurses to share their thinking and judgments about ETS in direct practice. These methods, congruent with the general tenets of naturalistic inquiry [72–77], resulted in real-time information about nursing judgments and cognitive processes related to ETS. Concurrent verbalization, collected through think aloud activities during direct clinical practice, "accesses both the information that is acquired from the clinical environment (e.g., clinical cues) and knowledge gained previously which is stored in the long-term memory" [78]. To address potential sources of informant bias, retrospective thought processes (recorded as the semi-structured interview responses) were verified with observations of the situation and of participants' behaviors (recorded as field notes) and with concurrent thought processes (recorded as think aloud audiotapes) [79].

The study examined the practice of seven expert pediatric critical care nurses. The inclusion criteria, derived from the nursing judgment literature [6,20,45], were nurses: (1) with at least 3 years of pediatric critical care experience, (2) who were recognized by peers and supervisor as being a highly skilled clinician who is able to recognize and communicate thought processes, (3) who demonstrated skill in being attuned to the needs of patient and family, (4) who were recognized as able to make rapid judgments about a patient's condition based on well-developed physical assessment skills, (5) who demonstrated care involving independent decisions about nursing interventions that may cross boundaries between another discipline and nursing, and (6) who paid attention to the outcomes of nursing care. The unit nurse educator identified potential participants who met these criteria. Nurses indicated their interest in participating to the unit nurse educator, and written informed consent was obtained. Data were collected as participants worked in direct practice caring for critically ill children whose ages ranged from 4 days to 7 months. During the observation periods, the researcher noted the nurses' actions, listened to their verbalizations, and made field notes using a focused observation guide. For the collection of concurrent verbalized data, participants wore a lapel microphone connected to a small cassette recorder that was carried in a fanny pack attached around the waist. Participants were directed to turn on the recorder and think aloud anytime they considered ETS. All nurses quickly demonstrated comfort and initiative with using the recorder. The tape-recorded semi-structured interviews that were conducted by the researcher were completed on the day of observation. The sample size of seven was determined following a review of the tapes of the last two participants in which data saturation occurred with the sixth and was confirmed with the seventh participant. Data was collected during seven day shifts with the average duration of participant observation of 7.65 hours (range, 7.5 to 10 hours). A total of 27 suctioning episodes were noted for the seven participants. Duration of think aloud recording ranged from 11.5 to 25.5 minutes; duration of interview audio recording ranged from 9.25 to 16.75 minutes per participant.

Data analysis followed an interpretive content analysis strategy [80]. The verbatim transcriptions of verbalizations and the typed field notes constituted the 181 pages of analyzed text. The process of understanding the data came from multiple focused readings of the transcripts. NUD*IST (Non-numerical Unstructured Data-Indexing, Searching and Theorizing) software was used to code documents and sort ideas. Coding document reports, which represented the categories and themes that emerged from the data, were printed and re-examined to identify relationships between and among the categories and themes. Comprehensive journal entries related to context as well as methodologic and analytic decisions constituted the audit trail for this study. Study rigor was enhanced by peer debriefings and member checks.

Results

Cue use emerged as the process that nurses performed when considering the need for and the ways to suction an intubated child. Cue use consisted of two core components: (a) cue recognition and (b) weighing the evidence. Cue recognition was the sensing of cues that nurses saw, heard, felt, or knew in the patient and the situation. Weighing the evidence was the thinking about the cues that were sensed. The cognitive activities of cue recognition and weighing the evidence formed a foundation for the nurses' judgments about the ways to implement the skill of ETS. The skilled performance of suctioning was the doing and was interwoven closely with the processes of cue recognition and weighing the evidence as illustrated in Fig. 1. Cue use was not a unidirectional process that started with cue recognition and proceeded to weighing the evidence before the enactment of the suctioning event. The components of cue recognition and weighing the evidence were interrelated and interconnected. Elements of one component influenced, and in turn, were influenced by, the elements of the other component. The multiple dimensions of cue use that emerged from the data

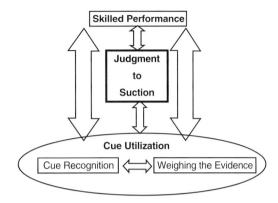

Fig. 1. Cue use in making clinical judgments.

attested to the complexity of the judgments related to suctioning made by the participants.

Cue recognition

Two elements of cue recognition emerged from the data: perceptual awareness and knowing. Perceptual awareness consisted of the cues related to the senses of seeing (visual), hearing (auditory), and feeling (tactile). Knowing was based on the cues nurses identified from knowledge of this type of patient, this particular patient, and this practice environment.

Perceptual awareness

Perceptual awareness is the process of sensing patient cues that nurses identified as they were making judgments related to ETS. Three categories of cues, related to the senses of seeing, hearing, and feeling, emerged from the nurses' words and action.

Perceptual awareness: visual cues
Nurses noted visual cues, including patient activity, color changes, breathing patterns, the nature of secretions, and monitoring patterns. These groupings of cues seemed to trigger the nurse to look for additional cues to confirm or discount a singular cue.

> "As soon as I walked into the room, I saw her sats were eighty nine. So that was kind of a trigger that maybe she was decompensating a little bit, so what I did was look at her breathing."

Patient activity (distress; moving; and coughing before, during, and after the suctioning episode) seemed to be meaningful for the nurses in determining not only the need to suction, but also the ways in which the suctioning should be done, how long to suction, and what adjunct interventions to implement. The cue of patient coughing was verbalized in combination with other cues, including desaturation and ventilator alarms. While the child was coughing, nurses would auscultate the chest, look for the presence of secretions in the endotracheal tube, and evaluate color and saturation readings simultaneously. Visual cues for suctioning related to pattern of breathing, included asymmetrical chest movement or paradoxical movements, and changes in rate, rhythm, and effort.

> "...her breathing has a little bit of a shudder to it, where she is taking some breaths and then just sort of does an extra one that can also to me indicate that she might have some secretions...presently the pattern of her breathing has changed from my first assessment and I suspect I'm going to have to suction."

At times, secretions visible in the endotracheal tube emerged as a cue that nurses considered singularly as an indication for suctioning.

> "I didn't listen to his chest because he needed to be done. You could see the secretions."

Nurses considered the amount, color, and tenacity of secretions in relation to the patient's condition and response to suctioning. Nurses visually noted changes in color, oxygen saturation levels, and monitored vital signs in conjunction with other cues. Desaturations always were considered in making the judgment to suction in conjunction with other perceived cues. Of interest, oxygen saturations less than 92% were noted to precede suctioning in only 6 of the 27 suctioning episodes.

> "The sats are also trending downwards, they're in the low nineties versus above 95, so based on how she sounds and how's she's looking, I will [suction]."

Perceptual awareness: auditory cues

Auditory cues were perceived during respiratory assessments at the beginning of shift, as well as after suctioning procedures. The skill of auditory discrimination required to differentiate breath and adventitious sounds heard on chest auscultation was evident in the nurses' descriptions.

> "...just going to have a listen to the chest and see what's going on. (Pause). Oh, squeaks. Yep, that sounds awful. Big squeaks, probably warrants a suctioning. (Pause). Okay, so time to suction."

Nurses noted auditory cues to confirm perceived visual and tactile cues and to evaluate the outcome of suctioning. Nurses used expressions including, "all clear," "much better," and "sounds all gone," to indicate that suctioning had been successful. The participants compared the sounds of their patients before and after suctioning as part of determining the outcome, the need to suction again, or the need to institute an adjunct intervention, such as inhaled bronchodilators or instillation of saline.

Ventilator alarms, including high pressure, minute ventilation, and tidal volume, presented additional auditory cues. Of interest, no nurse considered a ventilator alarm independent of other cues as an indication for suctioning. Sounds of secretions, audible while the patient was attached to the ventilator as well as when the patient was being manually ventilated, were additional auditory cues. Preoxygenation and manually ventilating (bagging) were identified as strategies to prevent transient hypoxemia and to enable the nurse to feel and hear secretions.

> "I'm just going to start bagging him...oh, you can hear the secretions down there, there's quite a lot...sound quite loose."

Perceptual awareness: tactile cues

Tactile cues indicating a need for suctioning were considered to be important. Touching the child's chest enabled the nurse to feel the vibrations that were caused by secretions within the chest that indicated a need for suctioning.

> "You could actually feel it on the chest without even listening to it that time."

Nurses also identified that they could feel the presence of secretions when manually ventilating the patient, and used this indicator to monitor the suctioning procedure. Nurses described tactile perceptions of feeling secretions and resistance as part of their ongoing assessment of the need for ETS.

> "You can just feel the pressure on the end of the catheters. So even as I moved it back a little bit to take it out, you could just feel the pressure on the end. So you know, it's down there but you're just not getting it."

Knowing

Knowing, the second element of the process of cue recognition, described the cues nurses identified from three aspects of knowledge- knowing this type of patient, knowing this particular patient, and knowing this practice environment.

Knowing: this type of patient

Cues associated with knowledge of this type of patient were related to the normal expectations for the patient condition and the general risks of ETS. Knowing this type of patient was based on knowledge of pathophysiology and clinical therapeutics. For example, knowing the potential complications for children with small endotracheal tubes was recognized as a cue that indicated a need for close nursing assessments related to suctioning.

> "He's only got a three and a half tube, a really tiny little tube. So some children... the slightest little bit of spit in there. And they become very panicky. He doesn't desat with it. His chest itself doesn't sound noisy, but it is obvious that it frustrates him."

Nurses explained that specific cues and actions based on knowing this type of patient also came from previous experiences in caring for similar patients as illustrated in this quote from an interview,

> "...because I look after cardiac patients a lot, looking after kids with a sternum dam, I know that if they've been lying there for a while, that the secretions are going to be thicker."

Knowing: this particular patient

Cues associated with knowing this patient included the noting of previous responses, identifying expected findings and outcomes, and forecasting planned procedures. Knowing this particular patient was based on knowledge derived from a nurse–patient relationship developed by noting patient rhythms and idiosyncrasies through direct "hands-on" experience. Knowing this particular patient required the nurse to develop a sense of the patient's responses to suctioning.

> "It felt smoother because I already know the child a little bit better. It's kind of like you get synchronized with the child and you get comfortable with using the bag for when they naturally want to draw breath. I don't try to fight the child. I let them kind of breathe, give her some good PEEP and even let her do some of the work. And it's the real feel part of the procedures. Ah, you work with the child, so it's not just you. You're not in total control, you have to work with the child."

Nurses were able to identify how a specific patient was like or unlike other similar patients. They described patient findings in comparison with the expected findings for similar patients; however, nurses modified the timing and method of suctioning based on an appraisal of this particular patient's unique responses.

> "Like in general, it would have been fine to leave him, but from knowing him, it just leads to more suctioning, more agitation, and more chance of encouraging that spot to bleed."

As nurses began to know this particular patient, identified cues became more patient specific. Nurses used documentation by others, verbal report, and suggestions from colleagues who had previous experience with the patient as sources of knowing until they had developed their own knowledge of this patient. Verbal shift report was an opportunity to share specific knowledge learned about this patient. This summary of care and patient responses was a two-way dialog as nurses asked questions related to the particular responses of this patient. As the shift progressed and nurses developed an awareness of this patient, they created their own sense of this patient that was used to refine their technique of suctioning.

> "So she's done well, that's three and I feel like I'm learning about her with each suctioning and she's working well with me."

Knowledge of this patient was derived from noting subtle changes and responses to treatments in this patient from day to day as well as over the shift. The participants used knowledge of procedures forecast for the patient, including chest closure, blood drawing, and chest radiograph, as a cue to be considered in determining the timing of suctioning.

> "...we will probably end up suctioning her because of the procedure that's going to be on at eleven. We'll do her probably before that at some point, I just didn't want to do her right before the blood work of course."

Knowing: this practice environment

Knowing this practice environment was another aspect of knowledge contributing to cue recognition. As with knowledge of this type of patient, knowing the practice environment developed over time and with experience in the unit. The participants' judgments about how and when they suctioned the patient were based on the recognition of cues related to specific equipment, unit routines, and scheduling of nurses' breaks. Knowledge of the type of equipment and ventilator system used at the bedside was a cue to implement specific suctioning procedures or to access assistance.

> "...for the first time I suctioned, just because of, of the mechanics of, turning the hypoxic mix to the bag from the ventilator. I probably would have had that other person standing there if the vent, if the RT had time she could have bagged."

Knowledge of specific unit routines was a cue in judging the need for suctioning in relation to planned extubation. Two nurses identified how suctioning before extubation was considered in response to patient condition as a measure to prevent problems after extubation, and because it was a unit expectation.

> "Well he sounds clear, no typical reason to suction, except that we were going to extubate. The protocol, we always do a suction before we extubate, just to make sure there is nothing sitting in the tube as we pull the tube up to fall into the lungs. So we always do one suction before extubation."

As well, participants discussed how they would determine the timing of suctioning in response to the availability of staff to cover their patient while they were away on break. Staff acknowledged the expectation that the nurse would ensure that other nurses would not be required to perform interventions that could have been done before the nurse's departure from the unit.

> "Baby has just waked up and sounds a little, um, like there are secretions in there. So, um, instead of break, I'm just going to go ahead and suction...at least I'll know that while I'm away at break that nobody will need to step in and intervene."

Weighing the evidence

The second component of cue use, weighing the evidence, represented the ways that nurses considered the cues that they recognized. Weighing the evidence represented the thinking activity, or mental dialog, that nurses used to formulate judgments related to suctioning. Two elements of this component emerged from the data: (1) determining the significance of perceptions—the way that the nurses attributed an importance to the perceived cues, and (2) corroborating impressions—the way that nurses sought to confirm or refute their thoughts about the importance of a cue to the patient situation. When nurses considered the cue to be important and was corroborated

with other cues, they regularly proceeded to suction the patient.

Weighing the evidence: determining significance

Determining the significance of the perception was based on a consideration of the relative importance and the fit of that cue with other recognized cues. Nurses did not respond to all recognized cues with the judgment to suction, even when the cue was congruent with the unit suctioning policy. This apparent paradox can be explained by the notion that the nurse determined the significance of cues in relation to other cues as part of the process of weighing the evidence. Cues that at one time resulted in the decision to suction also were associated with the decision not to suction the same patient at another time. It seemed that the nurse recognized a cue and then assigned that cue an importance, relative to an appraisal of patient cues and the clinical context. Some cues seemed to be considered more significant than others in certain situations. For example, the visual cue of secretions within the endotracheal tube and the auditory cue of hearing secretions when manually ventilating the patient were considered highly important in the decision to suction; however, not all cues were assigned a similar weighting. As a point of illustration, patient coughing was a visual cue of patient condition that was considered relevant, and prompted the nurses to suction at some times. At other times, coughing was interpreted as an effect of the suctioning procedure or patient moving and was discounted as an indicator to suction. In the following think aloud excerpt, the auditory cue of the ventilator alarm was not considered as important as the cues of patient activity, this type of patient, color, chest sounds, and oxygen saturations as the nurse made the judgment not to suction.

> "Oh, the ventilator is ringing off... but she's breathing quite nicely but sats were a little bit lower, dipped down to 95. She is pink, she is warm, she is well perfused. I think we just need to get that tube out. I'll have a quick listen of her chest and see if there's any change from when I went (pause). Oh, it sounds pretty good in there...I'm not going to suction...just going to leave things as they are and just sit and watch things."

The findings of this study suggest that nurses considered visual, auditory, and tactile cues in groupings that fit together as they weighed the evidence. The authors labeled this process of comparing and associating cues "creating a fit." When cues fit together, nurses created a mental image of a pattern of cues that seemed to be recognized readily and determined to be significant.

"The same pattern, I'm listening to her, feeling her, felt the resistance, heard the sounds."

Weighing the evidence: corroborating impressions

Corroborating impressions was an element of weighing the evidence that nurses performed when they sought verification of their assessments and judgments. Once the nurses had verified their impressions, they made a case for their judgments and confidently proceeded with the chosen nursing intervention. When cues did not fit with each other in a grouping that the nurse associated with the need for suctioning, nurses seemed to: (1) look for a rationale for the cue; (2) consult with other health care providers, such as respiratory therapist (RT); (3) consider research findings as a way of corroborating the impression.

"Okay, with the rate decrease the baby has just desaturated, so our RT is slowly bagging her because she seems to like that. I'm not sure exactly what's going on yet. Does it feel like she needs suction (to RT)?"

In summary, weighing the evidence appeared as the second component in the process of the cue use in making judgments about ETS. Weighing the evidence was the mental dialog of determining the significance of perceptions and corroborating impressions that was interconnected with cue recognition. Nurses continued to look for and recognize additional cues as part of the activities of seeking confirmation and creating groupings of cues to support the judgments to suction. Movement from cue recognition to weighing the evidence seemed to be an ongoing process.

Skilled performance

"Skilled performance" was the term used to characterize the ways that nurses performed the skill of suctioning. Skilled performance was derived from the process of cue use in the practice situation, and in turn, contributes to its process. It is evident in the data that nurses did not separate the sensing, thinking, and doing processes. The processes of cue recognition, weighing the evidence, and skilled performance were nonlinear, interwoven, and interrelated. Cues appraised during the procedure were used to create the nurse's sense of knowing the patient that was

important in making judgments about future suctioning interventions. The actual time spent in ETS was short, an average of 5 minutes; however, the considerations that nurses attended to in making judgments of when and how to suction were numerous, complex, and related to how the nurse was connected to the patient through sight, sound, and touch.

"...there was a distinct difference when I was bagging. I could hear it and I could feel it and that unfortunately is not something you can actually always, um, that's a feel thing that comes with time and it, it really is the connection of the brain to the hands and the ears, so it's a sensory process."

Nurses implemented specific strategies to facilitate this visual, auditory, and tactile connection with the patient. One nurse identified that the activities of surveillance were part of the suctioning procedure that may not be overtly visible, or even noted by the nurse.

So while that's going on, some of the other things that one has do, as well as being focused on the task of suctioning is how is the child tolerating, what's their color like, what's their breathing effort like and taking in the monitor so my head's moving and, and I'm probably not even aware of that.

Discussion

The findings of this study related to cue use were congruent with previously reported work about the process of clinical judgment in other nursing situations; however, this study also identified new knowledge that builds on our understanding of how nurses make judgments about suctioning critically ill children.

Nurses in this study did not perform ETS needlessly or routinely. All suctioning episodes were preceded by the judgment of patient need for the procedure. This finding was congruent with the suggestion that nurses should limit suctioning to when needed to minimize trauma associated with ETS [81]; however, the cues that nurses considered in determining the need for suctioning in this study were more numerous and complex than those suggested by Knox [81], who recommended that need for ETS be determined by assessment of chest and status of airway. Copnell and Fergusson [65] concluded that because most nurses in their study seemed to rely on a determination of patient deterioration as the need for suctioning, they were not using assessment skills to full advantage in caring for ventilated children; however, this current qualitative study—using a sample of expert nurses, multiple data collection methods, and thematic analysis—has revealed that expert nurses do use complex and multiple patient assessments in determining the need to suction. Portions of the cues recognized in this study were identified in a literature review examining the indications for suctioning [82]. Simmons [82] cautioned that the consideration of ventilator and technical parameters "must be assessed in conjunction with the clinical assessment of the patient." Yet, the specific clinical assessments that the nurse should consider were not described by Simmons. The findings of the current study provide further information about the specific visual, auditory, and tactile cues that expert nurses did consider in suctioning pediatric patients.

The cues that nurses used to judge the need for ETS are more numerous and diverse than those identified in the critical care nursing resources [83–86]. For example, the practice guidelines and texts do not identify visual cues, such as patient distress, patient coughing, or the quality of secretions (tenacity and color). Cues noted in this study, such as increased respiratory rate, "fighting" the ventilator, ventilator asynchrony, and changing breathing patterns, are not specified in the American Association for Respiratory Care (AARC) practice guidelines [66]. Cues related to context, such as the timing of nurses' scheduled breaks, and the availability of nursing staff or respiratory therapy personnel for two-person suctioning, were not identified previously in the literature. The finding that nurses considered cues in clusters to determine the significance of the cue before suctioning was not evident in the clinical practice guidelines or nursing texts. The AARC practice guidelines imply that any one criterion is indicative of the need for suctioning; however, the expert nurses in this study demonstrated that clinical decisions were based on a constellation of cues deemed relevant to a specific patient situation. This finding was congruent with the activity of coalescing of cues into clusters as inherent in pattern recognition based on tacit, or practical knowledge [87]. The finding of the interrelationship of the seeing, thinking, and doing in making judgments about suctioning also confirmed MacLeod's [88] research that identified three practice processes—noticing, understanding, and acting—that were "inextricably intertwined in a non-linear, non-sequential process."

Nurses made judgments based on the recognition of groups of cues, rather than acting on the basis of one cue alone, and their cue recognition was influenced by knowledge of this patient's condition and responses to suctioning. These findings are congruent with other critical care nursing research studies [1,2,45]. This study found that perceptual awareness required an engaged involvement with the patient. To assess, consider, and discriminate among multiple cues that were recognized in the patient situation, nurses developed a connectedness to the patient that contributed to knowing this particular patient. Evidence that the processes of perceptual awareness and knowing were interrelated emerged when nurses verbalized how they looked for and recognized different cues to make judgments about care as they began to develop knowledge and a sense of this particular patient. Knowing the patient has been identified as a crucial element in nurses' judgment processes [3,4,89–94]. In this study, as nurses began to know this particular patient, the cues they relied upon became more patient specific. Nurses' thinking activities moved from the general rules and expectations to a more specific approach when the unique characteristics of the patient were learned. In this study, the influence on clinical judgments by nurses' knowledge of the particular patient is congruent with other studies that suggest that as the nurse increases her understanding of the patient through an involved approach, the nurse provides care that is increasingly individualized [95,96].

The finding that nurses developed their knowledge of the patient from one suctioning episode to the next over the course of the shift, was congruent with previous findings that time spent with the patient was a factor that influenced the nurse's knowledge of the patient [4,5,20]. In this study, nursing actions illustrated how learning about this patient over time was relevant to how each nurse individualized interventions. Verbalizations included temporal and contextual information which suggest that as the nurses spent time with the patients, they were able to recall specific patient experiences and predict future responses.

The study participants verbalized cues that contributed to a multidimensional assessment of a patient's need for suctioning. Nurses did not consider patient signs in isolation of knowledge of the patient or of the practice environment. These experts did not implement a stepwise process of assessment, planning, implementing, and evaluating in making judgments about suctioning. The processes of cue recognition and weighing the evidence are iterative, dynamic, and ongoing throughout the judgment and performance of suctioning as was suggested previously in the judgment literature [26,27,34,39,97,98].

Nurse researchers have proposed that expert nurse judgments are based on a form of intuition, in which a consideration of a pattern of cues seems to generate outcomes without conscious awareness of the process [43,99,100]. The term "intuition" seems to have been used to explain expert nurses' use of unseen aspects of clinical knowledge, that although known by the nurse, can be described only vaguely. In contrast, the participants' concurrent and retrospective verbalizations in this study were replete with the identification of patterns of cues considered in making judgments. As well, not all of the cues that were recognized by participants during their think aloud sessions were remembered during the interviews that occurred immediately after the suctioning episodes. Think aloud is a research method that has been successful in bringing the unseen and unheard thought processes of experts into our understanding of judgment.

Recommendations

Nursing practice environments must continue to support strategies that enable nurses to develop a knowing or sense of the patient, such as verbal face-to-face report between nurses and higher proportions of full-time staff to promote consistent patient assignments. Nurse/patient ratios need to take into account the time that nurses need to appraise the unique attributes of the patient and to develop a sense of how this patient will respond to nursing interventions. "When nurses work in situations where it is impossible to know their patients sufficiently to see changing relevance, recognize early warning, or protect patients from violation of patient/family concerns or threats to their vulnerability, then the very ground for safe and astute nursing care is undermined" [87].

The complexity of the process of cue use in making the judgment to suction and in determining the method of performing that procedure mandate the knowledge and skills of a registered nurse; it is inappropriate to delegate this skill to nonregulated health care professionals. "Much nursing work is believed to be hidden from objective lay scrutiny, because of the subtle interpersonal nature of nursing interventions. Blindness to these aspects has led to nursing viewed as a series of tasks that can easily be delegated to less qualified personnel" [47]. As well, future practice guidelines should consider the clinical knowledge of experts drawn from qualitative studies in making recommendations for practice. It is apparent in this study that there are discrepancies between published guidelines and the ways in which expert nurses judged the need to suction and the methods of suctioning. Guidelines should be written in a way

that the characteristics of this particular patient and this type of patient are considered in addition to the theoretic aspects of the procedure and knowledge gained from randomized clinical trials.

The judgment processes of nurses who are not practicing at an expert level should be examined using a similar research design. Do novice critical care nurses use the elements of cue recognition and weighing the evidence in making clinical judgments similarly to expert nurses? As well, studies using the think aloud method must be conducted to continue to develop knowledge about the judgment process of nurses in direct practice. This study revealed that the think aloud method is feasible and effective in collecting data about nurses' judgment processes while providing complex patient care. It is imperative that the ways in which expert nurses protect the patient by assessing for and preventing complications be valued and described further.

Expert clinical nurses also need to be involved directly with the learning activities of novice critical care nurses. ETS is a skill that cannot be learned solely in a laboratory setting or by reading practice guidelines and unit procedures. Clinical bedside teaching by nurse experts is an essential strategy to enhance the development of clinical judgment skills [6,101]. The skilled performance demonstrated by the nurse participants was built on the judgments that nurses made using the process of cue use. As well, the recognition of the complexity of the underlying cognitive processes in performing similar nursing interventions must be incorporated into undergraduate nursing education when teaching clinical skills.

Summary

The findings of this study support the conclusion that judgments about ETS, made by expert pediatric critical care nurses, are dynamic, complex, and derived from a process of cue use. The process of cue use is made up of two elements—cue recognition and weighing the evidence—that are interrelated in an iterative relationship. The participants' words and actions attest that the "sensing" and "thinking" of the process of cue use are interwoven with, and integral to the skilled performance or "doing."

References

[1] Pyles S, Stern P. Discovery of nursing gestalt in critical care nursing: the importance of the gray gorilla syndrome. J Nurs Scholarsh 1983;15:51–7.

[2] Jacavone J, Dostal M. A descriptive study of nursing judgment in the assessment and management of cardiac pain. ANS Adv Nurs Sci 1992;15:54–63.

[3] Stannard D, Puntillo K, Miaskowski C, et al. Clinical judgment and the management of postoperative pain in critical care patients. Am J Crit Care 1996;5:433–41.

[4] Jenny J, Logan J. Knowing the patient: one aspect of clinical knowledge. J Nurs Scholarsh 1992;24:254–8.

[5] Jenny J, Logan J. Promoting ventilator independence: a grounded theory perspective. Dimens Crit Care Nurs 1994;18:29–37.

[6] Hanneman S. Advancing nursing practice with a unit-based clinical expert. J Nurs Scholarsh 1996;28:331–7.

[7] Matteson P, Hawkins J. Concept analysis of decision making. Nurs Forum 1990;25(2):4–10.

[8] Facione N, Facione P, Sanchez C. Critical thinking disposition as a measure of competent clinical judgment: The development of the California Critical Thinking Disposition Inventory. J Nurse Educ 1994;33:345–50.

[9] Facione N, Facione P. Externalizing the critical thinking in knowledge development and clinical judgment. Nurs Outlook 1996;44:129–36.

[10] Gordon J. Congruence between nurse educators and critical thinking experts on the conceptualizing of critical thinking. Diss Abstr Int 1995;57(09A):3842.

[11] Kataoka-Yahiro M, Saylor C. A critical thinking model for nursing judgment. J Nurs Educ 1994;33:351–6.

[12] Paul RW, Heaslip P. Critical thinking and intuitive nursing practice. J Adv Nurs 1995;22:40–7.

[13] Carnevali D. The diagnostic reasoning process. In: Carnevali D, Mitchell N, Woods C, Tanner C, editors. Diagnostic reasoning in nursing. New York: JB Lippincott; 1984. p. 25–57.

[14] Putzier D, Padrick K, Westfall V, et al. Diagnostic reasoning in critical care. Heart Lung 1985;14:430–7.

[15] Tanner C, Padrick K, Westfall V, et al. Diagnostic reasoning strategies of nurses and nursing students. Nurs Res 1987;36:358–63.

[16] Benner P, Tanner C, Chesla C. Expertise in nursing practice: caring, clinical judgment, and ethics. New York: Springer; 1996.

[17] Benner P. From novice to expert: excellence and power in nursing practice. Menlo Park (CA): Addison-Wesley; 1984.

[18] Miller M, Malcolm N. Critical thinking in the nursing curriculum. Nurs Health Care 1990;11:67–73.

[19] Tanner C. Provocative thoughts on critical thinking. J Nurs Educ 1994;33:339.

[20] Benner P, Tanner C, Chesla C. From beginner to expert: gaining a differentiated clinical world in critical care nursing. ANS Adv Nurs Sci 1992;14:13–28.

[21] Hammond KR, Kelly K, Schneider R, et al. Clinical inference in nursing: revising judgments. Nurs Res 1967;16:38–45.

[22] Kelly K. Clinical inference in nursing. Nurs Res 1966;15:123–6.

[23] Baumann A, Bourbonnais F. Nursing decision making in critical care. J Adv Nurs 1982;7:435–46.

[24] Baumann A, Bourbonnais F. When the chips are down: decision making in a crisis situation. Can Nurs 1983;79(5):23–5.

[25] Baumann A, Bourbonnais F. Rapid decision making in crisis situations: a case study approach for nurses. Toronto: McGraw-Hill Ryerson; 1984.

[26] Corcoran S. Decision analysis: a step-by-step guide for making clinical decisions. Nurs Health Care 1986;7:149–54.

[27] Corcoran S. Task complexity and nursing expertise as factors in decision making. Nurs Res 1986;35:107–12.

[28] Corcoran S. The planning by expert and novice nurses in cases of varying complexity. Nurs Res Health 1986;9:155–62.

[29] Grossman S, Campbell C, Riley B. Assessment of clinical decision making ability of critical care nurses. Dimens Crit Care Nurs 1996;15:272–9.

[30] Hansen A, Thomas D. A conceptualization of decision making: its application to a study of role and situation related differences in priority decisions. Nurs Res 1968;17:436–43.

[31] Hansen A, Thomas D. Role group differences in judging the importance of advising medical care. Nurs Res 1968;17:525–32.

[32] Henry S. Effect of levels of patient acuity on clinical decision making of critical care nurses with varying levels of knowledge and experience. Heart Lung 1991;20:478–85.

[33] Holl R. Characteristics of the registered nurse and professional beliefs and decision making. Crit Care Nurs Q 1994;17:60–6.

[34] Holzemer W. The structure of problem solving in simulations. Nurs Res 1986;35:231–6.

[35] Seldomridge EA. The influence of confidence, factual, and experiential knowledge on speed and accuracy of clinical judgment among novice and expert nurses. Diss Abstr Int 1996;57007(B):4303.

[36] Sims K, Fought S. Clinical decision making in critical care. Crit Care Nurs Q 1989;12:79–84.

[37] van den Berg R. The integration of patient cues, nursing knowledge and clinical judgments by Intensive Care Nurses in simulated situations of urgency [master's thesis]. Ottawa (Canada): University of Ottawa; 1996.

[38] Jenkins H. A research tool for measuring perceptions of clinical decision making. J Prof Nurs 1985;1:221–9.

[39] Fowler L. Clinical reasoning strategies used during care planning. Clin Nurs Res 1997;6:349–61.

[40] Tanner C. Teaching clinical judgment. Annu Rev Nurs Res 1987;5:153–73.

[41] Tanner C. Research on clinical judgment. In: Holzemer WL, editor. Review of research in nursing education. Thorofare (NJ): Charles B. Slack; 1987. p. 2–32.

[42] Benner P. Uncovering the knowledge embedded in clinical practice. J Nurs Scholarsh 1983;15:36–41.

[43] Benner P, Tanner C. Clinical judgment: how expert nurses use intuition. Am J Nurs 1987;87:23–31.

[44] Greenwood J. Critical thinking and nursing scripts: a case for the development of both. J Adv Nurs 2000; 31:428–36.

[45] Benner P, Hooper-Kyriakidis P, Stannard D. Clinical wisdom and interventions in critical care: a thinking in action approach. Philadelphia: WB Saunders; 1999.

[46] Cioffi J. Heuristics: servants to intuition in clinical decision making. J Adv Nurs 1997;26:203–8.

[47] Buckingham C, Adams A. Classifying clinical decision making: a unifying approach. J Adv Nurs 2000;32:981–9.

[48] Buckingham C, Adams A. Classifying clinical decision making: interpreting nursing intuition. J Adv Nurs 2000;32:990–8.

[49] Dreyfus H, Dreyfus S. Mind over machine: the power of human intuition and expertise in the era of the computer. New York: Free Press; 1986.

[50] Fisher A, Fonteyn M. An exploration of an innovative methodological approach for examining nurses' heuristic use in clinical practice. J Scholarly Inquiry 1995;9:263–76.

[51] Abrams C, Johnson B. Endotracheal suctioning of the neonate: an informal procedural study. Neonatal Netw 1984;3:18–21.

[52] Baun M. Physiologic determinants of a clinically successful method of endotracheal suction. West J Nurs Res 1984;6:213–28.

[53] Boothroyd A, Murthy B, Darbyshire A, et al. Endotracheal suctioning causes right upper lobe collapse in intubated children. Acta Paediatr 1996;85:1422–5.

[54] Brodsky L, Naviawala S, Stanievich J. A quantitative comparison of the early histopathological changes from tracheotomy and endotracheal intubation on the distal trachea in fetal lambs. Int J Pediatr Otorhinolaryngol 1987;12:273–82.

[55] Drew J, Padoms K, Clabburn SL. Routine instillation of saline down the endotracheal tube in infants with hyaline membrane disease. (abstract) Aus Pediatr J 1984;20:257.

[56] Ackerman M, Ecklund M, Abu-Jumah M. A review of normal saline instillation: implications for practice. Dimens Crit Care Nurs 1996;15:31–8.

[57] Brodsky L, Reidy M, Stanievich J. The effects of suctioning techniques on the distal tracheal mucosa in intubated low birth weight infants. Int J Pediatr Otorhinolaryngol 1987;14:1–14.

[58] Hagler D, Traver G. Endotracheal saline and suction catheters: sources of lower airway contamination. Am J Crit Care 1994;3:444–7.

[59] Hodge D. Endotracheal suctioning and the infant: a nursing care protocol to decrease complications. Neonatal Netw 1991;9:7–15.

[60] Kleiber C. Clinical implications of deep and shallow suctioning in neonatal patients. Focus Crit Care 1986; 13:36–9.

[61] Kleiber C, Krutzfield N, Rose E. Acute histological changes in the tracheobronchial tree associated with different suction catheter insertion techniques. Heart Lung 1988;17:10–4.

[62] Rivera R, Tibbals J. Complications of endotracheal intubation and mechanical ventilation in infants and children. Crit Care Med 1992;20:193–9.

[63] Wood CJ. Endotracheal suctioning: a literature review. Intensive Crit Care Nurs 1998;14:124–36.

[64] Wood CJ. Can nurses safely assess the need for endotracheal suction in short-term ventilated patients, instead of using routine techniques? Intensive Crit Care Nurs 1998;14:170–8.

[65] Copnell B, Ferguson D. Endotracheal suctioning: time worn ritual or timely intervention. Am J Crit Care 1995;4:100–5.

[66] American Association for Respiratory Care. Clinical practice guidelines: endotracheal suctioning of mechanically ventilated adults and children with artificial airways. Respir Care 1993;38:500–4.

[67] American Thoracic Society. Care of the child with a tracheostomy: the official statement of the American Thoracic Society. Am J Respir Crit Care Med 2000; 161:297–308.

[68] Brooks D, Solway S, Graham I, et al. A survey of suctioning practices among physical therapists, respiratory therapists and nurses. Can Respir J 1999;6: 513–20.

[69] De Carle B. Tracheostomy care. Nurs Times 1985; 81(40):50–4.

[70] Tolles C, Stone K. National survey of neonatal endotracheal suctioning practices. Neonatal Netw 1990;9:7–14.

[71] Brooks D, Anderson C, Carter M, et al. Clinical practice guidelines for suctioning the airway of the intubated and non-intubated patient. Can Respir J 2001;8:163–81.

[72] Sandelowski M. Whatever happened to qualitative description? Res Nurs Health 2000;23:334–40.

[73] Boyle J. Field research: a collaborative model for practice and research. In: Morse J, editor. Qualitative nursing research: a contemporary dialogue. Thousand Oaks (CA): Sage Publications; 1991. p. 273–99.

[74] Holxworth RJ, Wills C. Nurses' judgment regarding seclusion and restraint of psychiatric patients: a social judgment analysis. Res Nurs Health 1999;22: 189–201.

[75] Kuipers B, Moskowitz A, Kassier J. Critical decisions under uncertainty: representation and structure. Cognitive Science 1988;12:177–210.

[76] Rubin H, Rubin I. Qualitative interviewing: the art of hearing data. Thousand Oaks (CA): Sage Publications; 1995.

[77] Fonteyn M, Fisher A. Use of think aloud method to study nurses' reasoning and decision making in clinical practice settings. J Neurosci Nurs 1995;27: 124–8.

[78] Spence K, Greenwood J, McDonald M, et al. Processing knowledge in practice: preliminary find-

ings of a study into neonatal intensive care nursing. J Neonatal Nurs 1999;5(2):27–30.

[79] Johnson A, Sackett R. Direct systematic observation of behaviour. In: Bernard HR, editor. Handbook of methods in cultural anthropology. London: Atimira Press; 1998. p. 301–31.

[80] Burnard P. A method of analyzing interview transcripts in qualitative research. Nurs Educ Today 1991; 11:461–6.

[81] Knox A. Performing endotracheal suction on children: a literature review and implications for nursing. Intensive Crit Care Nurs 1993;9:48–54.

[82] Simmons C. How frequently should endotracheal suctioning be undertaken? Am J Crit Care 1997;1:4–6.

[83] Hazinski M. Nursing care of the critically ill child. 2nd edition. Toronto: Mosby Year Book; 1992.

[84] Curley MAQ, Thompson JE. Oxygenation and ventilation. In: Curley MAQ, Moloney-Harmon P, editors. Critical care nursing of infants and children. 2nd edition. Toronto: WB Saunders; 2001. p. 233–308.

[85] Henneman E, Ellstron K, St. John R. Airway management. In: Chulay M, Burns S, editors. Protocols for practice: care of the mechanically ventilated patients series. Aliso Viejo (CA): American Association of Critical Care Nurses; 1999. p. 18–20.

[86] Webster HF, Grant MJ, Slota MC, et al. Respiratory disorders. In: Slota M, editors. Core curriculum for pediatric critical care nursing. Toronto: WB Saunders; 1998. p. 82–6.

[87] Tanner C, Benner P, Chesla C, et al. The phenomenology of knowing a patient. J Nurs Scholarsh 1993;25:273–80.

[88] MacLeod M. "It's the little things that count." The hidden complexity of every day clinical practice. J Clin Nurs 1994;3:361–8.

[89] Jenks JM. The pattern of personal knowing in nursing clinical decision making. J Nurs Educ 1993;32: 399–405.

[90] Johnson JL, Ratner PA. The nature of knowledge used in nursing practice. In: Thorne SE, Hayes VE, editors. Nursing praxis: knowledge and action. Thousand Oaks (CA): Sage Publications; 1997. p. 3–22.

[91] Liaschenko J. Knowing the patient. In: Thorne SE, Hayes VE, editors. Nursing praxis: knowledge and action. Thousand Oaks (CA): Sage Publications; 1997. p. 23–37.

[92] Liaschenko J, Fisher A. Theorizing the knowledge that nurses use in the conduct of their work. Sch Inq Nurs Pract 1999;13:29–41.

[93] Radwin LE. Knowing the patient: A process model for individualized interventions. Nurs Res 1995;44: 354–70.

[94] Radwin LE. Conceptualizations of decision making in nursing analytic models and "Knowing the patient". Nurs Diagn 1995;6:16–22.

[95] Agan D. Intuitive knowing as a dimension of nursing. ANS Adv Nurs Sci 1987;10:63–70.

[96] Radwin LE. Knowing the patient: a review of research on an emerging concept. J Adv Nurs 1996; 23:1142–6.

[97] Brykcznski K. An interpretive study describing the clinical judgment of nurse practitioners. Sch Inq Nurs Pract 1989;3:75–104.

[98] Einhorn J. Expert judgment: some necessary conditions and an example. In: Connolly T, Arkes H, Hammond K, editors. Judgment and decision making: an interdisciplinary reader. Cambridge (UK): University Press; 2000. p. 324–35.

[99] Easen P, Wilcockson J. Intuition and rational decision making in professional thinking: a false dichotomy. J Adv Nurs 1996;24:667–73.

[100] Fonteyn M. Thinking strategies for nursing practice. New York: Lippincott; 1998.

[101] Rashotte J, Thomas M. Incorporating educational theory into critical care orientation. J Cont Educ Nurs 2002;33:131–7.

ELSEVIER
SAUNDERS

Crit Care Nurs Clin N Am 17 (2005) 341 – 347

CRITICAL CARE
NURSING CLINICS
OF NORTH AMERICA

Diabetic Ketoacidosis in the Pediatric ICU

Jennifer E. Bevacqua, RN, BSN, CCRN[a,b,*]

[a]Pediatric Intensive Care Unit, Emanuel Children's Hospital, 2801 N. Gantenbein, Portland, OR 97227, USA
[b]Pediatric Post-Anesthesia Care Unit, Doernbecher Children's Hospital, 3181 SW Sam Jackson Park Road,
Portland, OR 97239, USA

Diabetic ketoacidosis (DKA), a common diagnosis in the pediatric ICU (PICU), is a pathophysiologic, life-threatening process that results from uncontrolled diabetes mellitus (DM)-induced hyperglycemia. The most common types of DM include DM type 1, DM type 2, and gestational diabetes [1]. Infants and children can suffer the consequences of any of these three endocrine derangements; untreated DM types 1 and 2 lead to hyperglycemic states. Although DM type 2 can lead to DKA [2,3], this article discusses DKA as a consequence of DM type 1, which is the most common scenario.

This article reviews the pathophysiology, management, goals of treatment, and nursing implications of the child who is diagnosed with DKA. Within discussion of DKA pathophysiology, expected laboratory values and expected symptomatology are addressed.

Overview of insulin and glucose conduct

Glucose, the major product of carbohydrate digestion, supplies the body with its primary source of energy [4]. In the healthy child, six hormones regulate glucose concentration: insulin, glucagon, pancreatic somatostatin, glucocorticoids, epinephrine, and growth hormone. The latter five hormones (termed "counterregulatory hormones") oppose the action of insulin and increase serum glucose levels; however,

lack of these hormones also can decrease serum glucose. Thus, insulin is the only known endogenous agent that can decrease serum glucose levels by increasing its secretion. Without insulin, glucose cannot be used as substrate.

Insulin facilitates uptake, storage, and use of glucose by almost all tissues of the body [5]. Although the mechanism is not understood completely, insulin binds to its target cell which activates enzymes that lead to phosphorylation and glucose transport into the cell [5]. Brain cells do not require insulin mediation to use glucose [5]. In addition to carbohydrate metabolism, insulin also affects fat and protein (promoting fat and protein synthesis and storage) metabolism [5]. The lack of insulin can cause multiple metabolic difficulties. Furthermore, insulin secretion is not controlled solely by the plasma glucose concentration. Free fatty acids, amino acids, gastrointestinal hormones, and other factors contribute to the increase or decrease in insulin secretion [5].

Normal glucose concentration in the plasma is determined by the relationship between supply and demand. Dietary intake, glycogenolysis, and hepatic gluconeogenesis influence the supply of glucose, whereas the energy needs of the body influence the demand for glucose use [6].

Despite the complexity that is inherent in glucose metabolism and insulin regulation, the two often equilibrate well. With the proper balance of glucose and insulin, and normal interaction between the two, the serum glucose level should be 40 to 60 mg/dL for the 1-day old, 50 to 90 mg/dL for the infant (< 12 months), 60 to 100 mg/dL for the child, and 70 to 105 mg/dL for the adult [7]. Serum insulin levels are not measured routinely measured in the diagnosis or treatment of DKA.

* Pediatric Intensive Care Unit, Emanuel Children's Hospital, 2801 N. Gantenbein, Portland, OR 97227.
E-mail address: bevacqua@ohsu.edu

0899-5885/05/$ – see front matter © 2005 Elsevier Inc. All rights reserved.
doi:10.1016/j.ccell.2005.07.010

Pathophysiology of diabetic ketoacidosis

The pathophysiology of DKA is complex. Each pediatric patient also is complex in his or her individual insulin, glucose, hormonal, and metabolic needs [8]. Moreover, depending on the stage of this illness and the stage of treatment, a clinician can witness much variation in patient presentation and laboratory values while the patient remains critically ill. Understanding and remembering these peculiar facets will benefit the care of the child.

DKA begins with untreated DM. Deficiency of insulin, as is the case with DM type 1, prevents glucose from being used as substrate. The cascade of events starts with the lack of bioavailable substrate—glucose—for the body which leads to multiple problems. Lipolysis (catabolism of fats) begins to supply the body with another substrate to be used for fuel—FFAs. At the same time, the body recognizes the underuse of glucose and attempts compensation by increasing production of endogenous hormones that will make, release, or otherwise raise glucose levels. At this point, the patient is experiencing inappropriate production of FFAs, hyperglycemia that is due to lack of use, and increased counterregulatory hormone activity (Fig. 1).

Increased lipolysis

Without glucose, a product of fat breakdown will be used to fuel the body. Increased lipolysis results in the production of FFAs. In the liver, FFAs are converted into triglycerides (with carbon dioxide and water) or the ketoacids: acetoacetic acid and β-hydroxybutyric acid [6]. The diminished activity of insulin and the enhanced secretion of glucagon (both occur in uncontrolled DM) cause hepatocyte function to be "reset" to produce ketoacids preferentially over the triglycerides [6]. The ketoacids serve as an alternative and less efficient, source of energy while glucose is unavailable. As the situation progresses, ketoacids accumulate in the body. Acetoacetic acid is responsible for the fruity acetone breath of the patient who has DKA [1,9]. This ketoacid accumulation promotes an acidotic environment that denatures proteins and impairs cellular function [10] to an extent which corresponds with the degree of acidosis. Besides general cell dysfunction, two potentially lethal effects of acidosis include a decrease in cardiac contractility (a negative inotropic effect) [11,12] and arrhythmogenicity [13]. An increase in catecholamine (epinephrine and norepinephrine) levels secondary to acidosis may contribute to ar-

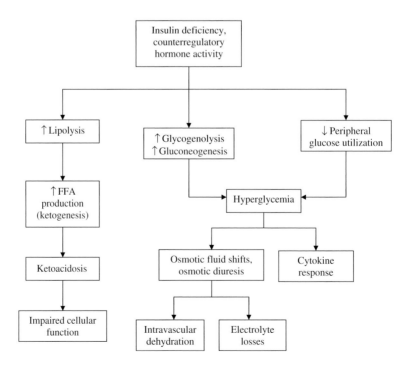

Fig. 1. Pathogenesis of diabetic ketoacidosis. *Adapted from* Goldberg PA, Inzucchi SE. Critical issues in endocrinology. Clin Chest Med 2003;24:586–606; with permission.

rhythmogenicity [14]. Although heightened vigilance is necessary in the PICU, cardiac effects are less common in children than in adults [15]. The ketoacidosis may contribute to nausea, vomiting, tachycardia, and abdominal pain [1]. DM most commonly is the result of an autoimmune, apoptotic (noninflammatory cell suicide) process, rather than a necrotic, inflammatory process [1]. As with any metabolic acidosis, the respiratory system attempts to compensate. Kussmaul respirations (rapid and deep) blow off carbon dioxide—a portion of carbonic acid—in efforts to normalize the pH of the serum and avoid the aforementioned sequelae of acidosis. These efforts are unlikely to compensate fully for the pH of the child who has DKA.

Hyperglycemia

Hyperglycemia is influenced by multiple factors in DKA. First, there is decreased peripheral glucose use. Ironically, although the body desperately needs glucose, the patient has excessive amounts in circulation that are unable to be used without insulin. Dietary intake likely will increase serum glucose levels. Second, as the body senses the underuse of glucose, it begins to form glucose in any way that it can. Normally, the extra glucose is stored in the form of glycogen, mainly in hepatic and muscle cells; however, with the type of glucose need that is seen in this situation, epinephrine and glucagon phosphorylate glycogen [5]. This action breaks glycogen into glucose, and thereby, increases serum blood glucose concentration. The body also compensates for this relative hypoglycemia by increasing gluconeogenesis. In gluconeogenesis, moderate quantities of glucose can be formed from various amino acids and glycerol (a portion of fat) [5]. Glucocorticoids (counterregulatory agents), such as cortisol, mobilize amino acids for this process [5].

Osmotic fluid shifts

Osmotic fluid shifts are one of the effects of the acute hyperglycemia (>200 mg/dL) that is seen in DKA. Glucose as an effective osmole leads to hypertonicity when increased in the extracellular space. Extracellular hypertonicity causes shifts between the extracellular fluid and intracellular fluid in an effort to equalize osmolarity. In addition, the kidneys are attempting to manage the hypertonic state. Once renal threshold is reached (~180 mg/dL) [1], glucose spills into the urine and leads to an osmotic diuresis with loss of water and electrolytes [16]. Polyuria, polydipsia, and dehydration will be evident, although if fluid intake is well maintained through polydipsia, dehydration may be minimal [15]. The combination of the effects of hypertonicity and the resultant urinary excretion of these nutrients can lead to an unbalanced state.

Sodium

Osmotic fluids shifts in DKA often result in a dilutional hyponatremia [15]. Most sodium (135–145 mEq/L) [17] is outside of the cell, and thus, the osmotic shifts may not change the actual amount of sodium in the extracellular fluid significantly. With the addition of water into the extracellular space in an attempt to equilibrate tonicity, a dilutional hyponatremia may result. To deduce the "true" sodium for a given glucose level that is greater than 100 mg/dL, use the following formula: [measured Na^+] + [(glucose − 100)/100] × 1.6 where glucose is measured in mg/dL [1,15]. Treatment of sodium should be based on this corrected value.

Potassium

Potassium is mainly an intracellular electrolyte. The extracellular concentration of potassium is 3.4 to 4.7 mEq/L for children [17]. Some sources claim that the metabolic acidosis that occurs in DKA drives some potassium out of the cell and into the extracellular fluid [4,17,18], whereas other investigators cite hyperglycemia [1,5] and the lack of insulin [6] as being responsible for depleting the cells of potassium. Regardless, in DKA there is a depletion of intracellular potassium, and this shift to increased extracellular potassium may or may not be evident in laboratory results, depending on the degree to which potassium has been excreted in the urine because of osmotic diuresis. Serum potassium levels may be low, normal, or high [19] although they most commonly are normal or high [1,20] in untreated DKA. Despite this, there is a whole body potassium depletion [9,15,16] because of the facets of osmotic shifts and diuresis. Insulin therapy is known to drive potassium into cells [1,20]; this underscores the importance of ensuring adequate potassium intake by way of intravenous fluids during therapy.

Phosphorus, magnesium, and calcium

Like potassium, phosphorus, magnesium, and calcium are depleted from the body during DKA [16]. The hypertonicity of the serum draws these electrolytes from inside cells to the extracellular space. They are excreted in the urine with the excess glucose, water, and other electrolytes. Normal magnesium levels are 1.7 to 2.1 mg/dL in children [17]. Serious arrhythmias and neurologic symptoms can arise with hypomagnesemia; however, the current literature does not comment on magnesium replacement in DKA. Hypomagnesemia may be "clinically insignificant" [21] in this case. Normal phosphorus levels are 4.5 to 5.5 mg/dL in children [17]. Replacement of phosphorus is not without risk of hypocalcemia and hypomagnesemia [22]. Normal ionized calcium levels are 1.10 to 1.38 mmol/L (4.40–5.52 mg/dL) in children [17]. Generally, calcium replacement is not indicated with DKA therapy. As with potassium, correction of acidosis and insulin therapy will begin to resolve the imbalances.

Cytokine milieu

DKA alters the cytokine milieu of the body [23–25]. It is not known definitively if hyperglycemia or another derangement in DKA is responsible for the increase in proinflammatory cytokines. Hoffman and colleagues [25] postulated that the time frame for the proinflammatory cytokine increase correlates with the progression of subclinical and clinical cerebral edema.

Increased counterregulatory hormone activity

The counterregulatory hormones increase serum glucose levels. In DKA, the body increases the levels of the counterregulatory hormones in an effort to remedy the relative hypoglycemia. During times of illness, stress, or infection these hormones often are elevated [4,15], and possibly precipitate DKA. These increases perpetuate metabolic decompensation by: (1) impairing insulin secretion (epinephrine) [1]; (2) antagonizing the action of insulin (epinephrine, cortisol, growth hormone) [1,4]; and (3) promoting glycogenolysis, gluconeogenesis, lipolysis, and ketogenesis (glucagon, epinephrine, growth hormone, cortisol) [1,4,20] while decreasing glucose use [1,4,20] and glucose clearance (epinephrine, growth hormone, cortisol) [1]. Somatostatin (also known as growth hormone inhibitory hormone) is a weak agent with contradictory effects [5]. In one study, octreotide, an analog of somatostatin, reduced the duration of ketonuria significantly [26]; this underscores the possibilities that counterregulatory hormone activity may have in the future treatment of DKA.

Diagnosis of diabetic ketoacidosis

The signs and symptoms for DKA can be straightforward or nonspecific [27]. Polyuria, poly-

dipsia, polyphagia with Kussmaul respirations, weight loss, abdominal pain, and nausea are common histories for the older child who has DKA [1,19]. Laboratory values show hyperglycemia (generally >200 mg/dL), metabolic acidosis, low bicarbonate, and hyperosmolality [19]. The child's primary care practitioner may discover possible DKA through urine laboratory results when evaluating the ill child.

Anion gap

Evaluating the anion gap can be helpful in narrowing the differential diagnosis of a patient who has metabolic acidosis. The anion gap is the difference between the unmeasured cations and the unmeasured anions in the blood, and can be calculated using the formula: $[Na^+] - ([Cl^-] + [HCO_3^-])$. There is no true anion gap in the blood because the body continually works to balance cations and anions. Thus, the anion gap formula was created only to be of diagnostic assistance. The normal anion gap using the above formula is 5 to 11 mEq/L [6]. In a pathophysiologic state of increased unmeasured anions, bicarbonate would be decreased without a concomitant increase in chloride. This would produce an "increased anion gap" per the formula, and would inform the practitioner that there are unmeasured anions in the blood. Many causes of increased anion gap exist: lactic acidosis, ketoacidosis, renal failure, ingestions (salicylate, methanol/formaldehyde, ethylene glycol, paraldehyde, toluene, sulfur, isoniazid overdose, iron overdose, ethanol), and rhabdomyolysis [6,28]. Metabolic acidosis with a normal anion gap indicates that there is a hyperchloremic acidosis. In this case, the amount of unmeasured anions is the same as normal (no metabolic acidosis) blood; however, the level of bicarbonate is decreased, whereas the level of chloride is increased. Diarrhea, renal tubular acidosis, renal failure, hypoaldosteronism, and ammonium chloride ingestion are some causes of hyperchloremic metabolic acidosis [6,28]. Because the negative charges on plasma proteins account for most of the unmeasured anions, hypoalbuminemia invalidates the above formula [6].

Complications of diabetic ketoacidosis

Acute complications of DKA and its treatment include hypoglycemia, persistent acidosis, hypokalemia, fluid overload, mucormycosis (an opportunistic fungus) infection [19], thrombosis [29,30], cerebral edema [19], as well as some rare complications, such as rhabdomyolysis [31] and ischemic intestinal necrosis [32]. Intensive care with evidence-based treatment of the patient who has DKA prevents most of these complications.

Cerebral edema is an especially worrisome complication of DKA; it occurs in at least 1% of cases of pediatric DKA [33]. It is more common in children than in adults [20,34] which might reflect the unique fluid and electrolyte needs of the child. There are multiple theories on the cause of cerebral edema in the patient who has DKA. Although there is agreement that cerebral edema in DKA involves an osmotic shift that results in intracellular swelling, the exact mechanism has yet to be identified. Prominent theories include overhydration, vasogenic edema, or postischemic changes [15,19,33–35]. Multiple investigators claim that cerebral edema has occurred before treatment; this suggests that the mechanism that causes cerebral edema is not due to simple overhydration with hypotonic fluids and subsequent intracellular edema [33,36]. Symptoms of cerebral edema may include decreased or altered level of consciousness, headache, abnormal pupil findings, sudden hypertension or hypotension, seizures, incontinence, bradycardia, and respiratory arrest [15,20]; these highlight the need for neurologic assessments in the care of the child who has DKA. CT scan may not detect subtle, but physiologically significant edema [34]. Risk factors for development of cerebral edema include lower initial partial pressures of arterial carbon dioxide, higher initial serum urea nitrogen concentrations, and the lack of increase in serum sodium during therapy when compared with random and matched control groups [33]. Standard treatment for cerebral edema is 20% mannitol, although hypertonic saline (3%) has shown promise [37], and theoretically, seems to be more physiologically appropriate than a diuretic. Until more is known about the pathogenesis of cerebral edema, treatments will be experimental.

Basic treatment of diabetic ketoacidosis

Fluid and electrolyte therapy

Insulin therapy along with fluid and electrolyte replacements are the mainstay of DKA treatment. The appropriate type and rate of fluid management in pediatric DKA has been controversial. Because of the dehydration that is inherent in the DKA process and the potential dangers of rapid correction, practitioners generally agree that this is a "touchy" situation [21,38] and that a conservative approach

is best [39]. Current recommendations for initial fluid therapy are 10 to 20 mL/kg 0.9% normal saline or lactated ringers over an hour, repeated once only if necessary [20,40]. The risk of neurologic complications is greater if the patient receives more than 50 mL/kg during the first 4 hours of therapy [36]. Recommendations for continued fluid therapy are less than or equal to 4 L/m^2/24 h [41] or 1.5 times the 24-hour maintenance requirements [20], although it is essential to remember to individualize each patient assessment, because the patient could be on either end of the hydration spectrum [42]. Continued fluid therapy should contain 0.45% to 0.9% normal saline [19–21,39,43], and maintain a fine balance between free water for re-expansion of extracellular space, but with enough sodium to maintain proper tonicity of serum and avoid hyponatremia. Polydipsia and composition of oral intake can differ widely and impact dehydration status. Recommendations for glucose and electrolytes can be found in Table 1. There is some disagreement about when phosphorus replacement is appropriate or necessary. Phosphorus replacement is indicated only if levels are low (< 3.0 mg/dL) [44] by one investigator, whereas another investigator [9] and the American Diabetic Association [20] advocate phosphorus replacement only in patients who have hypophosphatemic symptoms or a serum concentration of less than 1.0 mg/dL. Further research on these treatment regimens is needed.

Table 1
Recommendations for continued fluid and electrolyte therapies in pediatric DKA

Additive	Recommendation	References
Sodium content	0.45–0.9% NaCl, depending on serum sodium concentration	[19–21, 39,44]
Potassium content	If K$^+$ <2.5 mEq/L, treat K$^+$ and hold insulin. If K$^+$ 2.5–5.0, administer 30–60 mEq/L as 1/3 KPO$_4$ and 2/3 KCl or Kacetate. Do not give intravenous K$^+$ if > 5.0.	[20]
Phosphorus content	Replace if symptomatic or PO$_4$ <1.0 mg/dL, use KPO$_4$ in potassium replacement.	[9,20,39]
	Replace if PO$_4$ <1 mmol/L (3 mg/dL)	[43]
Glucose content	Add 5% dextrose once serum glucose ≤ 250 mg/dL. Once serum glucose ≤ 150 mg/dL, add 10% dextrose to fluids.	[9,19,20]

Insulin therapy

Insulin therapy by continuous infusion is recommended in the pediatric patient who has DKA. No initial bolus is recommended in the pediatric population [20]. The usual dose is 0.1 units/kg/h starting from after the initial fluid therapy until subcutaneous insulin is given in the recovery period [20]. Insulin should not be stopped completely during therapy unless serum glucose decreases to less than 100 mg/dL [19].

With this combination of insulin and fluid therapy, the metabolic acidosis should resolve. Persistent acidosis calls for a reassessment and review of therapy for the child. Bicarbonate therapy rarely is necessary and is not recommended unless acidosis is severe (pH<7.0) [1,9,20].

Nursing care

Nursing care is pivotal in the treatment of the child who has DKA. Besides the standard and highly important care of any critically ill child (eg, airway, breathing, circulation, physical assessment, patient and family psychologic support), the child with DKA has unique needs. Nursing staff need to:

- Perform frequent vital signs (every 30 minutes to every 2 hours)
- Monitor serum glucose every hour while the child is on continuous insulin. Ensure that the specimen is not diluted with dextrose-containing fluids.
- Monitor blood gases, serum electrolytes, and serum osmolarities every 2 to 4 hours until stable (for at least 12 hours after start of therapies)
- Monitor serum and urine ketones, depending on practitioners' discretion
- Evaluate neurologic and cardiac status frequently
- Monitor weight, intake, and urine output. Enforce "nothing by mouth" status until patient is ready for subcutaneous insulin in the recovery period.
- Monitor for complications of DKA and DKA therapy

Summary

DKA is a medical emergency. The complex pathophysiology of this disorder is compounded by the complexity of the child. Even within the pediatric population there is infinite variety in growth and metabolic needs, hormone levels, and fluid require-ments. More research is needed on how these differences impact therapy and how complications, such as cerebral edema, can be averted. For now, thoughtfully attending to pathophysiology, understanding evidence-based management, and individualizing therapy of the child who has DKA is the standard of care.

References

[1] Alemzadeh RW, Wyatt DT. Diabetes mellitus. In: Behrman RE, Kliegman RM, Jenson HB, editors. Nelson textbook of pediatrics. 17th edition. Philadelphia: Saunders; 2004. p. 1947–72.

[2] Pinhas-Hamiel O, Dolan LM, Zeitler PS. Diabetic ketoacidosis among obese African-American Adolescents with NIDDM. Diabetes Care 1997;20(4):484–6.

[3] Valabhji J, Watson M, Cox J, et al. Type 2 diabetes presenting as diabetic ketoacidosis in adolescence. Diabet Med 2003;20(5):416–7.

[4] Siegel J. Diabetes mellitus. In: Copstead LC, Banasik JL, editors. Pathophysiology biological and behavioral perspectives. 2nd edition. Philadelphia: W.B. Saunders Co.; 2000. p. 920–44.

[5] Guyton AC, Hall JE. Textbook of medical physiology. 10th edition. Philadelphia: W.B. Saunders Co.; 2000.

[6] Rose DB. Clinical physiology of acid-base and electrolyte disorders. 4th edition. New York: McGraw-Hill; 1994.

[7] Nicholson JF, Pesce MA. Reference ranges for laboratory tests and procedures. In: Behrman RE, Kliegman RM, Jenson HB, editors. Nelson textbook of pediatrics. 17th edition. Philadelphia: Saunders; 2004. p. 2396–426.

[8] Franzese A, Valerio G, Spagnuolo MI. Management of diabetes in childhood: are children small adults? Clin Nutr 2004;23:293–305.

[9] Goldberg PA, Inzucchi SE. Critical issues in endocrinology. Clin Chest Med 2003;24(4):583–606.

[10] Felver L. Acid-base homeostasis and imbalances. In: Copstead LC, Banasik JL, editors. Pathophysiology biological and behavioral perspectives. 2nd edition. Philadelphia: W.B. Saunders Co.; 2000.

[11] Balnave CD, Vaughan-Jones RD. Effect of intracellular pH on spontaneous Ca2 + sparks in rat ventricular myocytes. J Physiol 2000;528(1):25–37.

[12] Takahashi R, Shimazaki Y, Endoh M. Decrease in Ca2+-sensitizing effect of UD-CG 212 Cl, a metabolite of pimobendan, under acidotic conditions in canine ventricular myocardium. J Pharmacol Exp Ther 2001; 298(3):1060–6.

[13] Orchard CH, Kentish JC. Effects of changes of pH on the contractile function of cardiac muscle. Am J Physiol 1990;258(6):967–81.

[14] Felver L. Acid-base balance and imbalances. In: Woods SL, Sivarajan-Froelicher ES, Underhill-Motzer

PC, editors. Cardiac nursing. 4th edition. Philadelphia: Lippincott Williams & Wilkins; 2000. p. 156–7.

[15] White NH. Diabetic ketoacidosis in children. Endocrinology and Metabolism Clinics 2000;29(4):657–82.

[16] Atchley DW, Loeb RF, Richards DW, et al. A detailed study of electrolyte balances following withdrawal and reestablishment of insulin therapy. J Clin Invest 1933; 12:297–326.

[17] Fischbach F. A manual of laboratory and diagnostic tests. 7th edition. Philadelphia: Lippincott Williams & Wilkins; 2004.

[18] Fleckman AM. Diabetic ketoacidosis. Endocrinology and Metabolism Clinics of North America 1993;22(2): 181–207.

[19] Craig J. Endocrine system. In: Slota MC, editor. Core curriculum for pediatric critical care nursing. Philadelphia: W.B. Saunders Co.; 1998.

[20] American Diabetic Association. Hyperglycemic crises in patients with diabetes mellitus. Diabetes Care 2003; 26(Suppl 1):S109–17.

[21] Hafeez W, Vuguin P. Managing diabetic ketoacidosis—a delicate balance. Contemp Pediatr 2000;17(6): 72–8.

[22] Zipf WB, Bacon GE, Spencer ML, et al. Hypocalcemia, hypomagnesemia, and transient hypoparathyroidism during therapy with potassium phosphate in diabetic ketoacidosis. Diabetes Care 1979;2(3):265–8.

[23] Iori E, Calo L, Ceolotto G, et al. Diabetic ketosis activates lymphomonocyte-inducible nitric oxide synthase. Diabet Med 2002;19:777–83.

[24] Kitabchi AE, Stentz FB, Umpierrez GE. Diabetic ketoacidosis induces in vivo activation of human T-lymphocytes. Biochem Biophys Res Commun 2004; 315:404–7.

[25] Hoffman WH, Burek CL, Waller JL, et al. Cytokine response to diabetic ketoacidosis and its treatment. Clin Immunol 2003;108:175–81.

[26] Yun YS, Lee HC, Park CS, et al. Effects of long-acting somatostatin analogue (Sandostatin) on manifest diabetic ketoacidosis. J Diabetes Complications 1999; 13(5–6):288–92.

[27] Harper DE, Waldrop RD. Infant diabetic ketoacidosis in the emergency department. South Med J 1996;89(7): 729–31.

[28] Greenbaum LA. Pathophysiology of body fluids and fluid therapy. In: Behrman RE, Kliegman RM, Jenson HB, editors. Nelson textbook of pediatrics. 17th edition. Philadelphia: Saunders; 2004. p. 191–252.

[29] Worly JM, Fortenberry JD, Hansen I, et al. Deep venous thrombosis in children with diabetic ketoacidosis and femoral central venous catheters. Pediatrics 2004;113(1):e57–60.

[30] Carl GF, Hoffman WH, Passmore GG, et al. Diabetic ketoacidosis promotes a prothrombotic state. Endocr Res 2003;29(1):73–82.

[31] Casteels K, Beckers D, Wouters C, Van Geet C. Rhabdomyolysis in diabetic ketoacidosis. Pediatr Diabetes 2003;4:29–31.

[32] DiMeglio LA, Chaet MS, Quigley CA, Grosfeld JL. Massive ischemic intestinal necrosis at the onset of diabetes mellitus with ketoacidosis in a three-year-old girl. J Pediatr Surg 2003;38(10):1537–9.

[33] Glaser N, Barnett P, McCaslin I, et al. Risk factors for cerebral edema in children with diabetic ketoacidosis. N Engl J Med 2001;344(4):264–9.

[34] Bohn D, Daneman D. Diabetic ketoacidosis and cerebral edema. Curr Opin Pediatr 2002;14:287–91.

[35] Glaser NS, Wootton-Gorges SL, Marcin JP, et al. Mechanism of cerebral edema in children with diabetic ketoacidosis. J Pediatr 2004;145:164–71.

[36] Mahoney CP, Vlcek BM, DelAguila M. Risk factors for developing brain herniation during diabetic ketoacidosis. Pediatr Neurol 1999;21:721–7.

[37] Kamat P, Vats A, Gross M, et al. Use of hypertonic saline for the treatment of altered mental status associated with diabetic ketoacidosis. Pediatr Crit Care Med 2003;4(2):239–42.

[38] Inward CD, Chambers TL. Fluid management in diabetic ketoacidosis. Arch Dis Child 2002;86(6):443–5.

[39] Kitabchi AE, Umpierrez GE, Murphy MB, et al. Management of hyperglycemic crises in patients with diabetes. Diabetes Care 2001;24(1):131–53.

[40] Moff I, Peterson R. Endocrinology. In: Gunn VL, Nechyba C, editors. The Harriet Lane handbook. 16th edition. Philadelphia: Mosby; 2002. p. 213–6.

[41] Duck SC, Wyatt DT. Factors associated with brain herniation in the treatment of diabetic ketoacidosis. J Pediatr 1988;113(1):10–4.

[42] Harris GD, Fiordalisi I. Physiologic management of DKA. Arch Dis Child 2002;87(5):451–2.

[43] Felner EI, White PC. Improving management of diabetic ketoacidosis in children. Pediatrics 2001;108(3): 735–40.

[44] Carroll MF, Schade DS. Ten pivotal questions about diabetic ketoacidosis. Postgrad Med 2001;110(5): 89–94.

ELSEVIER
SAUNDERS

Crit Care Nurs Clin N Am 17 (2005) 349 – 360

CRITICAL CARE
NURSING CLINICS
OF NORTH AMERICA

Death in the Pediatric ICU: Caring for Children and Families at the End of Life

Beverley Copnell, RN, RSCN, BAppSc, PhD[a,b,*]

[a]*Neonatal Unit, The Royal Children's Hospital, Flemington Road, Parkville, Victoria 3052, Melbourne, Australia*
[b]*Murdoch Childrens Research Institute, Melbourne, Australia*

Death in childhood has become a rare occurrence in developed countries; nevertheless, significant numbers of children continue to die each year. The need to improve the care of dying children has been emphasized in several publications [1–3]. Several studies in the United States, Canada, the United Kingdom, the Netherlands, and Australia found that most in-hospital deaths took place in the pediatric ICU (PICU) [4–12]. Hence, much of the onus for providing quality care at the end of life falls on PICU staff. Traditionally, the PICU has been associated with curative functions; the entire concept of "critical care" is predicated on the possibility of survival [13]. Hence, PICU clinicians may be ill-prepared, educationally and psychologically, to provide this care. Several sets of guidelines have been produced that may assist clinicians in this task [14–18]. The need for research to improve care is acknowledged, and directives have been produced in the areas of general pediatrics [2] and critical care [19]; however, no directives specifically address research in PICU end-of-life care. This article summarizes current research findings and suggests future directions for research to improve care in this important area. Only articles that focus on, or include care of, PICU patients are reviewed here; research confined to neonatal or adult patients in the ICU has been excluded.

* Neonatal Unit, The Royal Children's Hospital, Flemington Road, Parkville, Victoria 3052 Australia.
E-mail address: bev.copnell@rch.org.au

How do children die in the pediatric ICU?

In a highly technological environment, the concept of "natural" death is rendered virtually meaningless. Critical illness demands a decision to continue to provide full intensive care management, including the performance of cardiopulmonary resuscitation (CPR) in the event of a deterioration (which may be expected or unexpected) or to "allow" death to occur. On this basis, Anderson and colleagues [20] considered that deaths in the PICU could be classified as planned or unplanned. It is more usual, and perhaps more useful, to consider the mode of death as belonging to one of four categories: (1) death that occurs despite all efforts on the part of clinicians (herein called "failed CPR"); (2) declaration of death on demonstration of lack of brain stem function in accordance with local legislation ("brain death"); (3) death after a decision to withhold one or more therapeutic interventions or supports ("limitation"); and (4) death after a decision to withdraw one or more therapies or supports that already have been initiated ("withdrawal").

Seventeen studies were found that documented the modes of death of PICU patients [6,10,20–34]; these studies are summarized in Table 1. Comparisons between these studies are hampered by inconsistencies of categorization (eg, inclusion of all restrictions other than a "do not resuscitate" order in the same category as withdrawals [6,10,31,32]) and of patient selection (inclusion of deaths outside the PICU [6,24]). Nevertheless, there are several points of interest. The combined "planned" deaths (withdrawals and limitations) varied in these studies from 30% to 65% of

Table 1
Studies reporting modes of death in PICUs

Author [ref]	Location	No. of PICUs	Type of study	Patient selection	Total deaths	Mode of death (% of total deaths)			
						Failed CPR	Brain death	Withdrawal	Limitation
Mink & Pollack, 1992 [21]	USA	1	Prospective cohort study	Consecutive PICU deaths to achieve sample size	50	38%	30%	24%	8%
Vernon et al, 1993 [22]	USA	1	Retrospective chart review	All PICU deaths in 54-month period	300	19%	23%	32%	26%
Ryan et al, 1993 [23]	Canada	1	Retrospective chart review	All PICU deaths in 24-month period	73	29%	22%	34%	15%
Lantos et al, 1993 [6]	USA	1	Retrospective chart review	All hospital deaths in 12-month period	54 (incl. 2 deaths outside PICU)	46%	24%	13% (incl. limitations other than DNR)	17%
Levetown et al, 1994 [24]	USA	16	Prospective cohort study	All PICU admissions in 24-month period	265 (incl. deaths outside PICU)	Not stated	Not stated	15%	22% (11% DNR; 11% others)
Anderson et al, 1994 [20]	New Zealand	1	Retrospective chart review	All PICU deaths in 12-month period	25	36%	0	56%	8%
Balfour-Lynn & Tasker, 1996 [25]	United Kingdom	1	Retrospective chart review	All PICU deaths in 24-month period	89	18%	17%	50%	15%
Martinot et al, 1998 [26]	France	9	Prospective cohort study	All PICU deaths (excluding preterm infants) in 4-month period	92	26%	20%	27%	27%
van der Wal et al, 1999 [10]	Netherlands	1	Retrospective chart review	All hospital deaths in 48-month period (PICU-specific data reported)	134	28%	24%	36% (incl. limitations other than DNR)	12%

Study	Country	No.	Study type	Sample	N				
Goh et al, 1999 [27]	Malaysia	1	Retrospective chart review	All PICU deaths in 2 time periods (12 & 18 months)	148	41%	8%	5%	46%
Burns et al, 2000 [28]	USA	3	Prospective cohort study	Consecutive PICU deaths to achieve sample size	97	30%	15%	55%	0
Meert et al, 2000 [29]	USA	1	Retrospective chart review, interview	All PICU deaths in 42-month period	155	35%	14%	34%	17%
Devictor et al, 2001 [30]	France	33	Prospective cohort study	All PICU deaths in 4-month period	264	60%[a]		40%[a]	
Althabe et al, 2003 [31]	Argentina	16	Prospective cohort study	All PICU deaths in 12-month period	448	52%	11.5%	20.5% (incl. limitations other than DNR)	16% (DNR only)
Garros et al, 2003 [32]	Canada	1	Prospective cohort study	All PICU deaths in 8-month period	99	27%	13%	43%	16%
Devictor & Nguyen, 2004 [33]	Northern & Southern Europe (NE, SE)	39 NE=12 SE=27	Prospective cohort study	All PICU deaths in 4-month period	NE=68 SE=282 Total 350	32% 48%	21% 22%	47%[a] 30%[a]	
Zawistowski & Devita, 2004 [34]	USA	1	Retrospective chart review	Quasi-random selection of PICU deaths to achieve convenience sample of 50 that were preceded by withdrawal of intervention(s)	125	16%	19%	40%	25%

Abbreviations: DNR, do not resuscitate; incl, including.

[a] Combined data reported for these categories.

the total. There is some tendency for this figure to increase in later publications, particularly those that arise from the United States [6,21,22,24,28,29,34]; this finding may indicate an increasing willingness among clinicians to limit or withdraw aggressive treatment. There are insufficient studies from other individual countries to draw this comparison; however, it is worth noting that one French study [26] reported a higher rate than all subsequent European studies [10,30,33]. These figures cast doubt on the notion of cultural factors dominating decision-making in this region [30,33]. Even allowing for inconsistent definition, there was considerable variation among studies in the extent to which active withdrawal was practiced in preference to limitation. Some investigators [27,31] acknowledged a lack of comfort with withdrawing interventions, whereas others offered no explanation. Finally, the reported instances of failed CPR, where figures were cited, varied from 18% to 52%, indicating that even in units where "planned" deaths predominate, substantial numbers of children continue to die in this manner. This mode of death requires a different approach in many ways, yet is largely neglected in the literature.

How decisions are made: clinicians' perspectives

Several studies have attempted to document some aspect of the decision-making process in end-of-life care, by retrospective review [20,22,23,27] and prospectively by physicians documenting their practice [21,24,30–33]. Because retrospective reviews are limited by the information documented in the patients' notes, the accuracy of the data cannot be guaranteed. Prospective studies have the advantage of being able to elicit specific and detailed data.

All studies suggested that physicians took the major role in decision-making, initiating discussions about withdrawing or limiting interventions in most cases. Parents were reported to initiate such discussions in 5% to 24% of cases [21,24,31,32]. Most studies described parents being involved in negotiating management options with the medical team, with the final decision sometimes being a compromise between potentially conflicting stances (eg, placing limits on aggressive treatment or withdrawing ventilation or vasoactive agents gradually instead of extubating the child) [20–23,27,32]. Goh and colleagues [27] described continuing full support when the parents were unable to accept any restrictions on management; Garros and colleagues [32] discussed honoring parents' refusal of specific therapies on religious grounds. The process of reaching a mutually

acceptable consensus was described as taking between 2 and 48 hours [20], and as requiring 1 to 10 discussions [24], and one to three formal meetings [20,32]. Garros and colleagues [32] found that difficulty in achieving a consensus was associated with families' religious affiliation, but with no other personal or clinical factors. In a Malaysian study, Goh and colleagues [27] reported the involvement of the extended family in almost all discussions.

Prospective studies from Europe [30,33] and Argentina [31] described a unilateral decision-making process by medical staff. Althabe and colleagues [31] indicated that families were informed of the decision to limit therapy in 36% of cases; withdrawal of therapy rarely occurred. Devictor and colleagues [30] detailed a process in which the medical team participated in several meetings to reach a consensus on management options. Parents rarely were involved in the meeting, and were informed of the decision in only 19% of cases. Parents' opinions on the continuation of life support were documented in 72% of cases, but no details were given as to how these opinions were solicited. In a follow-up study, practices in northern and southern European PICUs were compared using the same study design [33]. The results indicated that a similar process took place in both groups of PICUs, although this impression may be a function of the tool that was used. In northern European PICUs, parents were more likely to be informed of the decision of the medical team than in southern units (95% versus 68%), and more likely to agree with the decision (100% versus 86%). These practices were attributed by the investigators to cultural and religious differences in these countries; however, critics noted that parents' opinions were not solicited and that there was little to suggest widespread public support for such practices [35,36].

Nurses' participation in decision making was mentioned in four studies, and was reported as occurring in 41% [27], 46% [30], 75% [32], and 100% [20] of cases. Other staff reported as participating in discussions included physicians from other specialties [20,30], junior medical staff [30,32], psychologists or psychiatrists [30], chaplains, and social workers [32].

Clinicians' perceptions of the decision-making process were elicited in a survey of nurses and physicians in three PICUs [37]. Doctors were seen by both disciplines as initiating discussions concerning withdrawal of life support in most cases, with family members doing so on few occasions. There was disagreement on the nurses' role, with 55% of nurses and 28% of doctors indicating that they believed that nurses initiated discussions. The disciplines also disagreed on other aspects of the decision-making process. Physicians were more likely than nurses to perceive that families were given sufficient information, that discussions took place among team members, and that physicians were involved at the bedside [37].

As critics have observed [35,36], these studies, while providing some useful data, have failed to capture the details of the decision-making process. Researchers conducting prospective studies in particular are seen to have missed valuable opportunities by limiting the amount and type of data that they collected [35]. There are several indications in the literature that decision making is a complex process. Two studies [27,31] described the ongoing management of patients who were declared brain dead; the authors of both papers commented that societal acceptance of this concept was limited. Similarly, respondents' comments in a survey of clinicians' attitudes [38] suggested that decision-making was a negotiated process, and could not be described or determined by reference to "rules." No studies have sought to examine this complexity.

Managing the dying process

Several studies have made reference to the management of children dying in the PICU, and two studies focused exclusively on this topic [28,34]. These descriptions were confined almost entirely to patients in whom interventions were withdrawn or limited, and mainly concerned descriptions of which interventions were withdrawn [20,24,28,31,34] and administration of analgesia and sedation [9,12,20, 28,32,34]. Only one study [20] made specific reference to children dying after CPR.

Treatment modalities that were withdrawn or limited invariably included mechanical ventilation and vasoactive drugs, either singly or in combination. Most studies reported extubation as the most common mode of withdrawing ventilation, with smaller numbers of patients undergoing a slow wean from ventilation [20,24,28,34]. Althabe and colleagues [31] reported limitation or withdrawal of inotropes as the most common mode, followed by weaning of ventilation; extubation rarely was undertaken.

Administration of analgesia and/or sedation during withdrawal of life support was mentioned briefly by Anderson and colleagues [20]—who stated that 50% of patients received morphine—and was described in detail in three other studies [28,32,34]. In all, narcotics were administered to all patients barring those who were comatose, with the baseline dose being increased in various numbers of patients. All three studies made reference to neuromuscular blockade being in effect in a small number of patients at the time of withdrawal of life support, their reported practices complying with published recommendations [39]. One retrospective study of all inpatient deaths—83% of which took place in the PICU—reported that 84% of children received opioids and 23% received nonopioid analgesia [9]. This study alone reported the use of complementary medications (three patients) and nonpharmacologic therapy (five patients); it was not stated whether these patients died in the PICU [9]. A similar study [12] reported that pain medication was ordered for 81% of patients who died in the PICU.

In addition to documenting practices, Burns and colleagues [28] surveyed physicians and nurses to ascertain their opinions of medication administration. There was agreement between doctors and nurses in most cases on the reasons for administering analgesia and/or sedation to specific patients, and the adequacy of the dose to ensure the child's comfort; however, several nurses were dissatisfied with the medication dose [28].

None of these studies indicated the basis for decisions regarding choice or dose of medications. There were no references to use of formal pain or comfort assessment tools in the PICU studies. Carter and colleagues [12] observed that pain assessment and management were documented in only 33% and 34% of nursing and medical notes, respectively, and that no formal tools were used. They also noted that other symptoms were documented poorly, and suggested that the lack of validated scoring systems for symptoms other than pain may contribute to the lack of documentation. McCallum and colleagues [9] noted that five oncology patients had formal pain assessment records in their charts but these records were used sporadically in the final week of life; again, the location of these deaths was not specified. No studies mentioned consulting other services, such as Pain Management or Palliative Care, to assist with managing symptoms. Carter and colleagues [12] reported the infrequent involvement of support services, such as child life, social work, and pastoral care, for end-of-life support in general for patients in the PICU.

The presence of family members at the time of death was mentioned in several studies, with actual figures reported as 74% and 76% in two American studies [32,34], and 64% and 46% in northern and southern European PICUs, respectively [33]. Reasons for absence were not recorded or not commented on. Other studies made reference to most families wanting to be present [21], and extended families being present whenever possible [20]. One study referred to children dying after CPR, and reported that eight out of nine sets of parents were present throughout resuscitation [20]. Two studies reported that 30% [34] and 78% [32] of parents held their children as they died. Anderson and colleagues [20] reported that 11 patients were taken to a laying-out room outside the PICU for grieving to continue, and documented formal follow-up and use of family support services. No further details of the dying process were recorded in any studies. Mink and Pollack [21] commented that withdrawal of life support can enable death to occur at a prearranged time suitable for family members, but provided no details. Zawistowski and DeVita [34] noted that environmental enhancement, such as music and the presence of familiar objects, may be used, but no details were recorded in the charts that they reviewed.

In summary, descriptions of end-of-life management in the extant literature provide useful snapshots of practice. Poor documentation is a recurring theme in all retrospective studies, and all studies indicate areas in which care could be improved; however, the information that these studies provide is limited. In restricting the data collected, prospective studies have failed to capture the total picture of end-of-life care, and a rather simplistic view of the process is presented. It is suggested that this view is inconsistent with the experiences of most clinicians [40].

Nurses' role in end-of-life care

There is little in the literature concerning the nursing role in end-of-life care of patients in the PICU. One commentary [41] described the role as supervision of the dying process and of the parents, and suggested that nurses perform this work mainly by intuition. The authors stated that nurses do not take responsibility for end-of-life decision-making; rather, their role is to support the decisions made by others—physicians and parents. They stressed the importance of team work in the process. Nesbit and colleagues [42] described a clinical pathway for traumatic deaths that was developed to provide a systematized approach to patient and family care. The pathway specified intermediate goals and clinical outcomes, was for use by all disciplines involved in the child's care, and was intended to be the plan and the record of care.

Only one research report was found that specifically addressed the nursing role [43]. This Australian study was undertaken to improve the care given to

families of culturally diverse backgrounds. Through a coparticipatory methodology, nurses came to see their practices as attempts to control families and to ensure their conformity to established routines and the values of the PICU staff. Practices, such as providing privacy for parents and encouraging them to hold the child after death, were seen as normal, but were revealed as culturally informed notions of the dying process. These norms often were deemed inappropriate by parents holding other cultural beliefs. Nurses found it difficult to communicate and develop relationships with parents who did not speak fluent English; hence, parents often were unable to convey their wants and needs. It was realized that some parents acted against their own cultural values simply to please the nurses. An unstated implication of this study is that a large component of the nursing role consists of developing relationships with families to encourage them to express their needs.

This point also was made in a study of nurses' experiences of treatment withdrawal in the PICU [40]. Although not addressing the nursing role directly, this study described nurses as demonstrating complex skills in the physical care of the child and in developing relationships with families. The study also highlighted the complexity of the lived experience, and contrasted its findings with the highly mechanistic approach that dominates a large proportion of the literature.

Clinicians' attitudes

Considerable variations in end-of-life practices are apparent in the literature. Most studies have attempted to correlate practice with clinical factors, such as diagnosis, prognosis, and presence of chronic or pre-existing conditions [20–27,30,31,33]. There is also recognition that clinicians' own values, attitudes, and experiences can influence their practice. Two surveys of physicians and nurses, each in a single PICU, found considerable divergence of opinion concerning which patients should have limitations placed on their management and which interventions should be limited [44], and which factors they considered to be important in decision making [38,44]. These findings suggest that patient management in an individual unit may depend on which clinicians are involved in care; however, no attempt was made in either study to relate attitudes to clinician characteristics.

Such an attempt was made in a survey of nurses and physicians in three PICUs [37], which included an assessment of clinicians' compliance with current guidelines and ethical standards. Almost half of the nurses and a quarter of the physicians believed that there was an ethical difference between withdrawing and withholding life support. Fourteen percent of nurses and 26% of physicians disagreed that narcotics should be given to most patients after withdrawal of life support, and 2% of each group believed that neuromuscular blocking agents should be added to the medication regimen at this time. Overall, 16% of respondents were judged as being reluctant to follow guidelines. In a multifactorial analysis, years of clinical experience was the only significant factor associated with this reluctance. Political and religious affiliation of individuals, and factors relating to the practice setting, were all nonsignificant [37].

Examination of caregiver experiences may also help to shed light on attitudes and practices, but there are few studies in this area. A survey of nurses in two American PICUs [45] found that patient deaths rated as the most important stressor. Stress ratings were correlated negatively with the number of years of total and ICU nursing experience. Nurses in both units overestimated the number of patient deaths. Two qualitative studies have examined nurses' experiences of withdrawal of life support [40] and of grief following patients' death [46]. Both studies highlighted the emotional aspects of nurses' work. Rashotte and colleagues [46] identified several coping strategies that nurses used, and found that nurses considered the effective management of grief to be an experiential learning process. Only one study has examined physicians' experiences; this study focused on working with families of children in the PICU rather than exclusively with patient deaths [47]. In describing their work, doctors constantly referred to the need for psychosocial and interpersonal skills in providing parents with emotional support; an undercurrent to the data was the stress imposed on the physicians themselves in carrying out this work. Less experienced physicians, in particular, found this aspect difficult.

Parental perceptions

There is relatively little research on parental perceptions of end-of-life care in PICU. Only three studies relating exclusively to the topic were found [29,48,49]. Four studies with a broader focus included parents of children dying in the PICU [5,11,50,51], whereas one study of parental decision-making in the PICU included parents of survivors and nonsurvivors [52]. One study [5] was conducted in the United Kingdom; all others were done in the United States.

Two survey studies have described parents' experiences of, and satisfaction with, the process; one included 78 parents whose children had died in a single PICU [29]. The other study included 56 parents whose children had died after withdrawal or limitation of life support in three PICUs [49]. Both found wide variation in parents' satisfaction with various elements of their experience. There also was considerable variability in the amount of input that parents believed that they had in decisions, and their satisfaction with this input. Meert and colleagues [29] found that low satisfaction overall was more likely if the child died after acute illness, or if the parents felt uninformed, did not understand the cause of death, had less contact with the unit staff after the child's death, or did not perceive the staff as sympathetic and kind.

Both studies included several disturbing findings. Meert and colleagues [29] found that 22% of parents surveyed believed that they had insufficient information to make decisions, 44% believed that they had insufficient time to do so, and 10% believed that the wrong decision was made. Three parents expressed concern that the decision to withdraw support was influenced by their lack of insurance. Of 27 parents who had not been present at the time of death, 17 regretted this circumstance. Most of this number were not allowed to be present during resuscitation or brain stem function tests. Meyer and colleagues [49] found that 55% of parents believed they had little or no control during their child's final days and 24% would have made decisions differently. The survey did not elicit details of what specific decisions they would have changed, or whether their sense of control could have been increased. In addition, only 55% of parents believed their child was comfortable during his or her final days.

This last concern was raised in a study of parents whose children died of cancer [11]. Children who died in the PICU were not analyzed as such; however, almost all deaths from treatment-related complications took place in the PICU and accounted for 88% of deaths in this location. This group was perceived by parents to suffer more symptoms, have less successful treatment of pain, and to have a poorer quality of life in their final days. Overall, parents reported symptoms occurring more frequently than did physicians; they were more likely to report a greater degree of pain if the physician was not actively involved in end-of-life care.

Factors involved in parental decision-making were addressed in both surveys described above [29,49]. Factors rated as most important were physicians' recommendations, expectation of neurologic recovery, and degree of the child's pain and suffering [29]. Parents in the Boston study [49] were less influenced by staff, and cited their child's quality of life, their chance of getting better, and their perceived pain and discomfort as the most important factors.

Decision making also was the focus of a qualitative study [52], in which 39 parents were asked about their decisions to initiate and continue life support; one third of the children survived. Decision making in this context was revealed as a complex process. Important themes included the desire to prolong life (even while recognizing the inevitability of death), minimizing pain and suffering, evaluation of their child's quality of life, recognition of and valuing the child as a separate person with his/her own wants and needs, and issues of family and spirituality. Parents indicated they desired to participate in decision making and continued to make meaning of their experiences over time.

No studies have investigated exclusively parental experiences of sudden death in the PICU; however, three studies [5,50,51] have included PICU deaths in broader studies and are relevant to this review. Dent and colleagues [5] attempted to survey all parents in a geographical area in the United Kingdom whose children had died suddenly and unexpectedly. Deaths in the PICU were not reported separately but almost half took place there. Several findings were of concern. More than 25% of parents believed that they were given inadequate information while their child was being treated. Only 25% were aware that they could wash the child after death and bring in siblings. Less than half were offered a photograph of their child, and only a small number was offered other mementos that parents indicated they would have liked to have received. Less than half received information on practical issues or were offered follow-up care at the hospital. Ongoing formal follow-up by community agencies was rare.

Perhaps the most disturbing findings arose from an interview study of parents whose children died in a trauma center [50]. Grieving was assessed as pathologic in 76% of the 29 parents who participated. The main factor associated with pathologic mourning was lack of a support system beyond the immediate family. Successful support was identified as taking active care of the parents and encouraging the expression of emotional pain. The investigators developed a set of indices to predict pathologic mourning at the time of death. Whether these indices are amenable to interventions to promote healthy grieving is unclear.

A later study from the same institution [51] found that although most parents were grieving appropri-

ately, some had ongoing issues. The investigators concluded that unanswered questions or misconceptions concerning brain death, organ donation, or the child's medical care affected the grieving process adversely.

Meert and colleagues [48] evaluated the effect of end-of-life care on initial and long-term bereavement outcomes. In a survey of 57 parents, they found that death after an acute illness was associated with a higher intensity of grief immediately and at 3 to 5 years after the child's death. The intensity of early grief was predicted by parents' physical coping resources and the emotional attitudes of the PICU staff. A higher intensity of long-term grief was associated with poor cognitive coping resources (parents' sense of self-worth), inadequate information provision, and parental perception of PICU staff as emotionally uncaring. The investigators were unable to determine what constituted an emotionally caring or uncaring attitude, but speculated that parental perceptions reflected the quality of staff–parent relationships. They concluded, therefore, that close relationships can influence parental grieving. One important limitation of this study is that most of the participants were mothers; it is possible that only maternal grieving has been described.

Bereavement programs

The need for long-term support of bereaved parents is well-recognized, and this support is being seen increasingly as the responsibility of hospital staff. Parents in one study [49] indicated that much of their help after the child's death was provided by PICU nurses and other hospital staff. Nurse-managed bereavement programs have been described in general pediatric settings [53–56] and in PICUs [42,57]. The programs had similar components, such as provision of mementos and written information at the time of death; cards, letters, and telephone calls for 1 to 2 years after the child's death; remembrance services; referral to other services as required; and evaluation of the program. Education of nursing staff also was seen as an integral part of the program. Several programs incorporated the appointment of a bereavement coordinator at the unit level [42,53,54]. One included community outreach activities to build relations with primary care providers [53].

Ernewein and colleagues [57] researched nurses' perceptions of the bereavement program in one PICU. Nurses believed that the program generally was beneficial to parents. They also believed that providing bereavement care at the time of death helped them manage their own grief and increased their confidence in caring for parents, which, in turn, increased the parents' confidence in them. They were less comfortable providing follow-up care, such as sending cards or letters and making telephone calls. This discomfort also was reported by Nesbit and colleagues [42], who suggested that education of nursing staff and support from the bereavement coordinator was crucial to nurses being able to fulfill this part of the program.

None of the cited articles described parental perceptions in detail, although feedback was reported as generally positive [42,53–55]. Parents were said to rank the program consistently as an important resource for support and information [55], and to find that the program brought a sense of completion and could elicit new coping strategies [53]. The only negative feedback was reported by Nesbit and colleagues [42]; who cited parents as indicating that they would like more contact with physicians.

Only one study was found that evaluated the impact of a bereavement program on parental grief [51]. This program was developed in a trauma center after an earlier study that emphasized the importance of support networks [50]. The program was led by hospital chaplains and differed from others described in the literature in that it included face-to-face contact outside the hospital setting—thus removing the need for parents to return to the hospital—and education of, and feedback from, the family's supporters. The program concluded with an interview 1 year after death, which included formal evaluation. Of the 54 parents who completed the program, 59% were assessed as grieving normally, compared with 24% in the previous study [50]. Hence, the program seems to have had a beneficial effect on the grieving process, although the potential influence of other factors cannot be discounted.

Improving end-of-life care: the way forward

As this article demonstrates, research into end-of-life care in the PICU is in its infancy. Most extant research is descriptive in nature; it is useful in highlighting particular areas of practice and revealing deficiencies in care provision, but there is little scientific knowledge on which to base practice [2]. Even descriptive research has fallen short of its objectives. Retrospective studies are dependent on the quality of documentation, and frequently noted to be inadequate, whereas prospective studies have recorded insufficient detail. There certainly is a place for more descriptive studies, documenting hitherto

neglected aspects of practice. In addition, testing of interventions is required to establish their ability to achieve desired outcomes. Although more research is required in all areas addressed in this article, specific gaps in knowledge also are apparent.

As several studies have revealed, quality end-of-life care depends on the ability of clinicians to engage with families while maintaining their own well-being. Interpersonal and coping skills are vital to this process, as well as knowledge of the principles underpinning care. The need for improved education for physicians and nurses is well-documented and suggestions for improvements have been put forward [58–60]. Anecdotal evidence suggests that formal and informal education is currently provided; documentation of this education would be a useful first step in extending its provision and evaluating its effectiveness.

Despite the provision of guidelines, the question of if and when aggressive management should be discontinued has not been resolved. There are many suggestions in the literature that decisions in this area are difficult and complex, and not easily addressed by recourse to ethical principles. Alternative approaches to ethical reasoning may be more appropriate in this context [61]. More studies of the decision-making process, in all its complexity, are required. Caregiver and parental experience, in particular, are under-researched topics.

Questions regarding who does and should make these decisions have been raised by extant research and debated by commentators, with opinions divided as to the amount of input parents should have. However, if parental satisfaction and well-being are accepted as primary outcomes, the question may well be less one of "absolutes" than of perceptions: whether parents perceive that the appropriate people made the decision, regardless of who "actually" does so. In this area, as in others, differences in perception between parents and caregivers, and between various professional groups, have been revealed in extant studies. Case study approaches, using ethnographic methods, would enable further examination of these different understandings and illuminate how they arise.

It is notable that most research has been conducted in the United States, with small numbers of studies in other western (Anglo-European) countries. Only one study from an Asian country [27] and one from Latin America [31] were found. Only one study has addressed potential conflicts between parents and caregivers in the context of a multicultural society [43]. The issue of cultural influences on end-of-life care requires urgent attention. An important development in this area is the establishment of a palliative care task force and a global research agenda by the World Federation of Pediatric Intensive and Critical Care Societies [62].

The need for research into symptom management has been well-documented [2,3,63]. A major deficit highlighted in this article is the lack of formal assessment tools. Existing pain scoring systems should be tested in this population, and the development of tools to assess other symptoms should be a priority.

Quality improvement principles have much to offer this area of practice. It is important to develop clearly defined goals of end-of-life care and to evaluate outcomes. The clinical pathway described by one center [42] is an important initiative in this area. Evaluating quality demands the development of key performance indicators. A minimum data set could be produced to improve and standardize documentation, and to permit comparison between institutions.

Finally, the provision of research funding is vital if the scientific basis of end-of-life care is to improve. The exposure given to this area of practice in recent times has prompted several initiatives, including a program announcement by the U.S. National Institutes of Health [3]. This program is operative until January 2007, and provides excellent opportunities to develop research in this area. Multi-center and international research, in particular, could be supported by this initiative.

Summary

This article has highlighted major gaps in extant research into end-of-life care in the PICU. Current research concerning end-of-life decision making and management of the dying process mainly is descriptive in nature and narrow in focus. Studies of parental perceptions are few, but have highlighted several concerns. There is urgent need for further research in this area. Differences between caregivers and parents are apparent and should be addressed in future studies. The Anglocentric focus of most literature on this topic is of concern; a global approach to research on this topic is desirable.

References

[1] Hynson JL, Sawyer SM. Paediatric palliative care: distinctive needs and emerging issues. J Paediatr Child Health 2001;37(4):323–5.

[2] Board on Health Sciences Policy. Institute of Medicine: When children die: improving palliative and end-of-life care for children and their families. Washington, DC: National Academies Press; 2003.

[3] National Institutes of Health. Program announcement: improving care for dying children and their families. Available at: http://grants1.nih.gov/grants/guide/pa-files/PA-04-057.html. Accessed July 20, 2004.

[4] Ashby MA, Kosky RJ, Laver HT, et al. An enquiry into death and dying at the Adelaide Children's Hospital: a useful model? Med J Aust 1991;154(3):165–70.

[5] Dent A, Condon L, Blair P, et al. A study of bereavement care after a sudden and unexpected death. Arch Dis Child 1996;74(6):522–6.

[6] Lantos JD, Berger AC, Zucker AR. Do-not-resuscitate orders in a children's hospital. Crit Care Med 1993; 21(1):52–5.

[7] Feudtner C, Christakis DA, Zimmerman FJ, et al. Characteristics of deaths occurring in children's hospitals: implications for supportive care services. Pediatrics 2002;109(5):887–93.

[8] Feudtner C, Silveira MJ, Christakis DA. Where do children with complex chronic conditions die? Patterns in Washington State, 1980–1998. Pediatrics 2002;109(4): 656–60.

[9] McCallum DE, Byrne P, Bruera E. How children die in hospital. J Pain Symptom Manage 2000;20(6):417–23.

[10] van der Wal ME, Renfurm LN, van Vught AJ, et al. Circumstances of dying in hospitalized children. Eur J Pediatr 1999;158(7):560–5.

[11] Wolfe J, Grier HE, Klar N, et al. Symptoms and suffering at the end of life in children with cancer. N Engl J Med 2000;342(5):326–33.

[12] Carter BS, Howenstein M, Gilmer MJ, et al. Circumstances surrounding the deaths of hospitalized children: opportunities for pediatric palliative care. Pediatrics 2004;114(3):e361–6.

[13] Lynaugh JE, Fairman J. New nurses, new spaces: a preview of the AACN history study. Am J Crit Care 1992;1(1):19–24.

[14] American Academy of Pediatrics Committee on Bioethics. Guidelines on foregoing life-sustaining medical treatment. Pediatrics 1994;93(3):532–6.

[15] American Academy of Pediatrics Committee on Bioethics. Ethics and the care of critically ill infants and children. Pediatrics 1996;98(1):149–52.

[16] American Academy of Pediatrics Committee on Bioethics and Committee on Hospital Care. Palliative care for children. Pediatrics 2000;106(2):351–7.

[17] Royal College of Paediatrics and Child Health. Withholding or withdrawing life saving treatment in children: a framework for practice. London: Royal College of Paediatrics and Child Health; 1997.

[18] Truog RD, Cist AF, Brackett SE, et al. Recommendations for end-of-life care in the intensive care unit: The Ethics Committee of the Society of Critical Care Medicine. Crit Care Med 2001;29(12):2332–48.

[19] Rubenfeld GD, Randall Curtis J, End-of-life care in the ICU Working Group. End-of-life care in the intensive care unit: a research agenda. Crit Care Med 2001;29(10):2001–6.

[20] Anderson B, McCall E, Leversha A, et al. A review of children's dying in a paediatric intensive care unit. N Z Med J 1994;107(985):345–7.

[21] Mink RB, Pollack MM. Resuscitation and withdrawal of therapy in pediatric intensive care. Pediatrics 1992;89(5 Pt 1):961–3.

[22] Vernon DD, Dean JM, Timmons OD, et al. Modes of death in the pediatric intensive care unit: withdrawal and limitation of supportive care. Crit Care Med 1993; 21(11):1798–802.

[23] Ryan CA, Byrne P, Kuhn S, et al. No resuscitation and withdrawal of therapy in a neonatal and a pediatric intensive care unit in Canada. J Pediatr 1993;123(4): 534–8.

[24] Levetown M, Pollack MM, Cuerdon TT, et al. Limitations and withdrawals of medical intervention in pediatric critical care. JAMA 1994;272(16): 1271–5.

[25] Balfour-Lynn IM, Tasker RC. At the coalface - medical ethics in practice: Futility and death in paediatric medical intensive care. J Med Ethics 1996;22(5):279–81.

[26] Martinot A, Grandbastien B, Leteurtre S, et al. No resuscitation orders and withdrawal of therapy in French paediatric intensive care units. Groupe Francophone de Reanimation et d'Urgences Pediatriques. Acta Paediatr 1998;87(7):769–73.

[27] Goh AY, Lum LC, Chan PW, et al. Withdrawal and limitation of life support in paediatric intensive care. Arch Dis Child 1999;80(5):424–8.

[28] Burns JP, Mitchell C, Outwater KM, et al. End-of-life care in the pediatric intensive care unit after the forgoing of life-sustaining treatment. Crit Care Med 2000;28(8):3060–6.

[29] Meert KL, Thurston CS, Sarnaik AP. End-of-life decision-making and satisfaction with care: Parental perspectives. Pediatr Crit Care Med 2000;1(2): 179–85.

[30] Devictor DJ, Nguyen DT, Groupe Francophone de Reanimation et d'Urgences, Pediatriques. Forgoing life-sustaining treatments: how the decision is made in French pediatric intensive care units. Crit Care Med 2001;29(7):1356–9.

[31] Althabe M, Cardigni G, Vassallo JC, et al. Dying in the intensive care unit: collaborative multicenter study about forgoing life-sustaining treatment in Argentine pediatric intensive care units. Pediatr Crit Care Med 2003;4(2):164–9.

[32] Garros D, Rosychuk RJ, Cox PN. Circumstances surrounding end of life in a pediatric intensive care unit. Pediatrics 2003;112(5):e371–9.

[33] Devictor DJ, Nguyen DT. Forgoing life-sustaining treatments in children: a comparison between Northern and Southern European pediatric intensive care units. Pediatr Crit Care Med 2004;5(3):211–5.

[34] Zawistowski CA, DeVita MA. A descriptive study of children dying in the pediatric intensive care unit after withdrawal of life-sustaining treatment. Pediatr Crit Care Med 2004;5(3):216–23.

[35] Hoehn S, Nelson RM. Parents should not be excluded from decisions to forgo life-sustaining treatments! Crit Care Med 2001;29(7):1480–1.

[36] Frader JE. Global paternalism in pediatric intensive care unit end-of-life decisions? Pediatr Crit Care Med 2003;4(2):257–8.

[37] Burns JP, Mitchell C, Griffith JL, et al. End-of-life care in the pediatric intensive care unit: attitudes and practices of pediatric critical care physicians and nurses. Crit Care Med 2001;29(3):658–64.

[38] Randolph AG, Zollo MB, Wigton RS, et al. Factors explaining variability among caregivers in the intent to restrict life-support interventions in a pediatric intensive care unit. Crit Care Med 1997;25(3): 435–9.

[39] Truog RD, Burns JP, Mitchell C, et al. Pharmacologic paralysis and withdrawal of mechanical ventilation at the end of life. N Engl J Med 2000;342(7):508–11.

[40] Way C. In their own words: paediatric intensive care nurses' experiences of withdrawal of treatment. Pediatric Intensive Care Nursing 2003;4(1):17–31.

[41] de Groot-Bollujt W, Mourik M. Bereavement: role of the nurse in the care of terminally ill and dying children in the pediatric intensive care unit. Crit Care Med 1993;21(9 Suppl):S391–2.

[42] Nesbit MJ, Hill M, Peterson N. A comprehensive pediatric bereavement program: the patterns of your life. Crit Care Nurs Q 1997;20(2):48–62.

[43] McKinley D, Blackford J. Nurses' experiences of caring for culturally and linguistically diverse families when their child dies. Int J Nurs Pract 2001;7(4): 251–6.

[44] Keenan HT, Diekema DS, O'Rourke PP, et al. Attitudes toward limitation of support in a pediatric intensive care unit. Crit Care Med 2000;28(5):1590–4.

[45] Benica SW, Longo CB, Barnsteiner JH. Perceptions and significance of patient deaths for pediatric critical care nurses. Crit Care Nurse 1992;12(3):72–5.

[46] Rashotte J, Fothergill-Bourbonnais F, Chamberlain M. Pediatric intensive care nurses and their grief experiences: a phenomenological study. Heart Lung 1997; 26(5):372–86.

[47] Bartel D, Engler A, Natale J, et al. Working with families of suddenly and critically ill children: physician experiences. Arch Pediatr Adolesc Med 2000; 154(11):1127–33.

[48] Meert KL, Thurston CS, Thomas R. Parental coping and bereavement outcome after the death of a child in the pediatric intensive care unit. Pediatr Crit Care Med 2001;2(4):324–8.

[49] Meyer EC, Burns JP, Griffith JL, et al. Parental perspectives on end-of-life care in the pediatric intensive care unit. Crit Care Med 2002;30(1):226–31.

[50] Oliver RC, Fallat ME. Traumatic childhood death: how well do parents cope? Journal of Trauma-Injury Infection & Critical Care 1995;39(2):303–7 [discussion: 307–8].

[51] Oliver RC, Sturtevant JP, Scheetz JP, et al. Beneficial effects of a hospital bereavement intervention program after traumatic childhood death. Journal of

Trauma-Injury Infection & Critical Care 2001;50(3): 440–6 [discussion 447–8].

[52] Kirschbaum MS. Life support decisions for children: what do parents value? ANS Adv Nurs Sci 1996; 19(1):51–71.

[53] Heiney SP, Hasan L, Price K. Developing and implementing a bereavement program for a children's hospital. J Pediatr Nurs 1993;8(6):385–91.

[54] Johnson LC, Rincon B, Gober C, et al. The development of a comprehensive bereavement program to assist families experiencing pediatric loss. J Pediatr Nurs 1993;8(3):142–6.

[55] Stewart ES. Family matters. Family-centered care for the bereaved. Pediatr Nurs 1995;21(2):181–4.

[56] Cox SA. Pediatric bereavement: supporting the family and each other. J Trauma Nurs 2004;11(3):117–21.

[57] Ernewein C, McLellan AM, Rashotte J, et al. Development and utilization of a bereavement program in a pediatric intensive care unit. CACCN 1997;8(2): 16–21.

[58] AACN. Peaceful death: recommended competencies and curricular guidelines for end-of-life nursing care. Available at: http://www.aacn.nche.edu/Publications/ deathfin.htm. Accessed November 18, 2004.

[59] Danis M, Federman D, Fins JJ, et al. Incorporating palliative care into critical care education: principles, challenges, and opportunities. Crit Care Med 1999; 27(9):2005–13.

[60] Sahler OJZ, Frager G, Levetown M, et al. Medical education about end-of-life care in the pediatric setting: principles, challenges, and opportunities. Pediatrics 2000;105(3):575–84.

[61] Truog R, Burns J, Rogers M. Ethics. In: Tibboel D, van der Voort E, editors. Intensive care in childhood: a challenge to the future. Berlin: Springer; 1996. p. 467–90.

[62] van der Voort E, Latour JM, Duncan AW. Report of the World Federation of Pediatric Intensive and Critical Care Societies. Pediatr Crit Care Med 2004;5(3): 302–3.

[63] National Institutes of Health. State-of-the-science conference statement: improving end-of-life care. Available at: http://consensus.nih.gov/ta/024/End%20of% 20Life%20Statement%20DRAFT%2012-08-04% 20at%20700pm.pdf. Accessed January 6, 2005.

ELSEVIER
SAUNDERS

Crit Care Nurs Clin N Am 17 (2005) 361–373

CRITICAL CARE
NURSING CLINICS
OF NORTH AMERICA

Pediatric Fluid and Electrolyte Balance: Critical Care Case Studies

Kathryn E. Roberts, MSN, RN, CRNP, CCRN

Pediatric Intensive Care Unit, The Children's Hospital of Philadelphia, 34th Street & Civic Center, Philadelphia, PA 19104, USA

The care of the critically ill infant or child often is complicated further by disruptions in fluid or electrolyte balance. Prompt recognition of these disruptions is essential to the care of these patients. This article uses a case study approach to provide an overview of the principles of fluid and electrolyte balance in the critically ill infant and child.

Fluid homeostasis

Body fluids are composed of water and solutes. These solutes are electrically charged electrolytes (eg, Na^+, K^+, Cl^-) and nonelectrolytes (eg, glucose, urea). Fluid and electrolyte homeostasis occurs when fluid and electrolyte balance is maintained within narrow limits, despite a wide variation in dietary intake, metabolic rate, and kidney function.

Water is one of the most significant components of the human body, and accounts for approximately 50% to 80% of total body weight. Total body water (TBW) varies from one individual to another. The percentage of TBW varies with age, gender, skeletal muscle mass, and fat content. In the average adult, water accounts for approximately 50% to 60% of total weight. The body weight of children who are less than 1 year of age has a significantly higher percentage of body water; premature infants and neonates have the highest percentages. At birth, TBW is 70% to 75% of body weight. This decreases dramatically in the first year of life. At puberty, more changes occur. Because of the lower water content of

adipose tissue, TBW as a percentage of body weight is less in women than it is in men.

TBW is distributed in two compartments: intracellular fluid (ICF) and extracellular fluid (ECF). In addition to the changes in the percentage of TBW as body weight, infants and young children have higher percentages of ECF as compared with adults. More than half of the newborn infant's body weight is ECF. This changes rapidly over the first 6 to 8 weeks of life. By 3 years of age, body fluid components more closely resemble those of the adult, with an ECF of approximately 20% to 23% and an ICF of 40% to 50% [1].

Fluid compartments

ICF is made up of all of the fluid contained within the membranes of the cells; it is the largest fluid compartment in the body. ECF is not one isolated fluid compartment. It is composed of interstitial fluid, plasma, and transcellular water. Adequate ECF volume—in particular intravascular volume—is essential for normal functioning of the cardiovascular system. In contrast to older children and adults, premature infants and newborns have a significantly higher percentage of body water making up their total body weight, and significantly more of this water is found within the ECF. This is one of the reasons why infants exhibit signs of cardiovascular compromise when dehydrated faster than older children or adults.

Selectively permeable membranes separate each fluid compartment. These membranes permit the movement of water and certain solutes from one compartment to another. The movement of fluids and

---

E-mail address: robertsk@email.chop.edu

Table 1
Key physiologic concepts

Physiologic concept	Description
Osmosis	Osmosis is the movement of H_2O across a semipermeable membrane from an area of lower solute concentration to one of higher solute concentration.
Diffusion	Diffusion is the movement of particles through a solution or gas from an area of higher concentration to one of lower concentration. The greater the concentration gradient, the faster the rate of diffusion.
Filtration	Filtration is the movement of H_2O and solute from an area of increased hydrostatic pressure to an area of low hydrostatic pressure. It plays an important role in moving fluids out of the arterial end of the capillaries.
Active transport	Diffusion cannot occur in the absence of a concentration gradient or favorable electrical gradient. Energy is required to move particles against a concentration gradient. This happens through the process of active transport. The Na–K pump is one example of active transport. Active transport plays a vital role in maintaining the unique composition of the ECF and ICF.

electrolytes is dependent upon osmolality and a functioning renal system. Fluids move constantly from one body compartment to another, and then remain in specific compartments until an inequality in concentration of electrolytes develops and movement occurs. Movement of fluids and electrolytes occurs through osmosis, diffusion, active transport, and filtration (Table 1).

Fluid imbalances

Typically, fluid volume deficit is defined as a negative body fluid or water balance. When volume depletion occurs in the extracellular space, circulatory collapse can result. Fluid volume deficit is a common problem in critically ill infants and children, and occurs as the result of excess loss of fluids and electrolytes (diarrhea or vomiting), shifts of fluids and electrolytes into nonaccessible third spaces (burns, post abdominal surgery), and decreased intake of fluid and electrolytes (impaired thirst mechanism, dysphagia, prolonged NPO status). Gastrointestinal water loss from diarrheal disease usually is the most common cause of excess fluid volume loss in infants and children.

In the critically ill child, fluid volume loss through "third spacing" is a common cause of fluid volume loss. Third spacing occurs when fluids and electrolytes are found in a space other than the usual spaces of the ICF and ECF ("third space") [2]. Third spacing develops in ascites, pancreatitis, burns, peritonitis, sepsis, and intestinal obstruction.

Fluid volume overload is the actual excess of total body fluid or a relative excess in one or more fluid compartments. It occurs as the result of increased sodium concentration and water volume because of retention or excessive intake; decreased renal excretion of water and sodium; or decreased mobilization of fluid within the intracellular space. The major causes of excess fluid volume in critically ill infants and children are cardiorespiratory dysfunction, renal dysfunction, and inappropriate secretion of antidiuretic hormone [1].

Case study #1

Jamal is a 5-kg boy who was admitted to the pediatric ICU (PICU) with respiratory syncytial virus (RSV) bronchiolitis. His mother reports a 2- to 3-day history of fever, increased work of breathing, and decreased oral intake. He is lethargic but arousable, tachycardic, and in moderate respiratory distress. While conducting an initial assessment, you note that his anterior fontanel is sunken, his mucous membranes are dry, and his peripheral pulses are diminished. Intravenous (IV) fluids are infusing by way of a 24-gauge peripheral IV at a rate of 20 mL/h.

Vital signs: temperature, 39°C, heart rate (HR), 188, respiratory rate (RR), 64; blood pressure (BP), 75/42 mm Hg.

Diagnostic studies: Na, 137; K, 3.8; Cl, 100; serum urea nitrogen, 24; creatinine, 1.3.

How severe is Jamal's fluid volume deficit?

The severity of a child's fluid volume deficit is determined on the basis of clinical manifestations, diagnostic studies, and weight loss. Jamal's clinical picture is consistent with a moderate to severe fluid volume deficit (Table 2).

Table 2
Severity of fluid volume deficit

Clinical manifestations	Mild fluid deficit	Moderate fluid deficit	Severe fluid deficit
Mental Status			
Infants and young children	Thirsty, alert, restless	Thirsty, restless or lethargic but irritable to touch	Lethargic, somnolent
Older children and adults	Thirsty, alert, restless	Thirsty, alert	Usually conscious, apprehensive
Radial pulse	Normal rate and strength	Rapid and weak	Rapid, feeble, sometimes impalpable
Heart rate	Normal or mild tachycardia	Tachycardia	Severe tachycardia that may progress to bradycardia
Respirations	Normal	Normal to rapid	Deep and rapid
Fontanel & eyes	Normal	Slightly depressed	Severely sunken
Systolic blood pressure	Normal	Orthostatic hypotension	Severe hypotension
Skin elasticity	Pinch retracts immediately	Pinch retracts slowly	Pinch retracts very slowly (>3 sec)
Tears	Present	Present or absent	Absent
Mucous membranes	Moist	Dry	Very dry
Urine output	Normal	Oliguria	Oliguria or anuria
Body weight loss (%)	3−5	6−9	≥10
Estimated fluid deficit (mL/kg)	30−50	60−90	≥100

Data from Friedman AL. Nephrology: fluids and electrolytes. In: Behrman RE, Kliegman RM, editors. Nelson essentials of pediatrics. 4th Edition. Philadelphia: WB Saunders; 2002. p. 680; and AACN Pediatric Critical Care Pocket Reference Card © 1998.

What will Jamal's initial management include?

Initial management of the critically ill infant or child who has a fluid volume deficit focuses on expansion of the ECF volume to treat or prevent hypovolemic shock. Typically, 10 to 20 mL/kg of an isotonic solution is administered by way of an IV line. Infants or children who have a severe fluid volume deficit may require as much as 60 mL/kg [1]. Peripheral perfusion, heart rate, blood pressure, and urine output are monitored continuously to determine the infant or child's response to therapy.

Following initial fluid resuscitation, ongoing management is directed toward definitive replacement of water and electrolytes. In isotonatremic or hyponatremic dehydration (Box 1), further fluid losses generally are replaced over a period of 24 hours to prevent overexpansion of the ECF [3]. The need

---

Box 1. Sodium imbalances and dehydration

Hyponatremic dehydration

  Na$^+$ is less than 135 mEq/L
  Fluid shifts from ECF to ICF
  Earlier signs of cardiovascular collapse

Isonatremic dehydration

  Na$^+$ is 135 to 145 mEq/L
  No fluid shifts

Hypernatremic dehydration

  Na$^+$ is greater than 145 mEq/L
  Fluid shifts from ICF to ECF
  "Masking" of symptoms

Box 2. Maintenance fluid calculations

Hourly method

  1 to 10 kg: 4 mL/kg/h
  11 to 20 kg: 40 mL/h + 2 mL/kg/h (for kg 11−20)
  More than 20 kg: 60 mL/h + 1 mL/h (for every kg >20)

Daily method

  1 to 10 kg: 100 mL/kg/d
  11 to 20 kg: 1000 mL/d + 50 mL/kg/d (for kg 11−20)
  More than 20 kg: 1500 mL/d + 20 mL/kg/d (for every kg >20)

Table 3
Electrolyte imbalances

Electrolyte imbalance	Causes	Clinical manifestations	ECG findings	Management
Hyponatremia Na^+ <135 mEq/L	Vomiting/diarrhea Nasogastric suction ↓ Na^+ intake Fever Excessive diaphoresis ↑ water intake Burns & wounds Renal disease SIADH DKA Malnutrition	Irritability Seizures Lethargy Disorientation Cerebral edema Coma Respiratory failure Muscle cramps Nausea/vomiting Vary with alterations in fluid status	N/A	Treat underlying cause Frequent neurologic assessments Fluid replacement ±Hypertonic saline Monitor Na^+ levels
Hypernatremia Na^+ >145 mEq/L	↑ Na^+ intake renal disease ↑ insensible water loss Diabetes insipidus	Irritability/agitation High-pitched cry Seizures Flushed skin Lethargy/confusion Seizures Coma Muscle weakness Muscle twitching Intense thirst Vary with alterations in fluid status	N/A	Treat underlying cause Frequent neurological assessments Strict I&O Slow correction of fluid deficit Monitor Na levels
Hypokalemia K^+ <3.5 mEq/L	↓ K^+ intake Starvation Malabsorption syndromes Gastrointestinal losses Diuresis Nephritis Alkalosis	Muscle weakness, cramping, stiffness, paralysis, hyporeflexia Hypotension Lethargy Irritability Tetany Nausea/vomiting Abdominal distention Paralytic ileus Irregular, weak pulse	Flattened, inverted T waves Presence of U waves PVCs	Treat underlying cause Monitor ECG Frequent neuromuscular assessments K^+ replacement Monitor acid–base status

Imbalance	Causes	Signs/Symptoms	ECG/Cardiac	Treatment
Hyperkalemia K$^+$ > 5.5 mEq/L	↑ K$^+$ intake Renal disease/failure Adrenal insufficiency Metabolic acidosis Severe dehydration Burns Crushing injuries Hemolysis	Muscle weakness Ascending paralysis Hyperreflexia Confusion Apnea N/V Diarrhea ↓ cardiac function	Tall, peaked T waves Widened QRS Prolonged PR interval Ventricular arrhythmias Asystole Cardiac arrest	Treat underlying cause Monitor ECG Administer IV fluids D/C K$^+$ containing fluids/meds IV calcium administration Insulin + glucose Albuterol Na bicarbonate Kayexalate Dialysis Monitor serum K$^+$ levels Evaluate acid–base status
Hypocalcemia Ca$^+$ < 8mg/dL iCa < 1.15	↓ dietary Ca Vitamin D deficiency Renal insufficiency Diuretics Hypoparathyroidism Alkalosis ↑ serum protein	NM irritability Tingling sensation Chvostek's sign Trousseau's sign Tetany Muscle cramps Lethargy Seizures Hypotension	Prolonged QT interval	Treat underlying cause Monitor ECG IV calcium supplements Monitor Ca & Mg levels
Hypercalcemia Ca$^+$ > 10.5 mg/dL iCa > 1.34	Acidosis Prolonged immobilization Kidney disease Hyperparathyroidism Excessive administration	Lethargy Stupor Coma Seizures Anorexia N/V Constipation NM hypotonicity	Shortened QT interval Bradycardia Cardiac arrest	Treat underlying cause Monitor ECG IV fluids Loop diuretics
Hypomagnesemia Mg$^+$ < 1.4 mEq/L	↓ intake (NPO) Malabsorption syndromes ↑ renal excretion	NM excitability Tetany Confusion Dizziness Headache Seizures Coma Respiratory depression Tachycardia	PVCs Ventricular arrhythmias	Treat underlying cause IV Mg replacement Monitor ECG Neuromuscular assessments

(continued on next page)

Table 3 (*continued*)

Electrolyte imbalance	Causes	Clinical manifestations	ECG findings	Management
Hypermagnesemia Mg^+ <1.4 mEq/L	Chronic renal disease ↓ GFR/↓ excretion ECF deficit ↑ administration of Mg containing drugs	Lethargy Muscle weakness Seizures ↓ swallow ↓ gag Tachycardia Hypotension	Prolonged PR interval Prolonged QRS Prolonged QT AV block	Treat underlying cause Monitor ECG Administer calcium IV hydration Dialysis
Hypophosphatemia PO_4 <3 mg/dL	Limited intake Shift of PO_4 from ECF to ICF ↓ GI tract absorption ↑ renal excretion	Irritability Disorientation Tremors Seizures Hemolytic anemia ↓ myocardial function Potential respiratory failure Coma	Premature ectopic beats	Treat underlying cause Slow PO_4 replacement Monitor for other electrolyte imbalances
Hyperphosphatemia PO_4 >4.5 mEq/L	Chronic renal failure Rapid cell catabolism Excessive intake Neoplastic disease Hypoparathyroidism	Tachycardia Hyperreflexia Abdominal cramps Nausea Diarrhea Muscle tetany	N/A	Treat underlying cause Monitor PO_4 and Ca Dietary restrictions Antacid administration Hydration Correction of hypocalcemia Dialysis

Abbreviations: AV, atrioventricular; D/C, discontinue; DKA, diabetic ketoacidosis; GFR, glomerular filtration rate; GI, gastrointestinal; iCa, ionized calcium; I&O, intake & output; NM, neuromuscular; N/V, ; SIADH, syndrome of inappropriate antidiuretic hormone.

for sodium replacement should be considered in hyponatremic dehydration. In hypernatremic dehydration, these losses may be administered more slowly, over a period of 48 to 72 hours. It is important that replacement fluids not be administered too rapidly in hypernatremic dehydration as this may lead to neurologic complications related to rapid changes in serum sodium levels. Replacement fluids are administered in addition to maintenance fluids (Box 2). Potassium chloride may be added to any maintenance fluids once Jamal is producing adequate urine output. The need to replace any ongoing fluid losses must be assessed as well.

What other factors may be contributing to Jamal's fluid loss?

Factors, such as hyperthermia, hyperventilation, increased metabolic rate/activity, and overhead warmers/phototherapy, can increase insensible fluid losses. Hypothermia or sedation may lead to a decrease in insensible fluid losses. It is important to consider potential causes of increased or decreased insensible fluid losses when assessing fluid balance in the critically ill infant or child.

Why do infants, such as Jamal, have an increased risk for developing a fluid volume deficit?

During early infancy, most body water is found in the ECF. This contributes to greater and more rapid fluid loss. If an infant has decreased intake or has excessive fluid losses, a fluid volume deficit or dehydration may develop rapidly. The resulting decrease in intravascular volume leads to a decrease in circulating blood volume and inadequate systemic perfusion. Other factors that place infants at increased risk for fluid volume deficit include an increased metabolic rate, relatively greater body surface area, immature renal function, and increased fluid requirements [4].

Electrolyte imbalances

See Table 3 for a summary of electrolyte imbalances in the critically ill infant and child.

Sodium balance

Sodium (Na^+) is the major cation of the extracellular compartment. It regulates the voltage of action potentials in skeletal muscles, nerves, and the myocardium. Sodium plays a role in the maintenance of acid–base balance, and maintenance of fluid balance in the ECF through maintenance of the osmotic pressure (osmolality). Consequently, imbalances in water and sodium often occur together and are equated with alterations in serum osmolality. Extracellular sodium concentration normally is 135 to 145 mEq/L. The major factors that influence sodium excretion are glomerular filtration rate and aldosterone. Alterations in the sodium levels in the body often are the result of clinical conditions that involve fluid volume excess or deficit.

Hyponatremia is defined as a serum sodium concentration of less than 135 mEq/L. Typically, it occurs as a secondary manifestation of another disease state. In the critically ill infant or child, hyponatremia may occur as the result of excess water retention in the ECF, sodium loss from the ECF, or a combination of the two [3]. Hyponatremia may occur in conjunction with hypovolemia, euvolemia, or hypervolemia.

A decrease in serum sodium results in a shift in water from the ECF to the ICF. This shift in fluids leads to a generalized cellular swelling or edema. Within the brain, where there is limited capacity for expansion, the development of cerebral edema can have catastrophic consequences (eg, cerebral herniation and death). Severity of clinical symptoms directly correlates with the severity and rapidity of onset of the sodium deficit [5]. Serum sodium levels of less than 120 mEq/L are associated with seizures and coma. Children who develop hyponatremia over several days to several weeks may be asymptomatic or may develop mild clinical manifestations.

Hyponatremia can occur in conjunction with hypervolemia, euvolemia, or hypovolemia. Water intoxication, nephrotic syndrome, cardiac failure, renal failure, and the syndrome of inappropriate antidiuretic hormone (SIADH) are causes of hypervolemic hyponatremia. Hyponatremia in conjunction with hypovolemia may occur with renal (eg, osmotic diuresis, renal tubular acidosis) or extrarenal (eg, vomiting, diarrhea, burns) losses [3]. Other potential causes include excessive use of diuretics, osmotic diuresis, and adrenal insufficiency.

Case study #2

Marisa is a 16-year-old girl who was admitted to the PICU following a spinal fusion procedure.

Vital signs: temperature, 37.2°C; HR, 82; RR, 18; BP 110/68 mm Hg; spO$_2$, 97%.

Diagnostic studies: Na, 125 mEq/L; K, 3.5 mEq/L; Cl, 99; serum urea nitrogen, 10; creatinine, 0.3, serum osmolarity, 258.

On postoperative day 2, her urine output is noted to decrease from 1.5 mL/kg/h to 0.2 mL/kg/h.

What clinical condition might you suspect is occurring and how is this contributing to Marisa's hyponatremia?

SIADH develops as the result of excessive levels of circulating antidiuretic hormone (ADH). It is one of the most common causes of hyponatremia in children in a hospital setting [6]. SIADH associated with spinal surgeries has been reported in the literature [7]. Increased levels of circulating ADH result in the reabsorption of water that normally would be excreted in urine by the kidneys, and the development of fluid volume overload. This, in turn, leads to a dilutional hyponatremia and a decreased serum osmolality. The decreased osmolality causes a shift of fluid from the ECF to the ICF which can lead to the development of cerebral edema.

What causes the clinical manifestations that are associated with hyponatremia?

The clinical manifestations of hyponatremia are related to the cause of the hyponatremia and the rapidity of onset. Most of the symptoms occur as the result of the intracellular shift of water. Typically, the severe clinical manifestations of hyponatremia are not seen until the serum sodium decreases to levels of 120 to 125 mEq/L. At levels of less than 120 mEq/L, seizures, coma, and permanent neurologic damage may occur. Children often are at a higher risk for developing neurologic symptoms than are their adult counterparts.

What will Marisa's initial management include?

The first goal of management is to identify and treat/control the underlying cause of the hyponatremia. In Marisa's case, SIADH has been identified as the cause. In the child who has hypervolemia, management may include fluid restriction, administration of loop diuretics, and close monitoring of serum sodium levels. If serum sodium levels are increased too rapidly, cellular dehydration and neurologic damage may result. A general rule of thumb is that the serum sodium should increase no faster than 0.5 to 1.0 mEq/L/h. Other monitoring includes strict intake & output (I & O), urine specific gravity, serum electrolytes and serum osmolality (4–6 h), and daily weights.

In some cases, hypertonic saline may be considered to elevate serum sodium levels to 120 to 125 mEq/L. In the child who has hypovolemia, fluid and sodium losses must be replaced. This may or may not be done with a hypertonic saline solution.

Hypernatremia is defined as an excess of sodium in the ECF. It exists when serum sodium levels exceed 145 mEq/L. Hypernatremia may occur as the result of a pure sodium excess (eg, administration of large amounts of sodium bicarbonate) or as the result of a water deficit. Conditions that may lead to hypernatremic fluid deficit in the critically ill infant or child include diabetes insipidus, diabetes mellitus, increased insensible water loss, diarrhea, and dehydration.

The body normally responds to an increase in serum sodium with the release of ADH and stimulation of the thirst mechanism in an attempt to retain water and decrease serum sodium; however, this compensatory mechanism may not be sufficient to prevent the serum sodium from continuing to increase in the critically ill infant and child. Additionally, those patients who are unable to produce or respond to ADH are at an increased risk for the development of hypernatremia. Patients who are at risk for developing hypernatremia should be identified early on in their admission and monitored for clinical symptoms. Hypernatremia initially causes a generalized shrinking of cells as fluid moves from the ICF to the ECF. This may lead to subarachnoid, intradural, or subdural hemorrhages. Permanent central nervous system dysfunction can result when serum sodium concentrations reach levels greater than 160 mEq/L [8].

Case study #3

Hannah is a full-term, 1-month-old girl who was found pulseless and apneic after being put down for a nap. Cardiopulmonary resuscitation was initiated by the family and she was resuscitated and transported to the Emergency Department by Emergency Medical Services. Her grandmother reports that she has been irritable and "colicky" with decreased oral intake for the past 7 to 10 days. Administration of approximately 1/2 teaspoon of baking soda each day was the home remedy that was used to treat her symptoms. She was transferred to the PICU from the Emergency Department.

Hannah's physical examination upon admission to the ICU is as follows: intubated and mechanically ventilated, unresponsive, tachycardic, slightly hypotensive, sunken anterior fontanel, and "doughy" skin. She received a normal saline bolus of 10 mL/kg while in the Emergency Department; a second bolus is now infusing.

Diagnostic studies: Na, 165; K, 4.2; Cl, 125; CO_2, 14; serum urea nitrogen, 14; glucose, 167.

What will Hannah's initial management strategies include?

Hannah has a significant hypernatremia and fluid volume deficit. The cause of the hypernatremia was the administration of baking soda (sodium bicarbonate) over a period of approximately 1 week. Any patient who has hypernatremia needs to be monitored for seizure activity. Following initial resuscitation and stabilization, an electroencephalogram reveals that Hannah is having frequent subclinical seizure activity. Appropriate antiepileptic therapy is initiated.

The hypovolemic child requires fluid replacement and a slow correction of her fluid deficit over 48 to 72 hours. Patients who have a serum sodium level of 150 to 160 mEq/L should receive replacement fluids over a 24-hour time period. Those who have a serum sodium level that is greater than 160 mEq/L should receive fluid replacement therapy over a greater period of time [8]. Hannah's fluid replacement was administered over 48 hours. The type of IV fluids administered will vary depending on the rate at which the serum sodium level is decreasing. Generally, the serum sodium level should decrease at a rate no faster than 0.5 to 1.0 mEq/L/h, because rapid correction of hypernatremia can lead to fluid shifts from the ECF to the ICF and the development of cerebral edema. Patients must be monitored for the signs and symptoms of cerebral edema throughout the course of their treatment. Typically, the hypervolemic child is managed with diuretics and restricted sodium administration.

Ongoing management includes frequent neurologic assessments, strict I/O to monitor fluid balance, and frequent monitoring of serum sodium levels. Depending on the severity of the neurologic manifestations, patients may require ongoing management of seizures and rehabilitation.

Potassium balance

Potassium is the body's primary intracellular cation. Potassium has four major functions within the body: maintenance of cells' electrical neutrality and osmolality, neuromuscular transmission of nerve impulses, skeletal and cardiac muscle contraction and electrical conductivity, and maintenance of acid–base balance [9]. Maintenance of intracellular osmolarity

is accomplished through the "sodium–potassium" (active transport) pump. The normal range of serum potassium is 3.5 to 5.5 mEq/L, with a concentration of 160 mEq/L inside the cell.

Hypokalemia is defined as a serum potassium concentration of less than 3.5 mEq/L. Hypokalemia occurs as the result of a true deficit of potassium or a shift in potassium out of the ECF (intravascular space) into the ICF. A true deficit of potassium may be caused by decreased intake; however, excessive renal secretion, excessive gastrointestinal losses, or excessive sweating are more common causes of a potassium deficit. Conditions, such as alkalosis, and the excessive secretion or administration of insulin are potential causes of a shift of potassium out of the intravascular space into the ICF.

Case study #4

Malaki is a 2-month-old boy with trisomy 21, reactive airway disease, who is status post a complete atrioventricular canal repair at 2 weeks of age. He was admitted to the PICU unit 2 days ago in significant respiratory distress. An RSV titer is pending. He is in a 60% oxygen tent and has received additional treatments over the course of the day. He also is receiving his maintenance doses of digoxin and furosemide.

Malaki's oral intake has decreased significantly over the past 12 hours, although his urine output remains 2 mL/kg/h. He is lethargic and intermittently irritable. Serum chemistries reveal the following: Na, 138; K, 2.5; Cl, 97; PO_4, 4.

What factors may be contributing to Malaki's hypokalemia?

Several factors are contributing to Malaki's hypokalemia. Malaki has received albuterol and furosemide during his hospitalization. Albuterol activates the sodium–potassium pump and forces potassium to move intracellularly. Furosemide, a thiazide diuretic, causes increased excretion of potassium in the urine. This, in combination with his decreased oral intake, may be a contributing factor. As a child with a history of congenital heart disease, Malaki is at increased risk for the cardiovascular complications of hypokalemia.

What other diagnostic studies would you expect to be done?

Hypokalemia can cause several EKG changes— flattened, inverted T waves; presence of U waves; and premature ventricular contractions (PVCs). A 12-lead EKG should be performed, and, if not already in place, the patient should be placed on an EKG monitor. Additionally, a digoxin level must be measured. Hypokalemia predisposes patients to digoxin toxicity, and it is important to monitor Malaki for this potential complication of his hypokalemia.

What will Malaki's initial management strategies include?

The underlying cause of the hypokalemia must be identified and controlled. In a case such as this, holding at least one dosage of his maintenance furosemide may be appropriate. He should be assessed for the development of a fluid volume deficit, and appropriate IV maintenance fluids should be administered. Additionally, ECG, cardiac function, and neuromuscular examination must be monitored closely. Typically, potassium supplements are administered when the serum potassium level is less than 3 mEq/L (Box 3). ECG, cardiac function, and serum potassium levels are monitored frequently until the cause of the hypokalemia has been corrected or controlled.

Hyperkalemia is defined as a serum potassium level of greater than 5.5 mEq/L [9]. Typically, hyperkalemia occurs as the result of altered renal excretion of potassium, impaired extrarenal regulation, a shift from the ICF to the ECF, or increased potassium intake. Alterations in renal excretion of potassium may result from a decrease in the glomerular filtration rate or a decrease in potassium secretion by the renal tubules [9].

Case study #5

Andrew is a previously healthy 14-month-old boy who was admitted to the ICU with a new-onset leukemia and suspected tumor lysis syndrome (TLS). He is lethargic and irritable. Initial diagnostic studies reveal a serum potassium of 7.2 mEq/L and the following arterial blood gas results: pH 7.30 pCO_2 35 pO_2 91 HCO_3 18. Intermittent PVC's are noted on his cardiac monitor.

Vital signs: temperature, 37.7°C; pulse, 174; respiration, 32; BP 80/54 mm Hg; spO_2, 99%.

What factors are contributing to Andrew's hyperkalemia?

TLS is a group of metabolic effects that is associated with rapidly growing tumors. The metabolic abnormalities that are seen in TLS include hyperkalemia, hyperphosphatemia, hyperuricemia, and hypocalcemia (as a secondary effect of the hyperphosphatemia) [10]. The metabolic acidosis also is a contributing factor. Acidosis results in a shift of potassium from the ICF to the ECF. Although there is not a change in total body potassium content, this shift into the extracellular space also results in the clinical manifestations of hyperkalemia. These clinical manifestations are related to alterations in neuromuscular and cardiac functioning.

What will initial management strategies include?

Treatment of hyperkalemia varies depending upon the clinical presentation. If the potassium level is less than 6.5 mEq/L and no ECG changes are noted, discontinuation of fluids and medications containing potassium, along with close monitoring of serum potassium levels, may be sufficient. Administration of polystyrene sulfonate (Kayexalate) to increase potassium excretion also decreases potassium levels. Kayexalate can bind to calcium and magnesium in addition to potassium; therefore, it is important to monitor these electrolyte levels. Additionally, patients must be monitored for the clinical manifestations of hypocalcemia and hypomagnesemia. Potassium levels greater than 6.5 mEq/L or those that produce ECG changes require immediate treatment. Calcium gluconate (60–100 mg/kg) is administered to reduce the cardiac toxicity that is associated with hyperkalemia. The onset of action of calcium occurs within minutes

---

Box 3. Administration of potassium supplements

Treatment of hypokalemia:

   Two to 5 mEq/kg/d in divided dosages
   Intermittent infusion by way of syringe
pump or infusion pump

Maximum concentration

   Peripheral: 0.08 mEq/mL
   Central: 0.4 mEq/mL

Maximum administration rate

   1 mEq/kg/h and monitor EKG for dosages greater than 0.3 mEq/kg/h

and the effects last for approximately 30 minutes. Additionally, IV fluids are administered to expand ECF volume and to decrease the concentration of potassium in the ECF; however, this may not be a viable option in the child who has hyperkalemia and renal failure.

Redistribution of potassium from the ECF to ICF is necessary to decrease the elevated serum potassium level. Administration of insulin (0.1 unit/kg) stimulates the sodium–potassium pump and results in increased cellular uptake of potassium. Insulin should be administered in conjunction with dextrose (0.5–1 g/kg). A decrease in serum potassium should begin within 15 minutes and lasts for approximately 60 minutes [11].

The administration of sodium bicarbonate (1–2 mEq/L) also causes an intracellular shift of serum potassium; however, it may take up to 60 minutes for the sodium bicarbonate to decrease serum potassium levels [11]. The effects will last for several hours. Acid–base status is monitored closely in children who are receiving this therapy. Children who have respiratory failure are evaluated carefully, because sodium bicarbonate increases CO_2 production and may worsen respiratory acidosis if CO_2 cannot be excreted by the lungs. The development of hypernatremia is another potential complication of this therapy.

Albuterol, a β_2 adrenergic agonist, activates the sodium–potassium pump and stimulates the pancreas to release insulin, thereby shifting potassium into the cells [9]. It is administered by way of inhalation or IV infusion. It also has been recommended that albuterol be administered in conjunction with insulin because of the additive effect of the two drugs [9,11].

Calcium balance

Calcium, in conjunction with phosphorus and magnesium, plays an important role in nerve transmission, bone composition, and regulation of enzymatic processes. Homeostasis of these three electrolytes occurs through intestinal absorption and renal excretion. Most calcium is stored in the bones and teeth, and the remainder is found in soft tissue and serum. Of the calcium that is found within the serum, approximately 50% is bound to the protein or anions and is unavailable for use by the body. The remaining 50% is ionized and is available for the essential bodily functions of cardiac function, muscular contraction, nerve impulse transmission, and clotting. The ionized calcium level is of greatest physiologic significance, and direct measurement of ionized calcium is essential during a clinically important situation in which calcium levels may play a role.

Hypocalcemia is defined as a decrease of calcium in the ECF; it exists when serum calcium levels are less than 8 mg/dL in full-term infants and older children, and when ionized calcium levels are less than 4 mg/dL or 1.15 mmol/L. There are numerous potential causes of hypocalcemia, including, but not limited to, hypoparathyroidism, hypomagnesemia, hyperphosphatemia, vitamin D deficiency, calcium deficiency, impaired renal function, malabsorption syndromes, anticonvulsant therapy, nephrotic syndrome, acute pancreatitis, and transfusion with citrate-preserved blood [1,12].

Case study #6

Matthew is an 11-day-old boy who is postoperative day #2 following a tetralogy of Fallot repair. His course has been complicated by issues with postoperative bleeding and seizures. He has had no seizure activity over the past 12 hours; however, he required transfusion of multiple blood products overnight and continues to have moderate amounts of bloody drainage via his chest tube.

Vital signs: temperature, 37.5°C; pulse, 180; respiration, 20; BP, 66/31(45). A recent blood gas reveals an ionized calcium of 0.92 mmol/L.

Based on the above information, what is the most likely cause of Matthew's hypocalcemia?

The hypocalcemia most likely is related to the multiple blood products that were administered overnight. Citrate, a commonly used preservative in blood products, binds with calcium, and makes it unavailable for use by the body.

Why would you be especially concerned about hypocalcemia in this patient?

He already is at increased risk for compromised cardiac function following his surgery. Adequate levels of serum calcium are necessary for optimal cardiac function. Hypocalcemia is associated with arrhythmias, such as prolonged QT interval. This patient also has been having issues with bleeding, and calcium plays a role in the activation of clotting mechanisms. Additionally, he already has had problems with seizures postoperatively and hypocalcemia is a known cause of seizure activity.

What will initial management strategies include?

Acute management of hypocalcemia involves treating the cause and administering calcium supplements as needed. Patients must be monitored for cardiac, neurologic, and neuromuscular dysfunction. Concurrent conditions (eg, hyperphosphatemia, hypomagnesemia, respiratory alkalosis) must be identified and treated as needed [1].

Acute hypocalcemia in the child who is at risk for impending cardiovascular or neurologic failure must be treated immediately through restoration of ionized calcium levels. This is accomplished through the IV administration of calcium gluconate (100 mg/kg) or calcium chloride (10–20 mg/kg). While administering calcium supplements, monitor for arrhythmias. Rapid administration of calcium salts has been associated with bradycardia and asystole [13].

Hypercalcemia occurs as the result of an excess of calcium in the ECF, and the total serum calcium level is greater than 10.5 to 11 mg/dL. Generally, symptoms are not seen until the serum calcium level is greater than 12 mg/dL. Levels greater than 15 mg/dL may be life-threatening. Hypercalcemia is not a common occurrence, but may be seen in the critically ill child. In this population, it typically is associated with hyponatremia, hyperkalemia, resolution of chronic renal failure, and prolonged immobility.

Case study #7

John is a 17-year-old boy who has acute myelogenous leukemia and received a bone marrow transplant 77 days ago. He developed acute respiratory distress syndrome following his transplant, and was intubated and mechanically ventilated in the PICU for approximately 2 months. He spent a substantial portion of this time period heavily sedated and receiving neuromuscular blockade. A tracheostomy tube was placed 5 days ago and his mechanical ventilation is being weaned aggressively. His serum calcium levels have been climbing gradually over the past 7 to 10 days, and his current level is 13.2 mEq/L. Other electrolyte levels are within normal limits. He is lethargic and complains intermittently of nausea.

What is the most likely cause of John's hypercalcemia?

Prolonged immobility is the most likely cause of the hypercalcemia. During prolonged immobility, calcium moves from the bones, teeth, and intestine into the bloodstream to compensate for hypocalce-

mia. Long-term complications of immobility include osteoporosis and osteomalacia; however, hypercalcemia may occur during early stages when calcium is moving out of the bones and into the serum [14]. This calcium influx into the ECF can overwhelm the calcium regulatory hormones (parathyroid hormone and vitamin D) and renal excretion mechanisms [1].

Protein and pH also affect calcium levels. Increased albumin levels result in increased serum calcium levels. A decrease in serum pH increases ionized calcium, because more calcium is removed from protein binding sites and is available for participation in chemical reactions.

What will initial management strategies include?

Patients who have hypercalcemia and those who are at risk for the development of hypercalcemia must be identified and monitored for the related clinical manifestations. Particular attention should be paid to ECG monitoring and neurologic and gastrointestinal examinations. Calcium levels of greater than 15 mg/dL may be life-threatening and must be treated immediately. The goal of treatment is to reduce the amount of calcium in the ECF. This is accomplished through administration of IV fluids and loop diuretics. Thiazide diuretics are contraindicated because they restrict calcium excretion.

In John's case, his calcium levels are less than 15 mg/dL, and he is not exhibiting significant clinical manifestations. His hypercalcemia may be managed by increasing his fluid intake, adjusting his diuretic schedule to increase calcium excretion, and monitoring serum calcium levels. It also is essential to coordinate his plan of care with occupational and physical therapy services to increase his mobility and prepare him for transfer out of the ICU setting.

Summary

This article has presented an overview of several fluid and electrolyte imbalances that may occur in the critically ill infant or child. Imbalances in magnesium and phosphorous have not been discussed in detail in this article; an overview of clinical manifestations and management can be found in Table 3.

References

[1] Roberts KE. Fluid and electrolyte regulation. In: Curley MAQ, Moloney-Harmon PA, editors. Critical

care nursing of infants and children. 2nd edition. Philadelphia: W.B. Saunders; 2001. p. 369–92.

[2] Stark J. A comprehensive analysis of the fluid and electrolytes system. Crit Care Nurs Clin North Am 1998;10(4):471–5.

[3] Friedman AL. Nephrology: fluid and electrolytes. In: Behrman RE, Kliegman RM, editors. Nelson essentials of pediatrics. 4th edition. Philadelphia: WB Saunders; 2002. p. 671–709.

[4] Rabin N, Reed T, Vallino LM. Balance and imbalance of body fluids. In: Hockenberry MJ, editor. Wongs's nursing care of infants and children. 7th edition. St. Louis (MO): Mosby; 2003. p. 1171–206.

[5] Jospe N, Forbes G. Fluids and electrolytes—clinical aspects. Pediatr Rev 1996;17(11):395–403.

[6] Moritz ML, Ayus JC. Prevention of hospital-acquired hyponatremia: a case for using isotonic saline. Pediatrics 2003;11(2):227–30.

[7] Amini A, Schmidt MH. Syndrome of inappropriate secretion of antidiuretic hormone and hyponatremia after spinal surgery. Neurosurg Focus 2004;16(4):E10.

[8] Hellerstein S. Fluids and electrolytes: clinical aspects. Pediatr Rev 1993;14(3):103–15.

[9] Chmielewski CM. Hyperkalemic emergencies: mechanisms, manifestations and management. Crit Care Nurs Clin North Am 1998;10(4):449–58.

[10] Sarnaik AP. Tumor lysis syndrome. Available at: http://www.emedicine.com/ped/topic2328.htm. Accessed January 29, 2005.

[11] Ahee P, Crowe AV. The management of hyperkalemia in the emergency department. J Accid Emerg Med 2000;17:188–91.

[12] Singh J, Moghal N, Pearce SHS, et al. The investigation of hypocalcaemia and rickets. Arch Dis Child 2003;88:403–7.

[13] Styne DM, Glaser NS. Endocrinology. In: Behrman RE, Kliegman RM, editors. Nelson essentials of pediatrics. 4th edition. Philadelphia: WB Saunders; 2002. p. 711–66.

[14] Bouska Lee CA, Barrett CA, Ignatavicius DD. Fluids and electrolytes: a practical approach. 4th edition. Philadelphia: FA Davis; 1996.

ELSEVIER
SAUNDERS

Crit Care Nurs Clin N Am 17 (2005) 375–383

CRITICAL CARE
NURSING CLINICS
OF NORTH AMERICA

Low Cardiac Output Syndrome: Identification and Management

Linda Massé, MScA, LLM*, Marie Antonacci, BScN

Pediatric Intensive Care Unit, Montreal Children's Hospital, McGill University Centre, 2300 Tupper Street, Room F-240, Montreal, Quebec, H3H 1P3, Canada

Low cardiac output syndrome (LCOS) refers to a decrease in cardiac output that is due to transient myocardial dysfunction, as seen in patients who have various disease processes, including shock, and those who have undergone cardiac surgery. To prevent morbidity that is associated with poor systemic perfusion, early identification of this physiologic state and its consequences, and prompt management to maintain oxygen and nutrient supply to the peripheral tissues are essential. This article aims at improving the pediatric critical care nurse's understanding of the principles that govern myocardial function, the etiology, the clinical and laboratory assessment, the diagnosis, and the management of the child who has LCOS.

Cardiac function

The heart functions as a pump to distribute sufficient oxygenated blood to meet the tissues' requirements [1,2]. This entails that in stressful situations, cardiac output is modified so that all organs' needs are satisfied. The diastolic phase of the cardiac cycle is essential, because it is during ventricular relaxation that coronary filling occurs providing myocardial oxygenation [3]. The heart rate affects diastole significantly; a rate that is too rapid prevents attainment of complete myocardial relaxa-

tion and perfusion [4]. Cardiac dysfunction could result from any structural (eg, residual cardiac anomaly) or functional cardiac disorder (eg, disturbances in ventricular filling or emptying or increased systemic vascular resistance) [5]. Cardiac dysfunction may be aggravated further by metabolic acidosis secondary to systemic hypoperfusion [6]. The hemodynamic instability that is associated with heart failure often is confused with other disease processes, such as neonatal sepsis or overwhelming pneumonia. The common finding of these disturbances is that cardiac output decreases and leads to imbalances between metabolic cellular requirements and oxygen delivery [7].

Cardiac output

Cardiac output is defined as the volume of blood that is pumped by the heart to the systemic circulation per minute [3,4,8]. It represents the total blood flow in the body [7,9]. Cardiac output is dependent on the heart rate and the stroke volume (cardiac output = heart rate × stroke volume). It is influenced by three interdependent components: preload, afterload, and contractility [3]. If one or more of these elements is affected, a low cardiac output state may occur [2,10,11].

The heart rate refers to the frequency of a full atrial and ventricular contraction or beats per minute. Children are highly dependent on their heart rate to maintain adequate tissue perfusion [12]. A heart rate that is too fast affects the atrial and ventricular chamber filling time, and thus, diminishes the amount of blood that is ejected to the pulmonary and systemic

* Corresponding author.
  E-mail address: linda.masse@muhc.mcgill.ca
(L. Massé).

circulation [1]. A slow heart rate is significant because of the limitation in manipulating the child's stroke volume [4,12]. The rhythmic component of each contraction also is crucial. Atrioventricular synchrony refers to the sequential contraction of the atria followed by the ventricle. Hence, better ventricular filling and stroke volume is achieved by the atrial kick, which represents 30% of the volume. Loss of atrioventricular synchrony (as seen in junctional ectopic tachycardia [JET] and third-degree heart block), represents atrial and ventricular rhythms where each is under the control of a separate pacemaker focus. It also occurs with slower junctional or nodal rhythms. If untreated, the outcome is compromised tissue perfusion secondary to inadequate stroke volume and cardiac output.

The preload refers to the amount of myocardial fiber stretch present before each contraction [4,12]. It represents the volume in the ventricle and is affected directly by intravenous volume administration. It is determined indirectly by measuring the right atrial (RA) or left atrial pressures or the central venous pressure (CVP). Conditions that cause capillary leakage or decreased venous return, such as sepsis, hemorrhage, aggressive diuresis, excessive airway pressure, and postoperative cardiac surgical states, lead to decreased preload that affects cardiac output [1,13]. The use of vasoactive agents also can increase venous capacitance which decreases preload [1]. Although adequate preload is necessary, overstretching the ventricle by administering excessive volume is detrimental to the cardiac output [1,4].

Afterload is the sum of all forces opposing ventricular emptying [3,4,12]. Simplistically, afterload reflects the amount of vasoconstriction or resistance against which the ventricle is ejecting [3]. Afterload increases the work of the myocardium, has a direct effect on the ejection fraction, and results in alterations in the cardiac output [1]. Systemic and pulmonary hypertension, or aortic coarctation are anomalies that illustrate this point. High afterload is tolerated only with myocardial hypertrophy that results from a chronic increase in pressure [1].

Contractility refers to the myocardial fiber shortening that is seen during systole, which could be defined as the force generated by the myocardium independent of preload and afterload [12]. It refers to the strength and efficiency of the contraction [4]. Contractility is expressed as the ejection fraction, and is evaluated most accurately by echocardiography. Electrolyte imbalances (hyperkalemia, hypocalcemia, hypomagnesemia), hypoglycemia, severe acidosis, hypoxia, or hypoxemia influence the contractile function of the myocardium [1,10,14].

Cardiac output and oxygen delivery

Cardiac output and hemoglobin play the largest roles in oxygen delivery. The latter determines the availability of oxygen for tissue consumption, which emphasizes the importance of maintaining sufficient perfusion to the extremities [15–17]. During high metabolic requirements (as in exercise or disease states), cardiac output increases to meet the oxygen demands [18]. Inflammatory states and sepsis can alter the tissues' oxygen extraction capabilities, despite appropriate perfusion; this results in cells that are starving for oxygen and nutrients [7,19]. This triggers a switch to anaerobic glycolysis and leads to acidosis and increased serum lactate levels which are markers of diminished systemic perfusion [15,20].

The oxygen content represents the amount of oxygen carried by the blood to the cells. In healthy states, the oxygen delivered greatly exceeds the needs of the tissue. Therefore, if cellular metabolism increases in response to stress or physical activity, the body adapts by increasing its cardiac output. In conditions where cardiac output is impaired, the oxygen content should be maximized for adequate oxygen delivery [14]. Box 1 shows the relationship between systemic oxygen delivery, hemoglobin, and cardiac output.

Hemoglobin is the major vehicle for oxygen transport to the cells. The hemoglobin level represents the amount of red blood cells per volume of blood and indicates the oxygen-carrying capacity [4,14]. Hemoglobin levels may increase considerably in situations where hemoconcentration occurs

---

Box 1. Relationship between systemic oxygen delivery, arterial oxygen content, hemoglobin and cardiac output

Systemic oxygen delivery = arterial oxygen content × cardiac output

Arterial oxygen content = dissolved O_2 + oxy-hemoglobin

Arterial oxygen content = [PaO_2 × 0.0031] + [hemoglobin × 1.34 × % saturation]

Thus PaO_2 (dissolved O_2) is only a small contribution to oxygen content, so effectively:

Arterial O_2 content = hemoglobin × saturation

Systemic oxygen delivery = [hemoglobin × saturation] × cardiac output [7,18]

(eg, severe dehydration or shock) or decrease as a result of anemia, acute massive blood loss, or hemolytic reactions. Adjustment in hemoglobin levels is essential when perfusion and oxygen delivery cannot be optimized [3,10,11,19,21]. In children with "mixing" cardiac physiology and low arterial oxygen saturation, the hemoglobin must be maintained at a level that is optimal for adequate oxygen distribution [14]. When low cardiac output is present, the oxygen extraction is increased at the cellular level [3].

Etiology of low cardiac output syndrome

The causes of LCOS are multifactorial. LCOS may present in physiologic states that are affected by inadequate vascular volume (eg, decreased preload) or by increased systemic vascular resistance that leads to excessive afterload [3,10].

Examples of conditions that impair cardiac function are: (1) poor contractility, (2) valvular stenosis or insufficiency, (3) myocardial restriction or dysfunction resulting from irritation and edema associated with surgical resection, (4) an inflammatory process secondary to mediator release, and (5) tamponade [3]. These abnormalities may appear alone or in combination, and enhance the perfusion-uptake mismatch [3].

LCOS has been associated mainly with primary cardiac dysfunction following postoperative repair of congenital cardiac anomalies and congestive myopathies. All disease processes with impaired oxygen delivery and cardiac dysfunction that cause decreased tissue perfusion could lead to a low cardiac output state. For example, septic shock in children often is characterized by a low cardiac output state, where changes in systemic vascular resistance result in anaerobic metabolism, increased lactate production, and some cellular damage secondary to poor oxygen delivery and use [22].

Cardiac dysfunction leading to LCOS can derive from diastolic dysfunction originating from poor myocardial compliance or decreased cardiac relaxation [1,3,17]. This condition alters myocardial oxygenation and creates some degree of myocardial ischemia. In addition, the interdependence between both ventricles greatly affects the diastolic pressure. For example, an increase in right ventricular pressure interferes with the volume capacity of the left ventricle. As well, cardiac tamponade or high intrathoracic pressures restrict myocardial activity and impede venous return and end-diastolic ventricular filling, and thus, contribute to low cardiac output [1,10,23]. Myocardial dysfunction is noted within 4 to 6 hours after cardiopulmonary bypass and requires vigilant observation by the clinician during this time frame [24]. Signs of myocardial dysfunction include decreased peripheral pulses, cold extremities, oliguria, and low blood pressure [1]. In septic shock, the systolic and diastolic dysfunctions often are associated with alterations in the peripheral vascular tone modifying the ejection fraction of the myocardium [25]. When ventricular function is impaired, an increase in systemic vascular resistance worsens an already poor myocardial state which could result in cardiovascular collapse [3].

Cardiac impairment also may originate from rhythm disturbances. Causes of arrhythmias may include: (1) hypoxia [14,26]; (2) disturbances in impulse formation or impulse conduction; (3) reentry within the sinoatrial node and accessory pathways [6]; (4) surgical resection creating irritation, edema, or direct injury to the conduction system [6,8]; and (5) electrolyte imbalances and metabolic disorders [6,8,14].

Assessment of low cardiac output syndrome: clinical signs and symptoms

The level of risk for developing LCOS influences the extent of monitoring that is required in the pediatric ICU. Adequate monitoring implies a thorough initial and continuous assessment of the patient's hemodynamic status, the response to therapy, and evaluation of the changes noted in the physiologic status. Various clinical, laboratory, and physiologic variables are useful in determining the adequacy of the cardiac output and oxygen delivery. Systemic perfusion and cardiac output usually are assessed indirectly by monitoring vital signs, signs of systemic perfusion, and urine output. Signs and symptoms that are indicative of LCOS are shown in Box 2.

Box 2. Signs and symptoms indicative of low cardiac output syndrome [10,27]

Tachycardia
Hypotension
Narrow pulse pressure
Poor perfusion
    Cold extremities
    Weak pulses
    Slow capillary refill time
Oliguria or anuria

Table 1
Normal heart rate values according to age

Age interval	Heart rate (beats per minute; bpm)
Neonate less than 1 month	120–160 bpm (tachycardia greater or equal to 180 bpm)
1 month–1 year	100–160
1–3 years	98–163
3–5 years	65–132
5–8 years	70–115
8–12 years	55–107
12–16 years	55–102

Data from Curley MAQ, Bloeder Smith J, Moloney-Harmon PA, editors. Critical care nursing of infants and children. 2nd edition. Philadelphia: W.B Saunders Company; 1996; and Hazinski MF. Nursing care of the critically ill child. 2nd edition. St-Louis (MO): Mosby Year Book; 1992.

Vital signs

The heart rate encompasses a complete atrial and ventricular contraction whereby blood is ejected to the systemic and pulmonary vasculature permitting oxygen delivery. Normal heart rate values are listed in Table 1.

Tachycardia, especially if ventricular rate exceeds 180 to 220 beats per minute, compromises the ventricular diastolic and coronary artery filling time and results in diminished stroke volume, cardiac output, and poor myocardial perfusion [6,28]. Tachycardia develops in response to physiologic changes, such as pain, agitation, acidosis, hypovolemia, anemia, hypoxemia, fever, and low cardiac output. It also may appear as a compensatory mechanism to maintain systemic perfusion and cardiac output in the early phases of cardiac tamponade where adequate ventricular filling and emptying are restricted [4,10]. Electrolyte and metabolic disturbances also contribute to the manifestation of arrhythmias (eg, third-degree heart block may result from hypoxemia, metabolic acidosis, and electrolyte imbalances) [10]. Hypoxia, acidosis, hypocalcemia, hypomagnesemia, hypophosphatemia, hypokalemia or hyperkalemia, and hyperthermia are treatable causes of arrhythmias and should be investigated and corrected [10,19,22].

CVP represents the pressure in the great veins as blood returns to the heart. It is a reliable indicator of intravascular blood volume (preload) [3,11,14, 21,22]. Normal CVP values range between 8 and 10 mm Hg [1].

Blood pressure represents the conducting force of blood flow in organs and tissues. It entails two significant phases: systole and diastole. Systolic blood pressure is the pressure exerted within the arterial vasculature during ventricular contraction and is a reflection of the stroke volume. Diastolic pressure reflects blood volume and vascular tone (capacity). Blood pressure is an indicator of organ perfusion; however, it is an insensitive hemodynamic parameter because a drop in blood pressure will be seen only after all of the compensatory mechanisms (eg, catecholamine release with subsequent increase in heart rate and peripheral vasoconstriction) have failed to maintain cardiac output [20]. In certain congenital cardiac defects (eg, coarctation of the aorta), the blood pressure might be normal in the presence of compromised cardiac output if the systemic vascular resistance is elevated [3,28]. Usually, a high or normal systolic pressure with a low diastolic pressure is suggestive of systemic vasodilation with acceptable ventricular ejection, whereas a low systolic pressure associated with a high diastolic pressure is suggestive of poor ventricular ejection and systemic vasoconstriction [19]. Despite its limitation, monitoring blood pressure trends is helpful to evaluate the response to therapy. Normal blood pressure values are listed in Table 2.

Table 2
Normal blood pressure values according to age

Age	Systolic pressure (mm Hg)	Diastolic pressure (mm Hg)	Mean arterial pressure (mm Hg)
Birth (12 hrs, 3 kg weight)	50–70	25–45	33–53
Neonate (96 h)	60–90	20–60	33–70
Infant (6 mo)	87–105	53–66	64–79
Toddler (2 y)	95–105	53–66	67–79
School age (7 y)	97–112	57–71	70–85
Adolescent (15 y)	112–128	66–80	81–96

Data from Curley MAQ, Bloeder Smith J, Moloney-Harmon PA, editors. Critical care nursing of infants and children. 2nd edition. Philadelphia: W.B Saunders Company; 1996; and Hazinski MF. Nursing care of the critically ill child. 2nd edition. St-Louis (MO): Mosby Year Book; 1992.

Poor systemic perfusion

Capillary refill time refers to the number of seconds it takes for color to return after pressing on skin or nail beds. Normal value should be less than 3 seconds [12,29]. A prolonged refill time could result from decreased vascular volume or vasoconstriction; however, confounding factors, such as fever, ambient temperature, and use of vasoactive medication, must be ruled out before establishing a diagnosis of LCOS [3]. A capillary refill time of greater than 4 seconds is indicative of reduced stroke volume and peripheral perfusion.

Core–peripheral (toe) temperature gradient is the difference in degrees between body and skin temperature and is used as an indicator of perfusion [25]. Core or central temperature reflects the temperature of the blood flowing through the branches of the carotid arteries to the hypothalamus, and is measured most accurately by an esophageal probe. If unavailable, rectal temperature monitoring is acceptable. Toe temperature reflects skin temperature [19]. Generally, toe temperature trends are monitored; values greater than 34°C are considered a good sign, but when they approach ambient level (22° to 25°C), the presence of shock should be suspected [19]. Core–peripheral temperature gradient should be less than 3°C.

Urine output

Urine output is the volume of urine measured hourly. Infants and young children who have normal cardiac output void approximately 1 mL/kg/h, whereas older children and adults excrete 0.5 mL/kg/h (or 20–40 mL/h) [8]. Infants in cardiogenic shock lose the ability to maintain renal blood flow and glomerular filtration. Hence, this state of renal hypoperfusion is manifested by oliguria or anuria [3,10,13,21,30].

Diagnosis of low cardiac output syndrome

The clinical signs and symptoms that are used as indirect measures of cardiac output and systemic perfusion are insensitive markers. Cellular hypoxia and poor systemic perfusion may be present well before clinically apparent changes in cardiovascular responses are observed [16]. Supplemental laboratory testing is essential for prompt recognition of LCOS and implementation of appropriate therapy. Box 3 specifies the laboratory results associated with LCOS.

Box 3. Laboratory results indicative of low cardiac output syndrome [8,27,33]

Arterial-venous oxygen gradient $\geq 30\%$
Or metabolic acidosis (ie, an increase in the base deficit of > 4)
Or an increase in lactate of > 2 mmol/L on two successive blood gases

---

Arterial-venous oxygen gradient (A-V O_2) refers to the difference between arterial oxygen saturation and mixed venous oxygen saturation (Box 4). A-V O_2 represents the balance between oxygen delivery and consumption. Arterial-venous oxygen gradient is normally lower than 30% [8]. A-V O_2 changes correlate with variations in cardiac output when oxygen demands remain stable in the absence of hypoxemia and anemia. The combination of a high A-V O_2 and an elevated serum lactate level may indicate an inability to consume oxygen at the cellular level (ie, cellular metabolic dysfunction).

Mixed venous oxygen saturation (SvO_2) is defined as the oxygen saturation of hemoglobin in the pulmonary artery following mixing of the systemic venous circulation (originating from the superior and inferior vena cava) with the coronary venous circulation (draining by way of the coronary sinus). SvO_2 assesses the overall balance between oxygen transport and consumption, and thus, helps the clinician to evaluate how the patient's cardiac output meets the systemic oxygen demand [2]. Ideally, blood samples should be procured from a pulmonary artery or right ventricle line [3,14]. If these lines are unavailable, a specimen from a central venous site or RA catheter may be sent for analysis [9]. The sample must be measured directly by co-oximetry because the value cannot be determined solely by the arterial oxygen tension (PaO_2).

Normal values of mixed venous saturation range between 70% and 75%. An SvO_2 of less than 65% indicates an increased oxygen extraction by the cells which is suggestive of impaired tissue perfusion or increased metabolic rate [14]. SvO_2 values are influenced by cardiac physiology, oxygen consumption, and by changes in any of the four components of oxygen delivery: cardiac output, hemoglobin concentration, PaO_2, and arterial oxygen saturation (SaO_2) [7–9,14,16,21,29,31]. Therefore, mixed venous desaturation is caused by changes in one or more of these components leading to reduced oxygen delivery. An increase in oxygen consumption without a

---

Box 4. Determinants of arterial-venous oxygen gradient

A-V O_2 gradient = Arterial O_2 Saturation − Mixed venous O_2 Saturation
SaO_2 = *oxygen delivery SvO_2 = *oxygen consumption

	Result on arterial blood gas sample	Result on pulmonary artery/right ventricle/ central venous line or catheter or right atrial line or catheter

Normal arterial O_2 saturation: 95%
Normal mixed venous O_2 saturation: 75%
Normal A-V O_2 gradient: 20%−27%

* values apply to normal cardiorespiratory physiology

---

compensating increase in oxygen delivery also reduces mixed venous saturation [2,4,9,30].

The arterial blood gas is the most valuable diagnostic tool that is used to determine the acid–base balance and the oxygenation in the clinical setting [14]. Results can reveal the severity of hypoxemia and hypoperfusion (manifested by a metabolic acidosis). Normal arterial blood gas values are listed in Box 5.

Base deficit refers to the amount of base (in mmol) required to titrate 1 liter of whole blood to a pH of 7.40. It is a calculated value that estimates the metabolic component of blood pH, and reflects the degree of metabolic acidosis present at the peripheral level [18,25]. Base excess normally ranges between +2 and −2. A base deficit of greater than −5 mmol/L correlates with inadequate oxygenation and tissue perfusion, metabolic acidosis, and increased morbidity (eg, organ failure) [20].

Serum lactate level is a marker of the adequacy of tissue oxygenation, oxygen delivery, and oxygen extraction [22]. Lactate is produced when oxygen delivery is inadequate or when the tissues are unable to extract it appropriately [3,7,9,14]. In these situations, the cells turn to anaerobic glycolysis where glucose is metabolized to lactate [15,20]. Therefore, a serum lactate level represents a balance between its production and its elimination, and reflects the degree of tissue hypoxia and anaerobic cellular metabolism [13,21,22]. The normal lactate level in a healthy newborn usually is less than 2.5 mmol/L and in the adult, it approximates 2 mmol/L [29]. Increased lactate production usually is indicative of altered tissue perfusion but may result from any process that increases metabolic demand, such as hyperthermia and increased muscular activities (eg, seizures, shivering) [20,30]. Lactate is cleared primarily by the liver and kidneys, hence renal or hepatic failure can contribute to elevated levels [20,25]. Hyperlactatemia shortly after cardiopulmonary bypass may represent the extent of intraoperative or early postoperative tissue oxygen extraction, impaired lactate clearance, or both [21,31].

Serum lactate levels of between 4.5 and 6 mmol/L on admission and increasing levels in serial measurements are most predictive of morbidity and mortality [15,25,30]. Therefore, to evaluate the quality of systemic perfusion, admission and serial levels of serum lactate must be monitored [24]. Blood lactate levels will decrease within 60 minutes of initiating therapy aimed at increasing perfusion [19].

Box 5. Normal arterial blood gas values [8]

pH: 7.34−7.45
PaO_2: 80−100 mm Hg
$PaCO_2$: 35−45 mm Hg
SaO_2 saturation in acyanotic heart physiology: 95−97%
Saturation must be measured by co-oximetry

Management strategies

After a diagnosis of LCOS is established, appropriate interventions should be initiated to optimize cardiac function. The following strategies involve manipulation of the interdependent determinants of cardiac output, and are known to improve clinical outcome in the presence of myocardial dysfunction. Box 6 lists the goals for the management of LCOS.

Interventions should focus on minimizing oxygen consumption, which is achieved by decreasing meta-

Box 6. Goals of low cardiac output syndrome management [2,10,11,21,27, 28,31,33]

Optimize contractility/ventricular function
Improve diastolic dysfunction
Maintain adequate preload
Reduce afterload
Improve oxygen supply and demand
Allow time for ventricle to recover

bolic rate and demands. Included among these interventions are: (1) maintaining the patient normothermic or mildly hypothermic; (2) administering appropriate dosages of analgesia and sedation (caution is recommended to prevent respiratory and cardiovascular depression often seen with these agents) [2,3,6,10]; (3) initiating mechanical ventilation to decrease the work of breathing [3,19]; and (4) preventing or treating tachyarrhythmias promptly.

Arrhythmias, electrolyte disorders, and acid–base disturbances should be corrected to prevent further cardiac instability [10]. Inotropic support often is required, but careful titration is essential to avoid excessive myocardial efforts. Appropriate fluid repletion will help to restore effective tissue perfusion and re-establish the equilibrium between oxygen delivery and consumption [8,22]. Adequate preload obtained by administration of colloids or crystalloids should precede the use of inotropic agents [10,13].

Arrhythmias should be treated [10]. Sedation and hypothermia may help to slow the rate of nodal firing in tachyarrhythmias. Supraventricular tachycardia requires additional measures, such as vagal and Valsalva maneuvers, gag reflex, abdominal compression, or rectal stimulation; however, these techniques often are insufficient and pharmacologic agents, such as adenosine and amiodarone, often are necessary to convert this rapid narrow QRS complex arrhythmia [6]. Cardioversion should be considered for hemodynamically unstable patients [6]. At the other extreme, bradycardia associated with hypotension requires treatment with medication that stimulates heart rate (eg, isoproterenol or epinephrine) after preload is optimized. External or epicardial cardiac pacing may be necessary to attain an adequate heart rate [2, 12,14]. Atrio-ventricular pacing is required for arrhythmias involving atrioventricular asynchrony (eg, JET, slow junctional rhythm, third-degree heart block) and is prioritized over the use of inotropic support [11,28].

Pharmacotherapeutic agents should be considered after an adequate preload is obtained, and correction of electrolytes and blood gas abnormalities is achieved [7,8,10,29,32]. Their effects are dose-related and serve to augment cardiac output and improve myocardial contractility; however, prolonged usage or high doses may have detrimental adverse reactions, including: (1) arrhythmogenesis, (2) excessive chronotropy (increased heart rate), (3) increased myocardial oxygen consumption, (4) downregulation of β-adrenergic receptors, (5) increased afterload, and (6) hypertension [27]. Elevated hydrogen ion concentration—associated with persistent metabolic acidosis—may interfere with the inotropic effects of catecholamines and further depress myocardial contractility [27,31]. Sodium bicarbonate may be beneficial in this situation [6].

Dopamine primarily promotes myocardial contractility, but also improves splanchnic, cerebral, and coronary blood flow at low doses [1,14,19,33]. Its effect on renal arterial perfusion is believed to enhance renal function and output although this continues to be controversial [10,28,33]. In pediatric patients who have hypotension that is refractory to fluid resuscitation, dopamine remains the preferred treatment because of its alpha effects at high doses [8,9,13,22,33].

Dobutamine has gained popularity for its multifaceted actions that improve myocardial performance: chronotropy, contractility, and vasodilatory effects [14,28]. Another advantage is that it is less arrhythmogenic than other inotropic agents [33]. Although its vasodilatory properties reduce afterload, cardiac output may be improved without an increase in blood pressure which requires another inotrope in case of severe hypotension [6,14,19,28]. The synergistic action of dobutamine and milrinone is to increase cardiac output by altering afterload and increasing contractility, promoting their use in the treatment of elevated systemic and pulmonary vascular resistance.

The positive actions of epinephrine are that it increases heart rate and systolic pressure, and enhances stroke volume [22,29]. Despite these desired effects, the counterpart is the augmentation in metabolic rate and temperature, myocardial oxygen consumption, pulmonary and systemic vascular resistance, and lactate production. These side effects could impair peripheral organ perfusion further, which suggests that only low doses should be used in combination with other inotropic agents [19,22].

Milrinone is a phosphodiesterase III inhibitor that combines inotropic activity with afterload reduction [2,27,33]. It improves left ventricular relaxation and compliance and results in increased stroke volume and cardiac output [25]. Its vasodilatory effect decreases systemic vascular resistance [10]. It maintains favorable myocardial oxygen supply/demand ratio. Milrinone is recommended strongly when low cardiac output is associated with high vascular resistance, as seen in some septic shock states [11].

Vasodilatory agents are used for afterload reduction. Sodium nitroprusside, which is a smooth muscle relaxant that dilates arteries and veins, has a rapid onset of action and short half-life. Its peak effect is attained in 2 minutes and dissipates within 3 minutes of stopping the infusion, which facilitates its administration. It decreases atrial pressure (preload), and pulmonary and systemic vascular resistance (afterload). The dose starts at 0.5 µg/kg/min up to 5 to 10 µg/kg/min; however, it becomes more toxic at levels greater than 10 mg/dL. Prolonged period of infusion results in the formation of thiocyanate and cyanide [14]. These agents create toxicity that is more prevalent after 72 to 96 hours of infusion. Monitoring thiocyanate levels daily is essential. Its most common adverse effect is hypotension. Doses must be titrated carefully to obtain desired effects without adverse reactions because it can lead to pulmonary vasodilatation that results in increased intrapulmonary shunting and decreased PaO_2, and cerebral vasodilatation that may increase intracranial pressure. It also can inhibit platelet function [22].

Inhaled nitric oxide (NO) is an endothelium-derived relaxing agent that is produced in lung capillary cells. Following administration by inhalation, exogenous NO diffuses into adjacent vascular smooth muscle [28]. NO is indicated for treatment of pulmonary hypertension or low cardiac output associated with high pulmonary vascular resistance. It selectively decreases pulmonary vascular resistance and dilates pulmonary arteries near the best-ventilated alveoli, which improves the ventilation-perfusion match [17,28]. Therapeutic doses of inhaled NO have no effect on systemic circulation because NO is metabolized rapidly or bound to hemoglobin and neutralized [34]. Toxic levels of methemoglobin (ie, combination of NO with hemoglobin)—exceeding 20% of total hemoglobin—are responsible for critically reduced arterial oxygen content and episodes of severe, acute pulmonary injury with pulmonary edema, and may lead to death.

Summary

LCOS implies a transient decrease in systemic perfusion due to myocardial dysfunction. The outcome of this critical clinical state is inadequate oxygen delivery to meet cellular oxygen demand. Establishment of a clinical diagnosis requires a thorough and vigilant assessment of hemodynamic, electrophysiologic, and laboratory variables. Monitoring arterial-venous gradient, mixed venous oxygenation, and serial lactate levels provide the most accurate diagnostic information. The goals of therapeutic interventions aim at improving cardiac output by optimizing preload, minimizing afterload, enhancing contractility, and ensuring adequate heart rate and rhythm. Reacting promptly to change is essential in the care of the child who has LCOS to minimize the morbidity and mortality.

Acknowledgments

The authors thank Dr. Sam Shemie for initiating the thinking process that led to this article. His answers to the authors' questions helped in the understanding of the physiologic processes that are involved in the low cardiac output syndrome.

References

[1] Graham TP. Disorders of the circulation: myocardial dysfunction. In: Fuhrman BP, Zimmerman JJ, editors. Pediatric critical care. 2nd edition. St-Louis (MO): Mosby Inc.; 1998. p. 261–71.

[2] Tibby SM, Murdoch IA. Monitoring cardiac function in intensive care. Arch Dis Child 2003;88:46–52.

[3] Carcillo JA, Field AI. Clinical practice parameters for hemodynamic support of pediatric and neonatal patients in septic shock. Crit Care Med 2002;30(6): 1365–78.

[4] Hazinski MF. Cardiovascular disorders. In: Hazinski MF, editor. Nursing care of the critically ill child. 2nd edition. St-Louis (MO): Mosby Year Book; 1992. p. 117–271.

[5] Klein L, O'Connor CM, Gattis WA, et al. Pharmacologic therapy for patients with chronic heart failure and reduced systolic function: review of trials and practical considerations. Am J Cardiol 2003;91(9A):18F–40F.

[6] Lee C, Mason LJ. Pediatric cardiac emergencies. Anesthesiol Clin North Am 2001;19(2):287–308.

[7] Vincent J-L. Determination of oxygen delivery and consumption versus cardiac index and oxygen extraction ratio. Crit Care Clin 1996;12(4):995–1006.

[8] Vincent J-L, Gerlach H. Fluid resuscitation in severe sepsis and septic shock:an evidence-based review. Crit Care Med 2004;32(11):S451–4.

[9] Beale RJ, Hollenberg SM, Vincent J-L, et al. Vasopressor and intropic support in septic shock: an evidence-based review. Crit Care Med 2004;32(11): S455–65.

[10] Hoffman TM, Wernovsky G, Atz AM, et al. Prophylactic intravenous use of milrinone after cardiac operation in pediatrics (PRIMACORP) study. Am Heart J 2002;143(1):15–21.

[11] O'Laughlin MP. Congestive heart failure in children. Pediatr Clin North Am 1999;46(2):263–73.

[12] Craig J, Bloedel Smith J, Fineman LD. Tissue perfusion. In: Curley MAQ, Bloeder Smith J, Moloney-Harmon PA, editors. Critical care nursing of infants and children. 2nd edition. Philadelphia: W.B Saunders Company; 1996. p. 131–231.

[13] Dellinger RP. Cardiovascular management of septic shock. Crit Care Med 2003;31(3):946–55.

[14] Wilson WC, Shapiro B. Perioperative hypoxia. Anesthesiol Clin North Am 2001;19(4):769–812.

[15] Deshpande SA, Ward Platt MP. Association between blood lactate and acid-base status and mortality in ventilated babies. Arch Dis Child 1997;76:F15–20.

[16] Duke T, Butt W, South M, et al. Early markers of major adverse events in children after cardiac operations. J Thorac Cardiovasc Surg 1997;114(6): 1042–51.

[17] Hakanson E, Svedjeholm R, Vanhanen I. Physiologic aspects in postoperative cardiac patients. Ann Thorac Surg 1995;59:S12–4.

[18] Breen PH. Arterial blood gas and pH analysis: clinical approach and interpretation. Anesthesiol Clin North Am 2001;19(4):885–906.

[19] Butt W. Septic shock. Pediatr Clin North Am 2001; 48(3):601–25.

[20] Takami Y, Ina H. Significance of the initial arterial lactate level and transpulmonary arteriovenous lactate difference after open-heart surgery. Surg Today 2002; 32:207–12.

[21] Munoz R, Laussen PC, Palacio G, et al. Changes in whole blood lactate levels during cardiopulmonary bypass for surgery for congenital cardiac disease: an early indicator of morbidity and mortality. J Thorac Cardiovasc Surg 2000;119(1):155–62.

[22] Parker MM, Hazelzet JA, Carcillo JA. Pediatric considerations. Crit Care Med 2004;32(11):S591–4.

[23] Andrew P. Diastolic heart failure demystified. Chest 2003;124(2):744–53.

[24] Charpie JR, Dekeon MK, Goldberg CS, et al. Serial blood lactate measurements predict early outcome after neonatal repair or palliation for complex congenital heart disease. J Thorac Cardiovasc Surg 2000;120(1): 73–80.

[25] Fenton KE, Sable CA, Bell MJ, et al. Increases in serum levels of troponin I are associated with cardiac dysfunction and disease severity in pediatric patients with septic shock. Pediatr Crit Care Med 2004;5(6): 533–8.

[26] Kao W, Surjancev BP. Management of acute heart failure exacerbation. Crit Care Clin 2001;17(2):321–35.

[27] Doyle RA, Dhir AK, Moors AH, et al. Treatment of perioperative low cardiac output syndrome. Ann Thorac Surg 1995;59:S3–11.

[28] Leonard SR, Nikaidoh H, Copeland MM, et al. Cardiothoracic surgery. In: Levin DL, Morriss FC, editors. Essentials of pediatric intensive care. 2nd edition. New York: Churchill Livingstone; 1997. p. 611–23.

[29] Wernovsky G, Hoffman TM. Pediatric heart failure: solving the puzzle. Crit Care Med 2001;29(10): S212–3.

[30] Hatherill M, Sajjanhar T, Tibby SM, et al. Serum lactate as a predictor of mortality after paediatric cardiac surgery. Arch Dis Child 1997;77:235–8.

[31] Roth SJ. Postoperative care. In: Chang AC, Hanley F, Wernovsky G, et al, editors. Pediatric cardiac intensive care. Baltimore (MD): Williams & Wilkins; 1998. p. 163–84.

[32] Rao V, Ivanov J, Weisel RD, et al. Lactate release during reperfusion predicts low cardiac output syndrome after coronary bypass surgery. Ann Thorac Surg 2001;71:1925–30.

[33] Tabbutt S. Heart failure in pediatric septic shock: utilizing inotropic support. Crit Care Med 2001;29(10): S231–6.

[34] Wessel DL. Managing low cardiac output syndrome after congenital heart surgery. Crit Care Med 2001; 29(10):S220–30.

ELSEVIER
SAUNDERS

Crit Care Nurs Clin N Am 17 (2005) 385 – 393

CRITICAL CARE
NURSING CLINICS
OF NORTH AMERICA

Nutritional Assessment and Enteral Support of Critically Ill Children

Erwin Ista, RN*, Koen Joosten, MD, PhD

Department of Pediatrics, Erasmus MC - Sophia Children's Hospital, P.O. Box 2060, 3000 CB Rotterdam, The Netherlands

Critical illness has a major impact on the nutritional status of children. Nutritional assessment is required as an integral part of patient care; however, during an intensive care stay, attention is focused mostly on the primary medical problem and not on the child's nutritional status. When the child stays in the ICU for longer than 5 to 7 days, the chance of developing serious nutritional deficiencies increases significantly [1]. As early as 1980, researchers demonstrated protein-energy malnutrition in 15% to 20% of children who were admitted to the ICU [2]. A recent study showed a high prevalence (24%) of acute or chronic malnutrition in critically ill children who were admitted to a pediatric ICU (PICU) [3]. Therefore, nutritional support after initial nutritional assessment should be an essential aspect of the clinical management of patients in the PICU. The diversity in clinical presentation and the various age groups dictate a patient-tailored approach.

Several common hospital practices have been identified that may cause the deterioration of nutritional status in admitted patients (Box 1). In general, the development of malnutrition during an ICU stay can be related to the disease, incomplete nutritional assessment or determination of the patient's nutritional needs, or lack of adequate nutritional support.

Widespread ignorance of the physiologic effects of different feeding routes and the composition of nutritional products results in the inappropriate use of routes of administration of enteral and par-

enteral feeds of uncertain composition or inadequate amounts.

Critical care nurses play an important role in the feeding of critically ill children. Many procedures and caregiving interventions, such as placement of feeding tubes, registration of gastric retention, observation and care of the mouth, and administration of nutrition (enteral or parenteral), are within the nursing domain. This article discusses nutritional assessment techniques and enteral nutrition (EN) in critically ill children.

Nutritional assessment

Definition

Nutritional assessment can be defined as the interpretation of data concerning an individual's intake and use of nutrients to determine his or her health status. Data must be obtained by different means, and interpreted together to perform a comprehensive nutritional assessment. These data includes:

- General evaluation (including dietary and medical history and physical signs)
- Severity of illness assessment
- Assessment of body composition
- Laboratory studies (including the estimation of energy requirements)

Nutritional assessment is necessary to: (1) identify patients who have, or who are at risk for developing, protein-energy malnutrition; (2) establish the degree of malnutrition and the risk of developing malnu-

---
* Corresponding author.
E-mail address: w.ista@erasmusmc.nl (E. Ista).

trition related complications; and (3) evaluate the effect of nutritional support [4]. Accurate assessment of nutritional status in children is complex because of ongoing growth, changing energy needs, varying body composition, and disease [5]. In critically ill children this phenomenon is more complex because of weight shifts that are caused by third spacing of fluid; this can result in inaccurate anthropometric measurements and inaccurate assumptions of true weight [1].

Techniques

General evaluation

    A full medical and dietary history is necessary for an extensive nutritional assessment. When the critically ill child has a history of chronic disease, the initial nutritional status at admission might be poor and the child may need extra attention. Physical signs of malnutrition usually do not appear until malnutrition had been prolonged and severe; however, the first impression of the child and subjective assessment of muscle and fat mass can help. Subjective global assessment is a clinical technique that assesses nutritional status based on features of the history and

physical examination [6]. On admission, a detailed history concerning nutrition can be performed by the nursing staff.

    It also is important to be alert for the development of malnutrition during admission. A study by Sermet-Gaudelus and colleagues [7] showed that 79% of hospitalized children lost weight (>2%) during admission. Using a pediatric nutritional risk score, they found that the patients' degree of stress (Box 2), food intake, and pain were associated with weight loss. They developed a pediatric nutritional risk score that identifies three classes of risk (low, moderate, and high) and recommendations for nutritional interventions (Table 1).

Anthropometry

    Classic anthropometry is a term that describes the measurement of body weight, body length, and head circumference. Additional anthropometric mea-

Table 1

Pediatric nutritional risk score and recommendations for nutritional intervention

Risk factors [coefficients]				
Pathology	Pain [1] Food intake <50% [1]	Score	Nutritonal risk	Nutritional intervention
Mild (grade 1) [0]	None	0	Low	None
Mild (grade 1) [0]	One	1	Moderate	Assess food intake and weight daily
Mild (grade 1) [0]	Both	2	Moderate	Refer to a dietitian
Moderate (grade 2) [1]	None	1	Moderate	Start oral nutritional support (NS)
Moderate (grade 2) [1]	One	2	Moderate	
Moderate (grade 2) [1]	Both	3	High	Measure ingested food precisely
Severe (grade 3) [3]	None	3	High	Refer to a nutrition team
Severe (grade 3) [3]	One	4	High	Consider enteral or parenteral NS
Severe (grade 3) [3]	Both	5	High	

Adapted from Sermet-Gaudelus I, Poisson-Salomon AS, Colomb V, et al. Simple pediatric nutritional risk score to identify children at risk of malnutrition. Am J Clin Nutr 2000;72(1):64–70; with permission.

surements concern circumferences (mid upper arm, calf, abdominal), skin fold thickness, and lower leg length (knemometry).

Weight

Weight is the most important parameter for nutritional assessment of the critically ill child; therefore, it is a gold standard [1]. The assessment of weight in this group is not easy and changes in weight cannot be ascribed only to growth, because edema plays an important role. In our practice we propose assessing weight on admission and daily during the PICU stay (except in chronically ill children) [3,8].

Length

Body length is difficult to measure and generally is of limited value as a nutritional assessment tool on the ICU, because changes in linear growth are hard to point out over a short period of admission. For newborn infants and children up to 24 months of age, the lower leg length measure is a promising method for measurement of short-term linear growth; it consists of a heel-to-knee measurement (knemometry) [9]. The tool is hand-held, can be used inside an incubator, and is less disruptive than making length measurements.

Head circumference

Head circumference is another important aspect of nutritional assessment in young children and should be included in the initial assessment and follow-up. In the PICU this parameter is used rarely; however, on admission it could signal a history of severe chronic malnutrition. Serial measurements in neonates can aid in detecting the development of malnutrition.

Body circumferences and skin fold thickness

Measurements of body circumferences (mid upper arm, calf, abdominal) and skin fold thickness are anthropometric measurements that can provide information on fat mass and fat-free mass. Mid upper arm circumference (MUAC) is a measure of muscle, fat, and bone. It has been used as an index of malnutrition in rapid nutritional surveys when weight and length measurements were not feasible. We advocate measuring the MUAC in all children because it is simple to perform on admission and follow-up and it is an easy screening tool for malnutrition.

Feasibility of anthropometry. One has to take into account that the feasibility to perform anthropometric measurements decreases with the severity of disease. The feasibility to perform anthropometric measurements routinely was investigated. For weight, 35% of ventilated children were weighed on admission; 84% of all children who were in the PICU for more than 48 hours were weighed [3,8]. This knowledge underlines the need for a patient-tailored approach in which measurements can be performed in the individual patient to detect malnutrition.

Indirect calorimetry

Measuring energy expenditure allows for a more accurate monitoring of the child's varying energy needs in the course of critical illness. Clinically, the measurement of energy expenditure by indirect calorimetry (IC) is applicable in critical care, and is more accurate than estimating individual energy expenditure from standard prediction equations. IC provides noninvasive, reliable, repeatable, and affordable measurements of actual energy expenditure (resting energy expenditure in nonventilated children and total daily energy expenditure in ventilated children) and the respiratory quotient (RQ).

RQ is a helpful parameter in nutritional assessment because it has been considered important in evaluating substrate use or nutritional support and in determining overfeeding and underfeeding [10,11]. Table 2 shows the RQ values related to the feeding status used in clinical practice. An RQ of greater than 1 indicates overfeeding, which most of the time is due to carbohydrate overfeeding; therefore, attention should be focused on the carbohydrate intake.

In the critically ill child, quantification of energy expenditure also is important from the diagnostic standpoint because it allows the detection of hyper- or hypometabolic conditions that are related directly to the individual prognosis. The greatest advantage of using IC is to design a nutrition regimen that exactly meets the patient's energy requirements and avoids the complications of overfeeding [12].

The IC in the ICU is valuable because not much other information is available for approximating the needs of the critically ill child [1]. IC to determine energy requirements is being used widely as a research tool. In most ICUs, limited space at the bedside, the cost of multiple metabolic carts, and the availability of trained staff to operate them limit its routine use.

For the practical use of IC in critically ill children, accurate measurement requires the following conditions:

- Fraction of inspired oxygen of less than 0.60
- Tube leakage of less than 10%. Tube leakage is determined by comparison of inspired and expired tidal volumes measured by the ventilator, assuming that there are no other leaks in the patient–ventilator circuit.

In one investigation, the feasibility of routine use of IC performed by the nursing staff was studied; it was possible in 70% to 80% of the eligible mechanically ventilated children [3,8].

Taken together, nutritional assessment is important in providing optimal care to critically ill children. A simple and integrated nutrition screening should be part of the admission procedure in the ICU. It has to be followed by an individual calculation of macro- and micronutrient needs. In addition, nutritional assessment should be repeated regularly to monitor changes in nutritional status, diagnoses, or conditions that might put the child at nutritional risk, and to monitor the efficacy of nutritional support. Fig. 1 shows a standard of nutritional assessment for the PICU population.

Nutritional support

The most important element in nutritional support in the intensive care setting is to have a standard feeding protocol in which three issues should be considered:

- When to feed: indications for nutritional support
- What to feed: composition of nutritional formula and enteral feeding
- How to feed: how to administer EN

Application of such a protocol is the most important step in treating the malnourished patient in the ICU. The working group on nutrition and metabolism of the European Society of Intensive Care Medicine published a practical approach in 1998 for EN for adult patients in the ICU [13]. These recommendations consisted of the supply of macronutrients, micronutrients, and immunomodulating agents, and recommendations for feeding and organ dysfunction, feeding preparations, and conditioning and routes of feeding. Such a practical approach has not been published for critically ill children; however, the concept of this working group should be translated for the critically ill child.

When to feed: indications for nutritional support

For assessing the total nutritional status of a patient, several parameters have to be evaluated. Souba [14] stated that identification of the malnourished adult patient at risk is important because besides established indications for the use of nutritional support, there is a list of unproven indications that requires further study. There are accepted guidelines for the time to start additional nutritional support for the adult patient who has a severe illness; these consist of items, such as the duration of the catabolic state, days without nutrition, and the presence of malnutrition on admission [15].

Compared with adults, children have less physiologic reserves of fat and protein and increased energy

Table 2
Feeding status related to respiratory quotient

Feeding status	Respiratory quotient
Underfeeding	< 0.85
Adequate feeding	0.85–1.0
Overfeeding	> 1.0

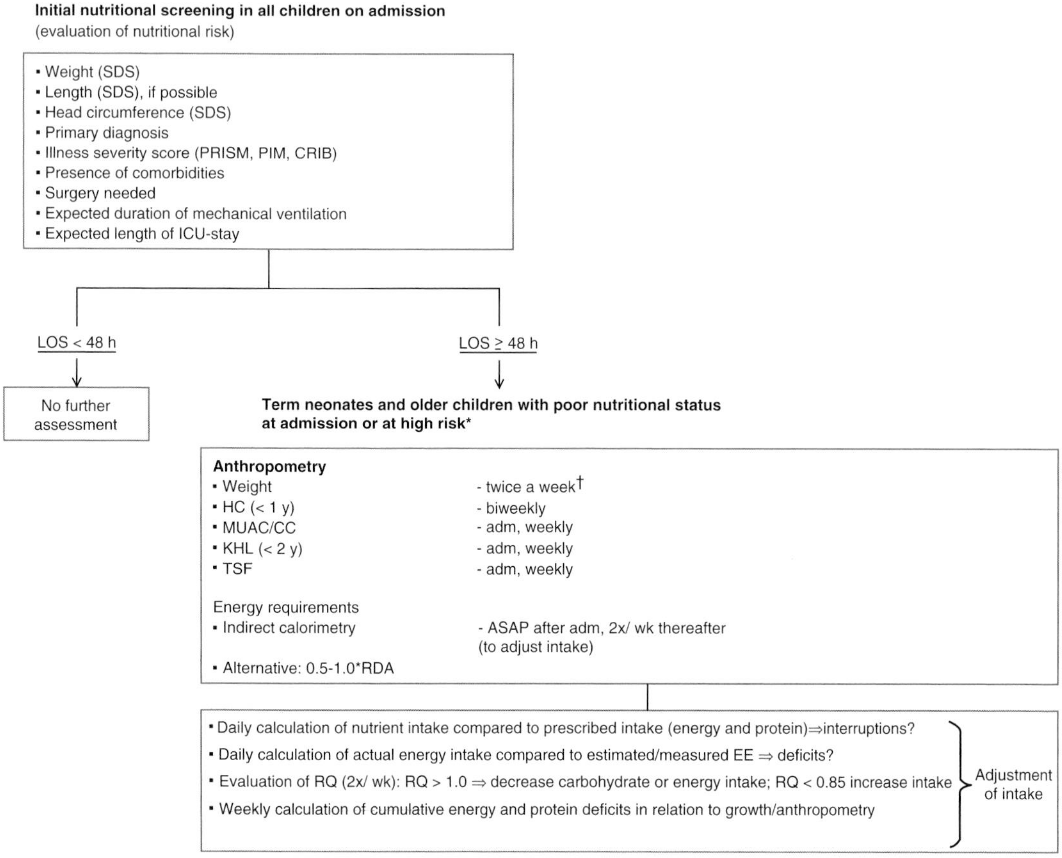

Initial nutritional screening in all children on admission
(evaluation of nutritional risk)

- Weight (SDS)
- Length (SDS), if possible
- Head circumference (SDS)
- Primary diagnosis
- Illness severity score (PRISM, PIM, CRIB)
- Presence of comorbidities
- Surgery needed
- Expected duration of mechanical ventilation
- Expected length of ICU-stay

LOS < 48 h

No further assessment

LOS ≥ 48 h

Term neonates and older children with poor nutritional status at admission or at high risk*

Anthropometry
- Weight   - twice a week[†]
- HC (< 1 y)   - biweekly
- MUAC/CC   - adm, weekly
- KHL (< 2 y)   - adm, weekly
- TSF   - adm, weekly

Energy requirements
- Indirect calorimetry   - ASAP after adm, 2x/ wk thereafter (to adjust intake)
- Alternative: 0.5-1.0*RDA

- Daily calculation of nutrient intake compared to prescribed intake (energy and protein)⇒interruptions?
- Daily calculation of actual energy intake compared to estimated/measured EE ⇒ deficits?
- Evaluation of RQ (2x/ wk): RQ > 1.0 ⇒ decrease carbohydrate or energy intake; RQ < 0.85 increase intake
- Weekly calculation of cumulative energy and protein deficits in relation to growth/anthropometry

Adjustment of intake

Fig. 1. Proposed standard of nutritional assessment in the pediatric ICU population. *Adapted from* Hulst JM. Nutritional assessment of critically ill children: the search for practical tools [master's thesis]. Rotterdam (The Netherlands): Erasmus University; 2004; with permission.
Abbreviations: Adm, admission; ASAP, as soon as possible; CC, calf circumference; CRIB, Clinical Risk Index for Babies; EE, energy expenditure; HC, head circumference; LFA, length for age; KHL, knee-heel length; LOS, length of stay; MUAC, mild upper arm circumference; PIM, Pediatric Index of Mortality; PRISM, Pediatric Risk of Mortality; RQ, respiratory quotient; SDS, standard deviation score; TSF, triceps skin fold; WFA, Weight for age; WFL, Weight for length.
* poor nutritional status: WFA-SDS or LFA-SDS or WFL-SDS <−2; risk groups: prolonged expected ICU-stay, prolonged duration of mechanical ventilation, children undergoing surgery, children with underlying growth-affecting disease such as children with major congenital malformations, cardiac anomalies, cystic fibrosis, Inflammatory bowel disease, HIV-infection.
† depending on age of child.

expenditure; therefore, children are at increased risk for malnutrition [16]. Furthermore, it seems appropriate to start nutritional support as soon as possible because children are in a state of growth, development, and organ maturation.

What to feed: composition of nutritional formulas

Current recommendations for nutritional support in critically ill pediatric patients are not based on randomized trials with feeding intervention studies. Knowledge concerning substrate intake and substrate use can be derived from adult studies and studies concerning primarily surgically treated newborn infants. Knowledge concerning energy expenditure can be derived from a few studies of mechanically ventilated children; however, some important conclusions can be drawn from these studies:

- There is a significant discrepancy between measured energy expenditure compared with calculated energy expenditure using predictive equations
- The total daily energy requirements can be higher or lower than values of resting energy expendi-

ture but in general the total daily energy requirements of the critically ill child will be lower than the total daily energy requirements for healthy children

- There is a considerable risk for overfeeding in the critically ill child for carbohydrate, fat and protein [11,17]
- There might be an individual maximum of oxidative capacity for carbohydrate, fat and protein
- Carbohydrate overfeeding can be determined by measuring the respiratory quotient; an RQ of more than 1.0 indicates overfeeding.
- Fat overfeeding can be determined by measuring plasma triglycerides levels or comparing fat intake with fat use.
- Protein needs can be determined by measuring urinary nitrogen excretion [11,18].
- Protein retention can be increased by a balanced glucose/fat solution [19].
- There might be an optimal nonprotein calorie: nitrogen ratio to enhance protein retention.

Energy requirements

The reference method to evaluate the energy need is IC. Some factors (eg, fever, injury, dialysis) cause an increase in energy expenditure, whereas other factors (eg, sedation or relaxation, decreased work of breathing, decreased loss of heat during mechanical ventilation) cause a decrease of energy expenditure.

A pragmatic estimate of energy requirements is given in Table 3, based on a percentage of the recommended daily allowances of healthy children. For growth of the infant for each 1 gram growth, 4 kcal growth should be added. One should account for 10% to 15% loss of energy when enteral feeding is supplied.

Protein requirements

The method to evaluate the protein need is to calculate urinary nitrogen excretion. Protein need can

range from 1 g/kg/d to 4 g/kg/d in the severely ill child. A recommendation is to start with enteral or parenteral protein of 1 g/kg/d, and to increase the amount depending on the need and level of blood urea. Proteins that are administered with fresh frozen plasma should not be taken into account. Standard enteral formulas can be administered because there is no evidence to use protein diet formulas.

Glucose requirements

Enteral or parenteral glucose should be administered at 4 to 6 mg/kg/min, depending on the severity of disease and the tolerance of the patient. The method to evaluate carbohydrate overfeeding is measuring a respiratory quotient with IC or to determine serum hyperglycemia or glucosuria. Insulin therapy is started for hyperglycemia, depending on the duration and the diagnosis, according to the current guidelines of intensive insulin therapy in adults [20].

Fat requirements

In general, the parenteral fat intake is less than the enteral fat intake because there is a maximum capacity to hydrolyze the administered parenteral fat emulsions. Furthermore, the absorption of enteral fat is 80% to 90%. When parenteral feeding, a low amount of fat—0.5 g/kg/d—is started in the acute phase of illness because of the risk of fat overloading. In general, a least 2% to 3% of calories should be linoleic acid to prevent fatty acid deficiency. The method to evaluate fat overload is to measure plasma triglycerides; fat intake should be adjusted depending on this level. The fat intake can be increased gradually to between 3 g/kg/d and 4 g/kg/d. When enteral feeding is supplied, fat in the amount of 1 g/kg/d to 1.5 g/kg/d should be given initially. This amount can be increased gradually to between 7 g/kg/d and 8 g/kg/d in small infants and to between 3 g/kg/d and 4 g/kg/d in older children.

Table 3
Nutrition schedule of early enteral feeding protocol

Age	Type of feeding[a]	Amount of feeding	
		Day 1 - half of RDA (kcal/kg/d)	Day 2 - total RDA (kcal/kg/d)
0–1 months	Nutrilon / breast milk	50	100
1–12 months	Infatrini / breast milk	47–100	95–100
1–6 years	Nutrini multi fiber	46	92
7–12 years	Tentrini multi fiber	35–42	70–84
>12 years	Nutrison multi fiber	25–30	49–60

[a] Nutricia, Zoetermeer, The Netherlands.

How to feed: administration of enteral nutrition

Although nutrition can be provided to critically ill children enterally or parenterally, the enteral route is preferred if there are no contraindications [21]. EN is the preferred method of nutritional support for pediatric patients when the gastrointestinal tract can by used. Advantages of EN are convenience, safety, and low cost. EN also is important in maintaining gastrointestinal mucosal integrity and immunologic function that may prevent bacterial translocation and multisystem organ failure in critically ill children [22]. Gastric and duodenal/jejunal feedings are the primary routes for EN administration in critically ill children. Gastric tubes usually are placed easily by bedside nurses with fewer complications. Nasoduodenal feeding tubes are recommended to reduce the risk of aspiration in the presence of delayed gastric emptying or reflux [22], and is a safe "way" when continuous enteral feeding of mechanically ventilated children is given.

Many strategies have been developed to increase the success rate for placement of feeding tubes in the small bowel/duodenum. Spalding and colleagues [23] tested the effectiveness of gastric insufflation as an adjunct to the placement of feeding tubes in the small bowel compared with the standard insertion technique. The investigators assumed that gastric insufflation is a technique for bedside insertion of a transpyloric feeding tube. Determination of tube position was done by a radiographic method. Other studies demonstrated that the transpyloric placement of feeding tubes using pH sensing is successful, but specialized equipment is required [24,25]. Chellis and colleagues described their experience with bedside placement method using metoclopramide (0.1 mg/kg, intravenously). Transpyloric placement was confirmed by absence of blue dye in nasogastric secretions as well as by an abdominal radiograph [26].

In the PICU at Sophia Children's Hospital, Rotterdam, The Netherlands, enteral feeding is given by a transpyloric route (duodenal feeding tube) in mechanically ventilated critically ill children. Transpyloric feeding was easy to establish within 24 hours after admission in most (44/46 [95%]) of the mechanically ventilated children of various ages and with various diseases [8] using a standard protocol.

The protocol for inserting a transpyloric feeding tube is as described:

A 6, 8, or 10 French enteral feeding tube of appropriate size for each patient is used.

Before insertion, the length of tubing needed to reach the stomach and the fourth part of the duodenum is determined.

The tube is placed in the stomach and the position is confirmed by injection of air with auscultation. Children are positioned right side down.

Before the feeding tube is advanced to the predetermined length, ice water is inserted to stimulate pyloric opening. The amount of ice water is related to the age of the patient (Table 4).

The position of a transpyloric feeding tube is determined by the use of a pH stick; if the pH is between 7.0 and 8.0 it can be concluded that the feeding tube is located transpyloric.

If this method is not successful after two attempts with ice water, erythromycin (10 mg/kg) is administrated intravenously for 30 minutes. Directly after infusion of erythromycin, a new attempt is executed. The use of erythromycin can be helpful in stimulating pyloric opening.

The bedside placement of pH-guided transpyloric small bowel feeding tubes can be done by nurses. In addition, it is a low cost method for determining the location of the feeding tube tip. Both of these are considered advantages of this particular method. If it is not possible to feed transpyloricly, continuous gastric feeding will be started and gastric motility agents (eg, motilium) will be added; however, it is not possible to give all patients EN. Gastric retention, diarrhea, and abdominal distention can limit the use of enteral feeding. If possible, the enteral route of feeding should be used, even with small amounts, unless it is absolutely contraindicated (eg, bowel obstruction, intractable diarrhea).

Early enteral nutrition

Zaloga and Roberts [27] reviewed the results of early EN in animal and human adult studies. Animal studies showed that early EN improved gut blood flow and gut mass, diminished the invasiveness of gut bacteria, protected the liver and prevented injury during shock, improved protein synthesis and the rate of wound healing, and increased survival after critical illness. More importantly, prospective, randomized trials in humans have indicated that early EN improved outcome during critical illness.

Table 4
Amount of ice water

Age child	Ice water
0–6 months	5 ml
6–12 months	10 ml
>1 year	1 ml/kg

Studies in premature and low birth-weight infants found that the lack of enteral feeding may result in an absence of the natural stimulus for growth of the intestinal mucosa, as well as diminished production of intestinal mucins, which acts as a barrier to bacterial translocation [28]. Further proof of the efficacy and safety of early enteral feeds was given in the form of case reports and case series of burn patients [29,30]. Chellis and colleagues performed a study in 42 critically ill children to evaluate the feasibility and safety of early enteral feedings. All patients were able to achieve caloric goals within 48 hours of beginning enteral feedings, and there were no documented complications, such as aspiration or abdominal distention [31]. A more recent retrospective study in 95 critically ill children showed that it was possible to start EN within 24 hours after admission in most children [32]. A limitation of both of these studies was the use of retrospective chart review for data collection.

A recent prospective analysis examined the use of an early enteral feeding protocol in critically ill children who were hemodynamically stable and who had not undergone abdominal surgery. The aim of the enteral feeding protocol was to feed critically ill children within 2 days after admission according to the total recommended daily energy intake (RDA) for healthy children. The type and amount of enteral feeding were based on the age category and weight of the child (see Table 3). On day 1 of admission, enteral feeding is started at 50% of the total RDA and increased to 100% of RDA on day 2. With this protocol, on day 1 and day 2, 90% and 89%, respectively, of the children received the type of feeding according to the protocol. In 10% and 11% of the cases, respectively, the caregivers deviated from the standard because of nutrition intolerance and logistical problems. Concerning the amount of the enteral feeding, on day 1 and day 2, 84% and 78% of the children, respectively, received the amount according to the protocol [8].

Despite the enthusiasm about enteral feeding, it is not possible to give all critically ill children the maximum required amount of enteral feeding according to RDA. Barriers for the adequacy of nutritional support in critically ill children are restriction of fluid intake, clinical interventions (extubation), administration of medications, gastrointestinal intolerance, and mechanical complications with the enteral feeding tube [32–34].

Enteral feeding in critically all children should be started as soon as possible. If critically ill children are hemodynamically stabilized—even if high doses of inotropics are necessary—small amounts of enteral feeding can be started. Because critically ill children suffer from gastric dysmotility and emptying difficulties, transpyloric tube feeding is the preferred route.

Total parenteral feeding is indicated when the gastric–intestinal tract is nonfunctional, when it is impossible to obtain enteral access, or when EN alone is not able to meet the child's energy requirements.

References

[1] Huddleston KC, Ferraro-McDuffie A, Wolff-Small T. Nutritional support of the critically ill child. Crit Care Nurs Clin North Am 1993;5(1):65–78.

[2] Pollack MM, Ruttimann UE, Wiley JS. Nutritional depletions in critically ill children: associations with physiologic instability and increased quantity of care. J Parenter Enteral Nutr 1985;9(3):309–13.

[3] Hulst JM. Nutritional assessment of critically ill children: the search for practical tools [master's thesis]. Rotterdam (The Netherlands): Erasmus University; 2004.

[4] Klein S, Kinney J, Jeejeebhoy K, et al. Nutrition support in clinical practice: review of published data and recommendations for future research directions. Summary of a conference sponsored by the National Institutes of Health, American Society for Parenteral and Enteral Nutrition, and American Society for Clinical Nutrition. Am J Clin Nutr 1997;66(3):683–706.

[5] Khoshoo V. Nutritional assessment in children and adolescents. Curr Opin Pediatr 1997;9(5):502–7.

[6] Detsky AS, McLaughlin JR, Baker JP, et al. What is subjective global assessment of nutritional status? J Parenter Enteral Nutr 1987;11(1):8–13.

[7] Sermet-Gaudelus I, Poisson-Salomon AS, Colomb V, et al. Simple pediatric nutritional risk score to identify children at risk of malnutrition. Am J Clin Nutr 2000; 72(1):64–70.

[8] Ista E, Joosten KFM. Successful early enteral feeding of critically ill children [abstract]. 15th ESPNIC Medical and Nursing Annual Congress; London; 2004. p. 103.

[9] Hermanussen M. Knemometry, a new tool for the investigation of growth. A review. Eur J Pediatr 1988; 147(4):350–5.

[10] McClave SA, Lowen CC, Kleber MJ, et al. Clinical use of the respiratory quotient obtained from indirect calorimetry. J Parenter Enteral Nutr 2003;27(1):21–6.

[11] Joosten KFM, Verhoeven JJ, Hazelzet JA. Energy expenditure and substrate utilization in mechanically ventilated children. Nutrition 1999;15(6):444–8.

[12] Brandi LS, Bertolini R, Calafa M. Indirect calorimetry in critically ill patients: clinical applications and practical advice. Nutrition 1997;13(4):349–58.

[13] Van den Berghe G, de Zegher F, Bouillon R. Clinical review 95: acute and prolonged critical illness as different neuroendocrine paradigms. J Clin Endocrinol Metab 1998;83(6):1827–34.

[14] Souba WW. Nutritional support. N Engl J Med 1997; 336(1):41–8.

[15] Revhaug A, Kjaeve J. Nutrition in the acute catabolic state. In: Revhaug A, editor. Acute catabolic state. Berlin: Springer-Verlag; 1996. p. 257–67.

[16] Cunningham JJ. Body composition and nutrition support in pediatrics: what to defend and how soon to begin. Nutr Clin Pract 1995;10(5):177–82.

[17] Chwals WJ. Overfeeding the critically ill child: fact or fantasy? New Horiz 1994;2(2):147–55.

[18] Mickell JJ. Urea nitrogen excretion in critically ill children. Pediatrics 1982;70(6):949–55.

[19] Nose O, Tipton JR, Ament ME, Yabuuchi H. Effect of the energy source on changes in energy expenditure, respiratory quotient, and nitrogen balance during total parenteral nutrition in children. Pediatr Res 1987; 21(6):538–41.

[20] Van den Berghe G, Wouters P, Weekers F, Verwaest C, Bruyninckx F, Schetz M, et al. Intensive insulin therapy in the critically ill patients. N Engl J Med 2001;345(19):1359–67.

[21] Curley MA, Castillo L. Nutrition and shock in pediatric patients. New Horiz 1998;6(2):212–25.

[22] Marian M. Pediatric nutrition support. Nutr Clin Pract 1993;8(5):199–209.

[23] Spalding HK, Sullivan KJ, Soremi O, et al. Bedside placement of transpyloric feeding tubes in the pediatric intensive care unit using gastric insufflation. Crit Care Med 2000;28(6):2041–4.

[24] Krafte-Jacobs B, Persinger M, Carver J, et al. Rapid placement of transpyloric feeding tubes: a comparison of pH-assisted and standard insertion techniques in children. Pediatrics 1996;98(2 Pt 1):242–8.

[25] Dimand RJ, Veereman-Wauters G, Braner DA. Bedside placement of pH-guided transpyloric small bowel feeding tubes in critically ill infants and small children. J Parenter Enteral Nutr 1997;21(2):112–4.

[26] Chellis MJ, Sanders SV, Dean JM, et al. Bedside transpyloric tube placement in the pediatric intensive care unit. J Parenter Enteral Nutr 1996;20(1):88–90.

[27] Zaloga GP, Roberts PR. Early enteral feeding improves outcome. In: Vincet JL, editor. Yearbook of intensive care and emergency medicine. Berlin: Springer-Verlag; 1997. p. 701–14.

[28] Wesley JR. Nutritional support in the pediatric intensive care unit. Curr Opin Gastroenterol 1994;10:210–7.

[29] Trocki O, Michelini JA, Robbins ST, et al. Evaluation of early enteral feeding in children less than 3 years old with smaller burns (8–25 per cent TBSA). Burns 1995;21(1):17–23.

[30] Engelhardt VJ, Clark SM. Early enteral feeding of a severely burned pediatric patient. J Burn Care Rehabil 1994;15(3):293–7.

[31] Chellis MJ, Sanders SV, Webster H, et al. Early enteral feeding in the pediatric intensive care unit. J Parenter Enteral Nutr 1996;20(1):71–3.

[32] Taylor RM, Preedy VR, Baker AJ, et al. Nutritional support in critically ill children. Clin Nutr 2003;22(4): 365–9.

[33] Adam S, Batson S. A study of problems associated with the delivery of enteral feed in critically ill patients in five ICUs in the UK. Intensive Care Med 1997; 23(3):261–6.

[34] Rogers EJ, Gilbertson HR, Heine RG, et al. Barriers to adequate nutrition in critically ill children. Nutrition 2003;19(10):865–8.

ELSEVIER
SAUNDERS

Crit Care Nurs Clin N Am 17 (2005) 395–404

CRITICAL CARE
NURSING CLINICS
OF NORTH AMERICA

Pediatric Poisonings: Recognition, Assessment, and Management

Maureen A. Madden, MSN, PNP-AC, FCCM[a,b,*]

[a]*Department of Pediatrics, Division of Critical Care Medicine, UMDNJ-Robert Wood Johnson Medical School,
100 Bayard Street, 3rd Floor, New Brunswick, NJ 08903, USA*
[b]*Pediatric Critical Care, Bristol-Myers Squibb Children's Hospital, 3rd Floor, 1 Robert Wood Johnson Place,
New Brunswick, NJ 08901, USA*

Poisoning represents one of the most common medical emergencies encountered in young children in the United States, and accounts for a significant proportion of emergency room visits for the adolescent population. Poisoning is a significant and persistent cause of morbidity and mortality in children and adolescents; 5% of all accidental childhood deaths are attributed to it. The scope of toxic substances involved in poisoning is broad, and requires health care providers to have an extensive knowledge of signs and symptoms of poisoning and specific therapeutic interventions and antidotes. There are multiple routes of exposure to toxic agents; ingestions account for most exposures [1]. Most children who ingest poisons suffer no harm; however, health care providers must recognize, assess, and manage those exposures that are most likely to cause serious injury, illness, or death and initiate appropriate management to minimize the physical injury that may occur. Those patients who are identified to be most at risk are likely to require management in an ICU setting.

The American Association of Poison Controls Centers collects and publishes an annual report detailing poison exposure data in the Toxic Exposure Surveillance System (TESS). The 2003 TESS report documented more than 2.3 million human exposures to toxins; 92.6% occurred in a residence. Children younger than 3 years of age were involved in 39%

of cases, and 52% of all toxic exposures happened in children younger than 6 years of age. Children younger than 19 years of age accounted for 66% of all combined pediatric and adult poisoning exposures; children younger than 6 years of age accounted for 79% of all pediatric exposures. There were 1106 reported fatalities for 2003. Although responsible for most poisoning reports, children under 6 years of age accounted for only 34 (3.1%) fatalities, and the younger than 19 years of age group accounted for 9.6% (106) of the total fatalities reported (Table 1). Despite having most poison exposures managed safely at home through the guidance of the poison control centers, these untoward events also result in a significant use of health care resources. Treatment in a health care facility was necessary in 21.9% of all toxic exposures. The percentage of patients treated in a health care facility varied greatly by age; only 23.2% of children younger than 13 years of age received treatment, as compared with 48.1% of adolescents [1]. More than 14% of all poisonings were admitted for management in the critical care setting.

Recognition

The TESS summary states that most poisonings can be classified as: acute; accidental or unintentional; occur in the home; and involve children younger than 6 years of age (Table 2). The primary goal of initial assessment is to discern which children are at clinical risk and treat them aggressively,

* Department of Pediatrics Division of Critical Care,
100 Bayard Street, 3rd Floor, New Brunswick, NJ 08903.
E-mail address: maddenma@umdnj.edu

doi:10.1016/j.ccell.2005.07.004

Table 1
Number of pediatric poison exposures in 2003

Age	Number of exposures	Percent of all exposures	Number of fatalities	Percent of all fatalities
Younger than 6 years	1,245,584	52%	34	3.1%
6–12 years	171,823	6.6%	7	0.6%
13–19 years	1,582,500	7.2%	65	5.9%

Data from Watson WA, Litovitz TL, Klein-Schwartz W, et al. 2003 Annual Report of the American Association of Poison Control Centers Toxic Exposure Surveillance System. Am J Emerg Med 2004;22:335–404.

when appropriate, while minimizing intervention in the population that has low risk of harm. The cornerstone of treatment includes a thorough evaluation of the ingestion episode, careful assessment of the patient, and application of basic supportive care when required.

The substances that are involved most frequently in human exposure are not those that are the most toxic substances, but are those that are the most accessible. Some of the more common agents that are seen in pediatric exposures include cosmetics and personal care products, cleaning substances, analgesics, foreign bodies, topicals, cough and cold preparations, and plants (Table 3). Toxic effects do not occur often with these agents because children usually do not ingest amounts sufficient to produce toxicity. Other substances that are ingested less frequently and do not require large amounts to produce toxic effects are alcohols, antidepressants, theophylline, barbiturates, cocaine, iron, clonidine, and caustics. The greatest number of hospitalizations, ICU admissions, and fatalities in pediatric poisonings occur with these agents. Although poisoning may be acute or chronic, most human toxic exposures were acute (91.7%); unintentional ingestions outnumbered intentional ingestions for all age groups [1]. Ingestion was the major route of exposure and accounted for almost 77% of cases; this is followed in frequency by dermal, inhalation, and ocular routes.

Table 2
Reason for human exposure by age

Reason	<6 years	6–12 years	13–19 years
Unintentional	61.1%	7.1%	4.2%
Intentional	0.4%	3.0%	27.8%
Other[a]	7.5%	10.3%	17.4%
Adverse reaction	8.2%	5.9%	8.1%
Unknown	5.1%	6.5%	15.0%

[a] Other includes: malicious, contamination or tampering, withdrawal.
Adapted from Watson WA, Litovitz TL, Klein-Schwartz W, et al. 2003 Annual Report of the American Association of Poison Control Centers Toxic Exposure Surveillance System. Am J Emerg Med 2004;22:335–404; with permission.

Although most exposures occur in young children, it is uncommon for poisoning in this age group to result in death. Most poisoning exposures in children younger than 6 years of age are unintentional, which imply that these exposures are not associated with malicious or suicidal intent. Poisonings in this age group usually involve only one substance that often is nontoxic or minimally toxic. The amount ingested usually is small and children usually present for evaluation soon after ingestion [2]. An alarming number of exposures in children younger than 6 years of age involve the ingestion of a grandparent's or elderly caretaker's medicine. These agents tend to be more toxic to children because they are dispensed often as sustained-release dosage forms. Reactions to toxic agents depend on the agent, the amount ingested, the size of the child, and the time lapse between exposure and treatment. The pharmacodynamics of children predisposes them to having an increased risk of adverse effects.

Most pediatric poisonings:

Involve toddlers or preschoolers
Are unintentional
Occur in or around the home
Involve a single substance
Involve small amounts ingested
Have no significant untoward effects

The general concept of the "one pill" rule states that a single adult therapeutic dose would not be expected to produce significant toxicity in a child. As a result, it is believed commonly that ingestion of one or two tablets by a toddler is a benign act and is not expected to produce toxicity of any significance. This is true for most agents; however, a small group of pharmaceutical agents and household products can create life-threatening effects when ingested in small quantities. A "sip or pill can kill," is a category of products with the potential to cause life-threatening toxicity or death in a child who is younger than 2 years of age, despite the ingestion of only one or two tablets or sips [3,4]. Approximately 24 agents have the potential to be fatal to individuals with small

Table 3
Pharmaceutical and non-pharmaceutical agents most frequently involved in pediatric exposures under age 6 years

Pharmaceutical agents	Percentage of exposures	Non-pharmaceutical agents	Percentages of exposures
Analgesics	7.8%	Cosmetics and personal care products	13.4%
Topicals	7.4%	Cleaning substances	9.7%
Cough and cold preparations	5.5%	Foreign bodies	7.4%
Vitamins	3.6%	Plants	4.6%
Antimicrobials	2.8%	Pesticides	4.1%
Antihistamines	2.6%	Art/crafts/office supplies	2.5%
Gastrointestinal preparations	2.4%		

Data from Watson WA, Litovitz TL, Klein-Schwartz W, et al. 2003 Annual Report of the American Association of Poison Control Centers Toxic Exposure Surveillance System. Am J Emerg Med 2004;22:335–404.

body mass. Nine of the most commonly ingested agents within this category are: calcium channel antagonists, camphor, clonidine and the imidazolines, cyclic antidepressants, opioids and opiates, Lomotil, salicylates, sulfonylureas, and toxic alcohols (methanol, ethylene glycol, and isopropanol) [3].

People of all ages are vulnerable to iatrogenic poisonings, environmental toxins, inadvertent ingestion of poisonous substances not stored in their proper containers, and idiosyncratic reactions to any pharmacologic substance. There are some age-related physiologic and behavioral factors that may predispose certain age groups to poison exposures; as a result, toddlers and adolescents have a high incidence of exposure to toxic substances.

Ingestions by children younger than 5 years of years, especially those aged 2 years and younger, typically involve unintentional behavior on the part of the child or caregiver. Normal developmental characteristics of the toddler increase the likelihood of ingestions in this age group. Toddlers are newly mobile, curious, and anxious to explore their environment through reaching, climbing, and tasting. Children may be attracted to potentially toxic substances based on color or appearance of the substance or the container, and mistakenly identify it as a candy or a beverage. Most agents are nontoxic because the intent is exploration rather than self-harm. Three prominent things typically put children at risk for toxic exposure: improper storage of substances in the home, children spending more time in other people's homes, and caregiver distraction [4]. Other factors that put children at risk include a chaotic or stressful home environment, an unemployed or single parent household, accessibility to toxic agents, lack of proper supervision, and desire to imitate adult behavior. In addition, as children develop greater mobility, there is a tendency for adults to misjudge the child's capabilities.

Several behavioral characteristics which are associated with adolescents differentiate their ingestions from those in younger children. Most adolescent ingestions occur in the home and are intentional rather than accidental. Adolescent ingestions frequently involve multiple substances; are a result of suicide attempts or substance abuse; and commonly involve a time delay between the actual ingestion and the seeking of medical attention, which associates them with worse outcomes. In addition, new and unfamiliar substances are being used for recreational purposes without any knowledge of their potential harmful effects. Therefore, it is important for the health care provider to be knowledgeable about the traditional causes of poisoning, new poisons and fads, and the new evidence for treating these pediatric poisonings [5].

New substances have emerged that have resulted in significant poisoning morbidity and mortality in the pediatric population. The new substances that are being abused by adolescents are producing acute and chronic toxicities. Some examples of these newer "club drugs" include "ecstasy," a designer amphetamine; gamma hydroxybutyrate; and ketamine, all of which have resulted in numerous deaths over the past 5 years. Over-the-counter medications, particularly those containing dextromethorphan (known as "dex"), have become popular recreational drugs among adolescents and have been responsible for at least five deaths [6].

Assessment and management

When a toxic ingestion is suspected, initial treatment is focused on stabilizing the patient's condition. The initial management concentrates on assessment and stabilization of airway, breathing, and circulation, the ABCs, which always are the priorities of resuscitation. The poisoned patient often presents in an acute-onset emergency and exhibits a broad range of multi-organ system pathophysiology. Attention should be given to the potentially urgent or emergent

Table 4
Toxidromes

Toxidrome	Symptoms	Causative agent
Sympathiomimetic (stimulant)	Restlessness Excessive speech and motor activity Tremor Insomnia Tachycardia Hyperthermia Mydriasis Hallucinations	Amphetamines Phencyclidine (PCP) Cocaine Other stimulants
Theophylline (specific sympathio-metic)	Tachycardia Hypotension Cardiac dysrhythmias Tachypnea Agitation Seizures Vomiting with epigastric pain	Theophylline
Sedative/hypnotic	Sedation Confusion Delirium Hallucinations Coma Paresthesia Diplopia Blurred vision Slurred speech Ataxia Nystagmus	Barbiturates Benzodiazepines
Opiate	Altered mental status Miosis Unresponsiveness Shallow respiration Bradypnea Bradycardia Hypotension Decreased bowel sounds Hypothermia	All narcotic agents Heroin Clonidine
Anticholinergic: (mnemonic) **Hot as a hare** **Dry as a bone** **Red as a beet** **Mad as a hatter** **Blind as a bat**	Fever Flushing Tachycardia Urinary retention Dry skin Blurred vision Mydriasis Decreased bowel sounds Ileus Myoclonus Psychosis Hallucinations Seizures Coma	Some mushrooms Cyclic antidepressants Antihistamines Atropinics Over-the-counter sleep preparations

Table 4 (*continued*)

Toxidrome	Symptoms	Causative agent
Cholinergic: (mnemonic) **SLUDGE**	**S**alivation **L**acrimation **U**rination **D**efecation **G**astrointestinal distress (diarrhea) **E**mesis Bradycardia	Organophosphates Insecticides Some mushrooms Severe black widow spider bites

concerns that are related to the stability and adequacy of the respiratory system and circulatory systems, when indicated. Supportive care, when indicated, particularly cardiorespiratory support, remains the mainstay of management in the poisoned patient. Supportive care includes airway monitoring, maintenance of normal oxygenation and ventilation, sustaining normothermia, correction of any hypotension or hypertension, correction of acid-base or electrolyte disturbances, EKG monitoring and recognition of dysrhythmias, identifying skin blistering and rhabdomyolysis, and keeping aware of current medical problems and medications.

In cases of poisoning, the letters D and E can extend the initial stabilization mnemonic to include Disability, Drugs, Decontamination, and ECG and exposure [7]. These are an important focus in the assessment and management of toxic exposures. A bedside assessment of serum glucose is indicated for any patient who presents with altered mental status or lethargy and for any patient who was exposed to agents that might cause hypoglycemia (eg, sulfonylureas) [2]. Hypoglycemia is one of the most easily detected and treatable untoward effects secondary to toxic exposures. ECG is a valuable tool in diagnosing cardiac effects that most commonly occur with agents, such as calcium channel blockers, tricyclic antidepressants, and antidysrhythmics.

After the ABCDEs have been addressed, the physical examination should focus on reassessment of vital signs and vital system functions. The clinical examination needs to be geared toward the central and autonomic nervous system; findings involving the eye and skin, oral, and gastrointestinal mucosa; and odors. These areas are the most likely to be affected in toxic syndromes. The secondary phase of evaluation and detoxification provides identification of clinical signs and symptoms that can help in the identification of the toxin, and possible initiation of appropriate treatment or antidote. The clinical syndromes, called toxidromes, make up a constellation of signs and symptoms that suggest a specific class of poisoning [8]. Toxidromes integrate initial vital signs, mental status changes, symptoms, clinical findings, and laboratory results to help identify the category of toxin. Correlation of clinical findings with the toxidrome category allows for incorporation of the toxidrome into clinical plans, and enables appropriate treatment to be initiated in a timely manner. The most common toxidromes are those for the sympathomimetic, theophylline, sedative/hypnotic, opiate, anticholinergic, and cholinergic agents (Table 4).

The goal of identification is to determine which patients are at risk for toxic effects. Bear in mind that approximately 40% of children who present with poisoning have not been exposed dangerously to the suspected toxin [9]. Therefore, it is imperative to look for clinical indicators of poisonous ingestion while providing supportive care, but before initiating antidote-type treatment. For most patients, the clinical condition, rather than the specific ingredients of the ingestion, directs the management. This approach does not preclude treating specific toxins or toxidromes, but rather reinforces the concept of basic clinical management and resuscitation techniques.

A thorough history needs to be obtained whenever there is suspicion of toxic exposure. This includes type and amount of ingestion (if known); the possibility of multiple agents; the time of ingestion; time of presentation; any history of vomiting, choking, coughing, or alteration in mental status; and any interventions performed before presentation at the medical facility. If suspected products or their containers are available, they should be brought with the child to the health care facility. In addition, past and current medical history should be ascertained as well as obtaining the profile of any medications that are taken on a regular basis. A complete physical examination and reassessment of the child needs to be performed, after stabilization of the ABCs.

Laboratory testing

After appropriate stabilization of the poisoned child occurs, the necessity for laboratory testing can be evaluated and tests can be ordered. The initial laboratory tests that are most beneficial are basic assessments that are not indicated uniquely for the poisoned patient [10]. Regardless of the substances that are believed be ingested by a child or adolescent, serum or urine toxicology screens may be necessary to rule out the possibility of additional unknown agents, as an adjunct modality in a child with an unknown diagnosis, or to confirm a toxic exposure

where abuse or neglect may be involved [5]. Recent studies that evaluated the usefulness of toxicology screening tests in pediatric patients concluded that it is costly and that indiscriminant use of toxicology screens does not impact the acute management of patients. Laboratory testing can be useful in a variety of settings to help confirm toxicologic diagnosis, guide decision making regarding specific management interventions, and confirm drug exposure. Appropriate laboratory studies include basic serum chemistry studies in symptomatic patients, confirmation of suspected toxins, and the determination for the need of specific antidotal therapy. The usefulness of antidotes is limited to a small sampling of drugs (Table 5). Serum chemistry tests that supply or enable the calculation of anion gap and blood gas analysis may be used in poisonings of unknown agents or in poisonings associated with substances that are known to cause a high anion gap metabolic acidosis. The differential diagnosis for an anion gap metabolic acidosis can be remembered easily using the mnemonic "MUDPILES," which stands for: methanol,

Table 5
Antidotes to common poisons

Poison	Antidote
Acetaminophen (Tylenol)	NAC (N-acetylcysteine)
Anticholinergics	Physostigmine
Anticoagulants	Vitamin K1, protamine
Benzodiazepines	Supportive care, flumazenil[a]
Botulism	Botulinum antitoxin, BIG (Botulism immune globulin)
Beta blockers	Glucagon
Calcium channel blockers	Calcium, glucagon
Cholinergics	Atropine, pralidoxime in organophosphate overdose
Carbon monoxide	Oxygen, hyperbaric oxygen
Cyanide	Amyl nitrate, sodium nitrate, sodium thiosulfate
Digoxin	Digoxin fab antibodies (Digibind)
Iron	Deferoxamine
Isoniazid	Pyridoxine
Lead	British antilewisite (Dimeracrol), edetate calcium disodium, 3-dimercaptosuccinic acid
Methemoglobinemia	Methylene blue
Opioids	Naloxone (Narcan)
Sulfonylureas (oral hypoglycemics)	Dextrose, octreotide
Toxic alcohols	Ethanol infusion, dialysis
Tricyclic antidepressants	Sodium bicarbonate

[a] Flumazenil may precipitate seizures when used with patients who are chronic benzodiazepine users or in situations, including tricyclic antidepressant overdose.

uremia, diabetic ketoacidosis, paraldehyde, iron/iso-niazid, lactic acidosis, ethylene glycol, and salicylates. Toxicologic analysis in children is most valuable in identifying serum drug levels [11]. For many poisons, the clinical effects and their toxicities correlate with the serum level of the drug. Management often is guided by the data provided by quantitative assays in these cases.

Toxicology screening is a term that typically is used to indicate laboratory detection of several commonly abused drugs or their metabolites, including amphetamines, barbiturates, benzodiazepines, cocaine, marijuana, opioids, and phencyclidine (PCP), to name a few. The toxicology screening assay only reflects the presence or absence of drugs or metabolites at or above a threshold concentration at the time the specimen is collected. It does not exclude the presence of drug or metabolite, only that the substance was not present at the minimal threshold quantity. Routine screening for drugs of abuse have been demonstrated to be unhelpful in the management of poisoned patients [10]. Suicide attempts require evaluation for unreported agents, including salicylates and acetaminophen, because of the widespread availability of these agents and the fact that most adolescents with suicidal intent are unreliable as historians. The use of specific therapies and techniques, such as antidotes and enhanced elimination techniques, are limited to cases where the expectation that a defined benefit outweighs the risk of the procedure is reasonable. There are limited data and information to distinguish lethal concentrations of certain drugs and toxic substances in children. Therefore, indications for the use of interventions in children usually are different from those in adults.

When the name or the amount of a poison ingested is unknown, the incident is not witnessed, or the history is vague, the child is treated aggressively as though a harmful substance was consumed. If ingestion has occurred, the dose potentially ingested should be calculated, assuming a worse case scenario—the maximal dose which could have been ingested [7]. When there is incomplete or inaccurate information about the toxic exposure, the physical examination, laboratory tests, and potentially a toxicologic screen, can be helpful in guiding management. If elements of the history provided are contradictory or questionable, it is especially important to rule out the possibility of trauma as a cause of the patient's clinical condition. Physical assessment focuses on the potential for unreported traumatic injuries, as well as significant details related to the ingestion and clinical presentation that suggests a toxidrome. The local poison control center or hospital pharmacist, if available, can provide details regarding the indications and guidelines for use of antidotes. Further management is guided by the principles of stabilization, diagnosis, and treatment simultaneously. If the substance is identified correctly, the management can be modified to specifically concentrate treatment for that specific toxin.

Gastrointestinal decontamination

Reducing the life-threatening potential of an ingested substance is an early management goal, and depends upon the effectiveness of several different treatment modalities. Further management focuses on removing the toxin physically from the body or decreasing the toxin's absorption availability. This is achieved by way of several methods, including gastrointestinal decontamination, altering metabolism to limit the production of toxic metabolites, increasing elimination of the ingested substance, administering a specific antidote, or implementing other suitable therapy in conjunction with continued supportive care. Four options are available for gastrointestinal decontamination: syrup of ipecac, gastric lavage, single or multiple dose activated charcoal, and whole bowel irrigation. Gastrointestinal decontamination, a well-established toxicology method for asymptomatic patients recently has fallen out of favor. Thereby, gastric lavage and syrup of ipecac, two long-standing treatments for poisonings recently have experienced a diminishing role in the management of acute poisonings, whereas newer antidotes are emerging [6,7,12]. Treatment recommendations continue to evolve because the preferred modality for gastric decontamination in the pediatric patient changes frequently.

There is no single preferred strategy for gastric decontamination in pediatric poisonings. If used at all, the decision regarding which gastric decontamination technique to use is largely dependent upon clinical status. Studies that investigated asymptomatic children showed no evidence of improved outcome following ingestion. Decontamination has been suggested to be beneficial for the asymptomatic child with a theoretical risk for significant toxicity [4]. If the pediatric patient has ingested a potentially life-threatening amount of a toxin and decontamination can be instituted promptly, gastric lavage, activated charcoal, or whole bowel irrigation may be considered because the benefits outweigh the risks involved. An individualized approach, based on the timing of ingestion, type of substance, and amount of the ingested substance, in conjunction with the clinical status, dictates treatment choices.

Historically, gastric emptying has been performed when a benefit is anticipated and one of the following conditions exist: the substance is not adsorbed by activated charcoal, the tablets are too large to be removed by gastric lavage, the window of opportunity to use activated charcoal is delayed or missed, or the child presents within 1 hour of ingestion without significant central nervous system symptoms. Unless dealing with a known anticholinergic overdose, gastric emptying has limited benefit if attempted more than 1 hour after ingestion, because most other toxins will have been absorbed or are no longer present in the stomach. Gastric-emptying methods include syrup of ipecac for forced emesis and gastric lavage.

Syrup of ipecac has been used in the home for forced emesis for more than 50 years. It has been the only recommended method of inducing emesis. Ipecac acts as a local gastric irritant and a central stimulant which triggers the vomiting center and results in emesis. Dosages of 10 mL for infants older than 6 months, 15 mL for children 1 to 12 years, and 30 mL for children older than 12 years usually produce emesis in 20 minutes. The amount of substance removed from the stomach is related inversely to the length of time from ingestion of the syrup of ipecac to emesis; however, research has demonstrated that even when ipecac is administered immediately after the ingestion of a toxic agent; it does not remove it completely from the stomach [13]. The results of several studies on the efficacy of syrup of ipecac have challenged the usefulness of this treatment for poisoning and the recommendations to keep it stored in the home. Studies suggest that there is no reduction in resource use or improvement in patient outcome from the use of syrup of ipecac at home [12]. The American Academy of Pediatrics (AAP) recommended ending the routine use of syrup of ipecac for unintentional ingestions, and suggested that health care providers advise parents to discard any ipecac kept for home use [13]. In addition, the removal of syrup of ipecac from the home environment will make it less readily available and potentially decrease the likelihood of intentional misuse of this emetic. Examples of people who abuse syrup of ipecac include adolescents with eating disorders and caregivers who are involved with Munchausen's syndrome by proxy [13]. Poison control centers have stopped recommending the routine use of syrup of ipecac in the home. It also is no longer favored in the clinical setting because its protracted vomiting effects are known to cause significant delay in the administration of activated charcoal.

Through the procedure of gastric lavage, the stomach is emptied, and decontamination in the presence of residual toxin within the stomach is augmented. The toxic substance is removed physically from the stomach by way of irrigation through a large-bore naso- or orogastric tube using room temperature fluids until the yield is clear. The large tube size that is required for effective lavage may not be possible to use in pediatric patients. Gastric lavage may not be an effective strategy in smaller children because pill fragments rarely can be removed with pediatric-sized gastric tubes. Because of its girth, the larger bore tubes only can be placed in the adolescent patient. To minimize the hazards of potential vomiting and aspiration, tracheal intubation must precede gastric lavage in patients whose gag reflex is diminished and whose ability to protect the airway is compromised.

Controversy surrounding the efficacy of gastric lavage exists in several studies; the use of gastric emptying in patients without life-threatening toxicity had no impact on patient outcome [7]. Although gastric lavage is no longer considered to be the routine standard of care in pediatric patients, it may play a role in selected situations. Therefore, gastric emptying should be considered for children in whom life-threatening toxic effects are exhibited or are expected, based on the history of the exposure or the clinical manifestation of untoward effects. Gastric lavage may be useful if the amount of toxin ingested is large, the substance is known to delay gastric emptying (barbiturates, anticholinergic drugs) or has been ingested within 1 to 2 hours of presentation, the substance may form a concretion, sustained release and insoluble compounds have been ingested, or if the agent is particularly toxic [4,14,15]. Gastric lavage is absolutely contraindicated with caustic and hydrocarbon ingestions.

There is increasing evidence that combination therapy of gastric emptying with gastric lavage, followed by the administration of activated charcoal, does not provide a clinical benefit [14]. Because complications associated with the two-step approach to decontamination are associated with a higher rate of intubation, aspiration, and ICU admission, gastric emptying, in addition to activated charcoal, cannot be considered the routine approach to patients. In most cases, the use of activated charcoal alone as a means of gastric decontamination is best. Activated charcoal reduces absorption of a toxin by the body by binding directly to toxins anywhere it comes in contact within the gastrointestinal tract. Most ingested toxins will adsorb to the activated charcoal, but it is ineffective with alcohols and glycols, hydrocarbons, caustics, heavy metals (eg, lead, mercury, lithium, arsenic) and agents with rapid onset. It is best administered by nasal or orogastric tube to small children, who may refuse to drink it because of its taste and gritty texture. It also may be administered as a flavored slurry. The addition of cola, chocolate milk, or cherry-flavored syrup improves the palatability and the ease of swallowing [4]. If the amount of ingested drug is known, a total charcoal dose determined by a (charcoal: ingestant) ratio of 10 g:1 g should be administered. This activated charcoal:drug ratio has been found to demonstrate optimal adherence of the toxin [14]. The total volume of fluid required to achieve this dose may necessitate that it be split into smaller aliquots (15–25 g in 75–120 mL) given every 1 to 2 hours. This multiple dosing regimen of activated charcoal also may provide increased efficacy in preventing absorption of sustained-release dosage form ingestions.

When the amount of the substance is unknown, a dose of activated charcoal of 1 g/kg is recommended. Commercial preparations of 15 g/75 mL, 25 g/120 mL, or 50 g/240 mL of activated charcoal are readily available. Administration of the entire premixed preparation which most closely approximates the child's weight is reasonable and often meets or exceeds the recommended 1 g/kg dose. At this time, the AAP does not support the routine administration of activated charcoal in the home because efficacy and safety have not been demonstrated [13].

Ideally, activated charcoal is administered within 1 hour of the ingestion because this is when the greatest benefit can be achieved. There are insufficient data to support or exclude its use 1 hour after ingestion [4]. The dose of activated charcoal is most effective in children when combined with a cathartic, such as sorbitol. Once bound to the charcoal, sorbitol propels the toxin rapidly through the intestinal tract, and decreases the transit time in the intestine. Coadministration with a laxative agent also prevents the charcoal from forming a concretion, especially when multiple dose activated charcoal is used. The presence of bowel sounds must be verified before administering charcoal. Charcoal is contraindicated in a patient with absent bowel sounds because it may indicate ileus or obstruction. Charcoal administration usually is followed by periods of vomiting, especially when its administration has been preceded by ipecac or when given with a large volume laxative, such as citrate of magnesia. The potential hazards of vomiting and aspiration are significant for patients who have a diminished ability to protect the airway, and intubation is indicated before administration of charcoal.

Whole bowel irrigation is a newer modality of gastric decontamination. It has the greatest usefulness for ingestions that involve sustained released, enteric-coated, or modified release preparations that have delayed or lengthened absorption. It also may be the preferred route of decontamination with patients who ingest drug-filled packets and substances that are not adsorbed to activated charcoal, especially heavy metals [4]. Whole bowel irrigation also enhances passage of whole pill fragments that have passed beyond the pylorus. Whole bowel irrigation has been shown to be effective when initiated within 4 hours after ingestion of enteric-coated preparations [4]. A polyethylene glycol–based isotonic electrolyte solution (GoLYTELY or CoLyte) will hasten evacuation of substances from the gastrointestinal tract without creating fluid and electrolyte shifts. The irrigating solution can be instilled orally or by way of a nasogastric tube at a rate of 500 mL/h for children up to 6 years of age, a rate of 1000 mL/h for children aged 6 to 12 years, and a rate of 1.5 to 2 L/h for children older than 12 years of age until the rectal effluent is clear [7]. The dose-limiting side effect of whole bowel irrigation includes gastrointestinal bloating and vomiting. These effects can be minimized by using slower rates of instillation and the adjunct use of antiemetics. Electrolyte abnormalities and fluid shifts have not been reported, and the bowel can be evacuated within 4 to 6 hours of initiation of therapy [4,7] Whole bowel irrigation is contraindicated with bowel obstruction, perforation, or ileus.

Enhanced elimination

In certain circumstances, efforts to adsorb and increase the enteric or renal excretion of a drug may improve patient outcomes. Two methods that can improve recovery are multiple dosing of activated charcoal and urinary alkalization. Multiple-dose activated charcoal (MDAC) has been shown to enhance elimination of certain agents. This is separate from its role of preventing absorption of the toxic agent through adsorption. Doses of activated charcoal are administered every 4 to 6 hours without cathartics, to avoid severe diarrhea, fluid shifts, and electrolyte abnormalities that could result in complications, such as hypernatremia and seizures. Repeated dosing was shown to enhance elimination by binding to toxins undergoing enterohepatic recirculation and preventing further absorption of the ingested drug; this results in an accelerated rate of drug clearance. In addition, MDAC continues adsorbing after the initial absorption or by way of the gastrointestinal dialysis effect by adsorbing toxins that are secreted across the gastric membrane into the bowel lumen [7]. This is well-described for theophylline, phenobarbital, salicylates, carbamazepine, and phenytoin. Drugs in a bound state adsorbed to activated charcoal are nontoxic. A dose of 0.5 to 1 g/kg every 1 to 4 hours in severe toxicities (especially theophylline SR) to 0.5 g/kg every 4 to 6 hours for less severe toxicities is recommended. Multiple doses should be administered only in patients who have an intact gag reflex or a protected airway, and with no evidence of ileus or mechanical bowel obstruction.

Excretion of a toxin by way of the renal system depends upon the ability of the drug to be trapped in the urine, and subsequently be eliminated by the body. Many toxic compounds that are excreted renally are weak bases or acids, and therefore, are dependent on the pH of the urine for ionization. Alkalinization of the urine to a pH of greater than 7.5 is effective in producing the ion-trapping mechanism. Ionized drugs are not reabsorbed and can be excreted. Enhanced elimination of a toxin is achieved with forced diuresis in association with alkalinization of the urine. It was found to be beneficial in the enhanced elimination of salicylates and phenobarbital. This method can be used when the child has a potentially life-threatening amount of drug, is hemodynamically stable, and has normal renal function and no evidence of cerebral or pulmonary edema. The goal is to keep the urinary pH greater than 7.5 [4]. This can be achieved by providing a continuous intravenous infusion of sodium bicarbonate combined with potassium chloride; levels are monitored by way of clinical and laboratory assessment. Potassium must be added to the intravenous fluid in an effort to prevent hypokalemia. Hypokalemia results in hydrogen ions being released to reabsorb potassium ions, and thereby, prevents alkalinization.

Summary

Pediatric poisonings account for a significant morbidity and use of health care resources each year in the United States. The treatment of children who have ingested substances, accidentally or intentionally, is a challenge to emergency and critical care providers. Being aware of the new recommendations and the constant development of new products and pharmaceutical agents makes this challenge especially difficult. An understanding of toxidromes and gastrointestinal decontamination techniques will help to improve the care that the pediatric patient receives. The early presentation and management of pediatric poisonings will help to improve patient outcomes and

decrease the incidence of preventable acute or permanent organ injury. The early recognition and differentiation of the pediatric patient who requires supportive care from the patient who requires further interventions is crucial and must be done on an individual basis. Appropriate supportive care entails the monitoring of vital signs and level of consciousness, airway control, ventilation and circulatory support, maintenance of normothermia, urine output, and acid–base balance. After these issues are addressed, further management that is directed at gastrointestinal decontamination and treatment with specific antidotes will complete the care. The primary goal is to discern which children are at clinical risk and treat them aggressively when appropriate, while minimizing medical interventions for the rest.

Acknowledgments

The author thanks Christine Jaderlund, Pharm.D for her invaluable help in the preparation of this manuscript.

References

[1] Watson WA, Litovitz TL, Klein-Schwartz W, et al. 2003 Annual Report of the American Association of Poison Control Centers Toxic Exposure Surveillance System. Am J Emerg Med 2004;22(5):335–404.

[2] Hoffman RJ, Osterhoudt KC. Evaluation and management of pediatric poisonings. Pediatr Case Rev 2002; 2(1):51–63.

[3] Michael JB, Sztajnkrycer MD. Deadly pediatric poisons: nine common agents that kill at low doses. Emerg Med Clin N Am 2004;22:1019–50.

[4] Bryant S, Singer J. Management of toxic exposure in children. Emerg Med Clin N Am 2003;21(1):101–19.

[5] Liebelt E. Pediatric poisonings in the new millennium: new poisons, new insights, new evidence. Curr Opin Pediatr 2001;13(2):155–6.

[6] University of Alabama. Clinical toxicology consultation service. Available at: http://www.health.uab.edu/4Docs/show.asp?durki. Accessed January 4, 2005.

[7] Abbruzzi G, Stork CM. Pediatric toxicologic concerns. Emerg Med Clin N Am 2002;20(1):223–47.

[8] Aks SE. Toxidromes. Available at: http://www.toxicon.er.uic.edu/toxidro.htm. Accessed January 10, 2005.

[9] Hwang CF. The utility of the history and clinical signs of poisoning in childhood: a prospective study. Ther Drug Monit 2003;25(6):728–34.

[10] Hoffman RJ, Nelson L. Rational use of toxicology testing in children. Curr Opin Pediatr 2001;13:183–8.

[11] Belson MG, Simon HK, Sullivan K, et al. The utility

of toxicological analysis in children with suspected ingestions. Pediatr Emerg Care 1999;15:383–7.

[12] Bond GR. Home syrup of ipecac use does not reduce emergency department use or improve outcome. Pediatrics 2003;112(5):1061–4.

[13] American Academy of Pediatrics Policy Statement. Poison treatment in the home. Pediatrics 2003;112(5): 1182–5.

[14] Bond GR. The role of activated charcoal and gastric emptying in gastrointestinal decontamination: a state of the art review. Ann Emerg Med 2002;39(3): 273–86.

[15] Liebelt EL, DeAngelis CD. Evolving trends and treatment advances in pediatric poisonings. JAMA 1999; 282:1113–5.

ELSEVIER
SAUNDERS

Crit Care Nurs Clin N Am 17 (2005) 405–416

CRITICAL CARE
NURSING CLINICS
OF NORTH AMERICA

Management of the Pediatric Postoperative Cardiac Surgery Patient

Dorothy M. Beke, RN, MS, CPNP*, Nancy J. Braudis, RN, MS, CPNP,
Patricia Lincoln, RN, MS

Cardiac Intensive Care Unit, Children's Hospital, 300 Longwood Avenue, Boston, MA 02115, USA

Optimal management of the postoperative pediatric cardiac surgical patient requires a thorough understanding of patient anatomy, physiology, surgical repair or palliation, and clinical condition. This necessitates a dedicated team of clinicians including skilled nurses, physicians, and respiratory therapists specialized in the care of patients who have complex congenital heart disease. Intraoperative events associated with cardiopulmonary bypass (CPB), surgical procedure, anesthesia, and medications have the potential to produce multisystemic effects. Postoperative care focuses on anticipating potentially deleterious events and instituting a proactive approach in managing patients. Intervention strategies are directed at preventing low cardiac output and avoiding adverse sequelae in major organ systems. Invasive hemodynamic monitoring, laboratory analysis, and clinical examination provide essential assessment information for effective management of the postoperative patient.

A comprehensive intraoperative report provides the necessary information for appropriate postoperative management and describes patient diagnosis, pathophysiology, surgical procedure, and intraoperative events. Details include time on CPB, duration of hypothermic arrest, aortic cross-clamp time, complications, hemodynamic status, and presence of invasive catheters, drains, and pacing wires. Immediate perioperative evaluation entails a clinical examination; assessment of vital signs and hemodynamic parameters; ECG analysis; assessment of arterial blood gas, hematocrit, electrolytes, and other pertinent laboratory data; and chest radiograph interpretation. Initial and routine chest radiograph assessment focuses on evaluation of endotracheal tube placement; lung fields; intracardiac, central venous, and arterial catheter positions; chest tubes; and drains.

Hemodynamic monitoring

Intravascular catheters are placed intraoperatively for postoperative hemodynamic monitoring, nontraumatic blood sampling, and the administration of vasoactive infusions, parental nutrition, and volume. Intracardiac catheter placement and function are validated by chest radiograph confirmation (Fig. 1), waveform assessment, and presence of blood return. Morbidity factors associated with catheter use include nonfunction, thrombus, and infection [1]. Left atrial (LA) lines are generally used for pressure monitoring because an air embolism or clot traveling into the coronary or cerebral circulation may be devastating to the patient. Catheters are removed after all desired information is obtained. This information may include right atrial (RA) and pulmonary artery (PA) saturations to evaluate systemic Vo_2 or presence of residual ventricular septal defects, LA tracing to demonstrate certain arrhythmias, and PA pullback

---
* Corresponding author.
  E-mail address: dorothy.beke@childrens.harvard.edu (D.M. Beke).

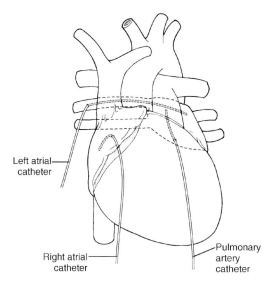

Fig. 1. Intracardiac catheter placement.

Left atrial catheter

Right atrial catheter

Pulmonary artery catheter

pressures to assess for residual obstruction. The most common problem encountered with the removal of these catheters is bleeding, occurring most often with LA and PA catheters [1,2]. Careful evaluation of hematologic status and assessment of hemodynamics, patency of chest tubes, and blood product availability before line removal may minimize complications and associated risks.

Right atrial pressure

Catheters placed directly into the right atrium or other central venous pressure location (such as the internal jugular or superior vena cava) are used to measure systemic venous return to the heart, preload, right ventricular (RV) function, and blood oxygen saturation. These catheters indicate RV end-diastolic pressure if the tricuspid valve is normal. The average normal range of RA pressure and central venous pressure is 1 to 5 mm Hg; however, these pressures may be slightly elevated in the postoperative cardiac patient (6–8 mm Hg) (Box 1) [3,4]. Accurate interpretation of saturations obtained from the RA

Box 1. Causes of elevated or decreased right atrial/central venous pressure

Elevated

Intravascular volume overload
↓ RV function, RV hypertrophy or failure
↑ RV afterload (↑ pulmonary vascular resistance)
Tricuspid valve stenosis, regurgitation, obstruction (thrombus)
Left ventricular to RA shunt
Cardiac tamponade
Arrhythmias
Catheter or transducer placement or malfunction

Decreased

Low intravascular volume
Inadequate preload
Systemic vasodilation
Catheter or transducer placement or malfunction

Data from Roth SJ. Postoperative care. In: Chang AC, Hanley FL, Wernovsky G, et al, editors. Pediatric cardiac intensive care. Philadelphia: Lippincott, Williams, and Wilkins; 1998. p. 169.

Box 2. Causes of elevated or decreased right atrial saturation

Elevated

LA to RA shunt
Anomalous pulmonary venous return
↑ O_2 delivery
↓ O_2 extraction
Catheter tip location (by renal veins)

Decreased

↑ O_2 extraction (low cardiac output)
↓ Arterial O_2 saturation with normal atrioventricular O_2 difference (single ventricle physiology)
Catheter tip location (by coronary sinus)

Data from Roth SJ. Postoperative care. In: Chang AC, Hanley FL, Wernovsky G, et al, editors. Pediatric cardiac intensive care. Philadelphia: Lippincott, Williams, and Wilkins; 1998. p. 171.

catheter is dependent on confirmation of catheter tip placement and patient anatomy (Box 2).

Left atrial pressure

LA pressure (LAP) is usually measured by a catheter threaded either across the right superior pulmonary vein or through the LA appendage into the left atrium. Normal LAP is typically 1 to 2 mm Hg greater than RA pressure; however, in the postoperative pediatric patient, a LAP less than 12 to 14 mm Hg is generally tolerated [3,4]. LAP monitoring provides information related to pulmonary venous pressure and left heart preload and function. LAP reflects left ventricular end-diastolic pressure in the absence of mitral valve pathology (Box 3). The normal oxygen saturation of LA blood is 100% [5]. Conditions

---

Box 3. Causes of elevated or decreased left atrial pressure

Elevated

↑ Left ventricular end-diastolic pressure
↓ Left ventricular function, left ventricular hypertrophy or failure
↑ Left ventricular afterload
Mitral valve stenosis, regurgitation, obstruction (thrombus)
Large right to left shunt
Intravascular volume overload
Cardiac tamponade
Tachyarrhythmias
Catheter or transducer placement or malfunction

Decreased

↓ Intravascular fluid status
Inadequate preload
Catheter or transducer placement or malfunction

Data from Roth SJ. Postoperative care. In: Chang AC, Hanley FL, Wernovsky G, et al, editors. Pediatric cardiac intensive care. Philadelphia: Lippincott, Williams, and Wilkins; 1998. p. 168.

Box 4. Causes of elevated or decreased pulmonary artery pressure

Elevated

Obstruction of the pulmonary circulation: anatomic defect, pulmonary embolus
Primary pulmonary hypertension
Pulmonary vascular obstructive disease
Inflammatory response to CPB
Mechanical obstruction of the airway: atelectasis, mechanical ventilation, effusion, pneumothorax
Reactive airway
Lung hypoplasia
Alveolar hypoplasia
Acidosis
Blood hyperviscosity
↑ LAP
Large left to right shunts
Persistent pulmonary hypertension of the newborn
Catheter or transducer placement or malfunction

Decreased

↓ Intravascular volume
Obstruction to pulmonary blood flow
↓ Cardiac output
Catheter or transducer placement or malfunction

Data from Roth SJ. Postoperative care. In: Chang AC, Hanley FL, Wernovsky G, et al, editors. Pediatric cardiac intensive care. Philadelphia: Lippincott, Williams, and Wilkins; 1998. p. 170.

---

resulting in RA to LA shunting or pulmonary vein desaturation may decrease LA oxygen saturation [3].

Pulmonary artery pressure

PA pressure (PAP) is usually monitored by a catheter threaded through the right ventricle, across the RV outflow tract, and into the main PA. This catheter may continue into the branch PAs. The PAP is monitored in terms of systolic, diastolic, and mean pressures. Mean PAP is normally 10 to 20 mm Hg in the pediatric patient, with an average value of 15 mm Hg [3,4]. In the postoperative cardiac patient, mean PAP may be greater than 15 mm Hg; however, it should be less than 25 mm Hg [5]. In comparison to arterial blood pressure, PAP usually measures approximately one fourth to one third of systemic blood pressure. Under usual circumstances, the systolic PAP is the equivalent of the RV systolic pressure, whereas the diastolic PAP is consistent with the LAP in the absence of pulmonary hypertension or mitral valve disease (Box 4). Oxygen saturation obtained in the PAs is usually less than 80% [5]. Values greater than this often indicate a significant left to right intracardiac shunt.

Cardiac output

Cardiac output is the amount of blood ejected from the ventricle into the systemic circulation. It is a function of heart rate multiplied by ventricular stroke volume. Stroke volume is impacted by preload, afterload, and contractility. Cardiac output is measured in terms of cardiac index, which is expressed as a fraction of body surface area (liters per minute per square meter) [3]. In comparison to an adult, cardiac output in the neonate is heart rate dependent and related to the neonatal myocardium's reduced diastolic compliance and decreased ability to increase stroke volume [6]. Frequent assessment of cardiac output is accomplished by monitoring heart rate, blood pressure, intracardiac filling pressures, peripheral perfusion, temperature, acid-base balance, systemic VO_2, and urine output.

Preload

Preload is the volume of blood in the ventricle during diastole and reflects circulating intravascular volume. Excessive fluid loss or insufficient volume replacement may decrease preload and may occur with postoperative bleeding, vasodilation with rewarming, and third spacing of fluids related to a systemic vascular response following CPB or diuresis [5]. Correction of abnormal coagulation factors may be accomplished with fresh-frozen plasma or cryoprecipitate, and active bleeding or decreased hematocrit is treated with packed red blood cells. Hypovolemia, unrelated to bleeding, may be managed with colloid or crystalloid fluid replacement. Fluid boluses are administered in conjunction with assessment of filling pressures, arterial pressure, liver distention, peripheral edema, and fontanel fullness.

Afterload

Afterload is resistance to ventricular ejection. Increases in pulmonary vascular resistance (PVR) or systemic vascular resistance (SVR) may be triggered by hypoxia, acidosis, hypothermia, or pain. SVR may increase as a compensatory mechanism of a low cardiac output state. Residual RV or left ventricular outflow tract obstruction also increases resistance. Elevated PVR may be associated with acute or chronic conditions. Newborns have extremely reactive pulmonary vasculature and are more susceptible to increased PVR. Treatment of increased afterload involves avoiding known etiologies and eliminating predisposing factors. Strategies include mechanical ventilatory manipulation to decrease PVR and administering vasodilating agents to decrease SVR.

Heart rate and contractility

Heart rate varies with patient age and size. Any abnormal heart rate or cardiac rhythm may potentially affect cardiac output. In the neonate, tachycardia up to 200 beats per minute is generally tolerated in an effort to increase cardiac output [7]. In the older child, increased heart rate may decrease cardiac output due to limited ventricular filling. Myocardial dysfunction or impaired contractility may impact cardiac output. Symptoms include decreased perfusion with increased filling pressures. Chronic impairment may result from preoperative pressure or volume overload in relation to a specific cardiac defect. Drugs, anesthesia, ischemia, acidosis, hypoxia, extensive ventriculotomy, myocardial resection, tamponade, or residual hemodynamic anomalies also depress contractility [7]. Except in cases of cardiac tamponade, treatment focuses on support of contractility with inotropic agents and afterload reduction.

Altered hemostasis in the postoperative period results from surgical trauma, dilution of clotting factors, inadequate heparin reversal, or destruction of platelets and blood products post CPB. Management involves replacement of blood products, avoiding hypertension, and correcting the underlying cause of bleeding. Chest tube drainage greater than 3 mL/kg/h for over 3 hours or greater than 5 mL/kg in an hour is cause for concern. Assuring patency of chest tube drains facilitates evacuation of blood and chest cavity fluids. Significant blood loss may necessitate surgical intervention.

Any abrupt cessation of chest tube output accompanied by tachycardia and increased filling pressures may be indicative of cardiac tamponade. Tamponade produces compression of the cardiac chambers, restricting venous return to the heart and limiting contractility. Narrowed pulse pressure and hypotension unresponsive to volume administration may occur. Prompt intervention including vigorous milking of chest tubes or chest exploration may be necessary to stabilize hemodynamics and achieve hemostasis.

Low cardiac output

Alterations in cardiac output are common during the postoperative phase. Potential sources of low cardiac output include (1) residual cardiac lesion; (2) myocardial ischemia secondary to circulatory arrest, hypothermia, aortic cross-clamp time, or reperfusion injury; (3) insufficient, intraoperative myocardial protection and cardioplegia; (4) inflammatory response triggered by CPB; (5) changes in SVR and PVR; (6) arrhythmias; (7) cardiac tamponade; and (8) ventriculotomy [7–9]. Echocardiography or cardiac catheterization may be warranted for further exploration of potential causes of low cardiac output. Low cardiac output syndrome (LCOS) due to any residual cardiac lesion is unlikely to improve with conventional medical management. Cardiac catheterization or surgical intervention may be necessary to correct any identified residual defect.

Measures to assess and treat LCOS are necessary to reduce time on mechanical ventilation, hospital length of stay, and overall mortality and morbidity [10]. Cardiac index may progressively decrease in the perioperative phase and is lowest at approximately 9 to 12 hours following CPB [11]. This progressive decline in cardiac index is usually associated with elevations in SVR and PVR. Anticipation or avoidance of factors contributing to LCOS is paramount to maintaining stability in the postoperative patient. Maintaining adequate preload, administering vasoactive infusions to improve cardiac contractility, and taking measures to reduce SVR and PVR are essential in managing LCOS.

Inotropic support with a dopamine infusion of 5 to 15 μg/kg/min may assist with cardiac contractility and treating hypotension associated with LCOS. After dopamine is titrated beyond 10 to 15 μg/kg/min, epinephrine may be considered as an additional therapy. The potent α_1 and β_1 effects of epinephrine initiated at 0.01 to 0.1 μg/kg/min are indicated in treating severe hypotension [3] (Table 1). The chronotropic effects of epinephrine and high-dose dopamine may be especially useful in treating hypotension in the neonate because cardiac output is heart rate dependent in this population. The catecholamine response produced by inotropic agents predispose the patient to arrhythmias and increased ventricular filling, with subsequent strain on diastolic function that may be deleterious to a recovering myocardium [8]. Milrinone, a noncatecholamine phosphodiesterase-inhibiting medication, has combined effects of inotropy and afterload reduction and may be used in combination with other vasoactive therapies in preventing or managing LCOS. A loading dose of 50 μg/kg/min followed by a continuous infusion was found to increase cardiac index in pediatric patients following CPB [12,13]. Hoffman and colleagues [9] reported a 64% relative risk reduction in patients developing LCOS who were placed on high-dose infusions of milrinone (0.75 μg/kg/min). For persistent low cardiac output, afterload-reducing agents such as nitroprusside may be considered after blood pressure has stabilized [8].

Factors that contribute to increased SVR and PVR, such as pain, hypoxia, and acidosis, are avoided. Adjunct therapies may include mechanical ventilation

Table 1
Cardiovascular receptors and receptor response to catecholamine vasoactive agents

Cardiovascular receptors			Receptor response					
Receptor	Location	Activity	Agent	α_1	β_1	β_2	DA$_1$	DA$_2$
α_1	Cardiac myocyte	+Inotropy	Dopamine	0–3+	2+–3+	1+	3+	3+
	Peripheral vasculature	Vasoconstiction	Dobutamine	0–1+	3+	1+	0	0
β_1	Cardiac myocyte	+Inotropy, chronotropy	Epinephrine	3+	3+	3+	0	0
β_2	Peripheral vasculature	Vasodilation	Norepinephrine	3+	3+	1+	0	0
DA$_1$	Peripheral vasculature	Renal vasodilation	Isoproterenol	0	3+	3+	0	0
DA$_2$	Peripheral vasculature	Peripheral vasodilation	Phenylephrine	3+	0–1+	0–1+	0	0

Abbreviations: DA$_1$, dopaminergic receptor type 1; DA$_2$, dopaminergic receptor type 2.
From Roth SJ. Pharmacologic manipulation of the cardiovascular system. Unpublished manuscript, 2002; with permission.

strategies, adequate patient sedation and analgesia, pharmacologic paralysis, and arrhythmia management. Atrioventricular (AV) synchrony may provide a critical advantage in the postoperative patient who has low cardiac output. Cardiac pacing or anti-arrhythmic medications may be indicated.

Extracorporeal membrane oxygenation (ECMO) may be a consideration for progressive myocardial dysfunction refractory to conventional therapies. This form of mechanical circulatory support is also indicated for failure to wean from CPB and for cardio-pulmonary failure causing profound low cardiac output, hypoxemia, and cardiac arrest [14,15]. Cardiac ECMO may be used (1) to provide short-term myocardial support until intrinsic cardiac ejection returns spontaneously or there is correction of the underlying cause or (2) for longer duration, as a bridge to cardiac transplantation. A system for rapid-deployment cardiac ECMO requires the appropriate resources and personnel including a skilled team of physicians, nurses, and ECMO perfusionists. Effective use of rapid-deployment cardiac ECMO decreases mortality in pediatric cardiac patients who have a reversible cause for hemodynamic decompensation and cardiac arrest [14,16].

Arrhythmias

The physiologic stress of cardiovascular surgery increases the incidence of arrhythmias in the postoperative period. Contributing factors include anesthesia, CPB, hypothermia, surgical incisions, hemodynamic instability, and increased circulating catecholamines [4]. Accurate diagnosis and immediate intervention are essential to the successful management of arrhythmias.

The incidence of arrhythmias identified at the Cardiovascular Intensive Care Unit at Children's Hospital, Boston, Massachusetts is approximately 80 per year per 1000 cases. The most common arrhythmias were supraventricular tachycardia (38%), ventricular tachycardia (22%), junctional ectopic tachycardia (21%), and complete heart block (17%). Ectopic atrial tachycardia (2%) was rarely found in the postoperative period.

Loss of AV synchrony accounts for a 20% to 30% reduction in cardiac output [7]. Poor heart rate variability in the face of clinical changes is an important finding in the identification of arrhythmias [17]. Cannon waves, visible on the LA tracing, provide important clues for early detection of abnormal rhythms. Arrhythmias should be treated only if the

patient's condition is compromised by a decrease in cardiac output or if the rhythm is suspected of deteriorating to a more harmful one.

Following repair of a congenital heart defect, pacing wires are often placed for temporary external pacing. An atrial wire tracing, performed with pacing wires, may be used as a diagnostic tool for rapid tachycardias when the P wave is not easily identified or obscured by the QRS complex [18]. These data provide more detail of the electrical activity from the atrial tissue.

Supraventricular tachycardia is a re-entry tachycardia that has an abrupt onset with a regular rate. Supraventricular tachycardia is often poorly tolerated in infants, although it usually responds to vagal stimulation, cardioversion, or overdrive burst pacing. In stable patients, adenosine is the first-line drug used to block the AV node and break the re-entry circuit [18]. A patient who has unstable hemodynamics should be treated with synchronized cardioversion.

Ventricular arrhythmias are uncommon in infants and children but occur with increased frequency in adolescents and adults. Conditions that predispose patients to ventricular arrhythmias include acidosis, low cardiac output, electrolyte imbalance, and myocardial ischemia [4]. There are two types of ventricular tachycardia: monomorphic ventricular tachycardia and torsades de pointes. Monomorphic ventricular tachycardia shows a wide QRS complex and is treated with lidocaine followed by procainamide or amiodarone in patients who have stable hemodynamics [19]. Acute management of the unstable patient who has monomorphic ventricular tachycardia is synchronized cardioversion. Torsades de pointes has a varying QRS morphology and twists around the baseline. It usually occurs in patients who have low magnesium and calcium levels; treatment includes the administration of magnesium sulfate and lidocaine [4].

Junctional ectopic tachycardia is the most common postoperative arrhythmia in infants and children less than 2 years old [18]. Echocardiography findings include a rapid ventricular rate with normal QRS morphology. The atrial rate is typically slower than the ventricular rate, and the P wave is usually inverted and may occur before, during, or after the QRS complex. The rapid ventricular rate and dissociated atrial contraction produce a reduction in blood pressure and a rise in atrial pressures. Treatment includes mild hypothermia, a reduction in exogenous catecholamines, pacing to restore AV synchrony, and the use of procainamide or amiodarone [20].

Third-degree heart block involves the complete dissociation of the atria and the ventricles. The atria and ventricles depolarize independently of each other, with the atrial rate being faster than the ventricular rate. Treatment for complete heart block is temporary external AV sequential pacing. Postoperative AV block is usually transient and often resolves within 10 days [18]. A permanent pacemaker is implanted in patients who have complete heart block that persists beyond 10 to 14 days after cardiac surgery [21].

Ectopic atrial tachycardia is an uncommon but difficult rhythm caused by automaticity from a single atrial focus [22]. Features include a heart rate of 100 to 280 beats per minute and an abnormal P wave. It often occurs with high levels of circulating cate-cholamines but rarely persists beyond the immediate postoperative period. Treatment includes lowering exogenous catecholamines, using digoxin to block the AV node, and using esmolol to control the ventricular response [18].

Thermoregulation

The general goal of temperature regulation is normothermia. Although temperature instability is common in the perioperative phase, extremes are avoided. A mild degree of induced hypothermia may be useful in treating certain tachyarrhythmias (such as junctional ectopic tachycardia); however, lower body temperature contributes to increased SVR and PVR, coagulopathy, and bleeding [4,5]. The neonate is particularly vulnerable to the adverse effects of low temperature because of decreased temperature regulation mechanisms and a larger ratio of body surface area to mass. Cold stress in the neonate triggers a sympathetic nervous system response, causing peripheral and pulmonary vasoconstriction, greater oxygen consumption, and increased brown fat metabolism. Resultant hypoglycemia, hypoxia, and acidosis may be detrimental to the postoperative patient. Temperature should be monitored closely, and gradual rewarming of the infant may be best accomplished with radiant warming devices.

Hyperthermia in the postoperative period results from activation of inflammatory markers produced by CPB or a state of low cardiac output. Elevated body temperature increases metabolic demand and oxygen consumption, exacerbates tachyarrhythmias, lowers seizure threshold [7], and may potentiate the risk of neurologic injury. In addition, brain temperature elevation persists for at least 6 hours following CPB [23]. Aggressive temperature management is crucial to avoid the adverse effects of hyperthermia and includes treatment with antipyretics and surface cooling.

Respiratory

Alterations in intrathoracic pressure produced by positive pressure ventilation and respiratory variation may exert effects on myocardial function, specifically on systemic venous return, RV function, PVR, pulmonary venous return, and cardiac output [5,7]. Ventilatory management focuses on optimal gas exchange and tissue oxygenation based on cardiac physiology and surgical repair. Measures to minimize pain, agitation, and ventilator asynchrony with the onset of spontaneous respirations may decrease potentially devastating effects on cardiopulmonary function. The subsequent stress response related to these factors may be especially detrimental in the patient who has minimal cardiac reserve [7]. Ensuring adequate levels of analgesia and sedation and providing strategies that enhance optimal mechanical ventilation improve level of comfort and reduce excessive work of breathing.

Inflammatory and ischemic effects of CPB have the potential to compromise cardiopulmonary function in the postoperative phase [6]. Excess pulmonary fluid, decreased lung compliance, pulmonary hypertension exacerbated by CPB, intracardiac shunting, pulmonary pathology, and diminished respiratory effort may complicate weaning from mechanical ventilatory support. The presence of a residual defect should be considered after attempts to wean and extubate a patient from mechanical ventilation have failed. These patients may require further evaluation by ECG or cardiac catheterization. Other sources of respiratory compromise may be related to phrenic nerve insult, metabolic imbalance, airway injury or obstruction, and poor nutrition [5]. Providing a diuretic regimen and maintaining a negative fluid balance as required may assist with cardiopulmonary function and weaning from ventilatory support. Continuous pulse oximetry, clinical examination, arterial blood gas analysis, end-tidal carbon dioxide, and monitored hemodynamic parameters provide essential data when assessing cardiopulmonary function.

Pulmonary hypertension

The effects of CPB, pulmonary leukosequestration, microemboli, and hypothermia have been implicated in altered function of pulmonary vascular endothelium and in elevated PVR with increased pulmonary vasoreactivity in the postoperative period [4,10]. Excessive pulmonary blood flow and left to right intracardiac shunts before and after CPB, elevated pulmonary venous pressure, lung pathology, blood products, and protamine are among the other risk factors for increasing PVR [10]. Dysfunctional pulmonary endothelium after CPB may be responsible for increased generation of pulmonary vasoconstricting mediators (including endothelin 1 and thromboxane A_2) [4] and for decreased endogenous nitric oxide production associated with vasodilation [24]. These multifactorial events predispose the patient to acute pulmonary hypertensive crisis or an acute rise in PAP (with resultant decrease in cardiac output, acidosis, hypoxemia) [4] and to increased RV afterload (worsening pre-existent RV dysfunction) [25,26]. Increased PVR is further exacerbated by hypoxia and hypoventilation, acidosis and hypercarbia, α-adrenergic inotropes, and environmental factors causing stress.

Anatomic obstruction causing decreased pulmonary blood flow is potentially reversible and should be differentiated from true pulmonary vasoconstriction that may be treated with pulmonary vasodilator therapy [26]. In the acute postoperative phase, measures to reduce PAP and avoid precipitating factors are instituted until the return of endogenous nitric oxide production and a decrease in pulmonary reactivity. These measures include maintaining alkalosis [27]; optimizing ventilation and oxygenation; supporting cardiac output and treating RV failure; providing optimal analgesia, sedation, and chemical paralysis; and eliminating environmental factors leading to stress. Intravenous afterload-reducing medications such as milrinone and nitroprusside may facilitate vasodilation of pulmonary vasculature; however, they are associated with increased intrapulmonary shunting and systemic hypotension [8]. Inhaled nitric oxide is a selective, rapid-onset pulmonary vasodilator that does not have the systemic effects of other intravenous therapies and may be therapeutic in reducing PAP and PVR [26,28]. The efficacy and safety of phosphodiesterase-5 inhibitors such as sildenafil citrate are currently being investigated in clinical trials and show promise in the treatment of rebound pulmonary hypertension [29].

Fluid and electrolytes

Assessment of fluid status is multifactorial and includes monitoring of heart rate, filling pressures, blood pressure, urine output, and acid-base balance. During the first 24 hours following CPB, intravenous fluids are administered at one half to two thirds of the maintenance rate. After urine output increases, fluids are generally advanced to full maintenance on the first or second postoperative day. For patients who do not require CPB, full maintenance fluids are initiated immediately after cardiac surgery.

Electrolytes are measured within the first hour following surgery and every 4 to 6 hours thereafter, depending on the degree of illness. Young infants have limited ability to maintain normal blood glucose levels due to decreased glycogen stores and increased metabolism [3]. Serum glucose is closely monitored in neonates because hypoglycemia may depress myocardial function or cause seizures. Mild hyponatremia may be treated with limiting diuretics and restricting free water; however, a serum sodium level less than 125 mEq/L is a risk factor for seizures and usually requires additional sodium supplementation [3]. Elevated serum sodium levels are unusual and may be associated with renal failure or excessive use of sodium bicarbonate.

Calcium acts as a positive inotrope, affecting contractility of cardiac muscle, vascular smooth muscle, and skeletal muscle. Hypocalcemia may occur as a symptom of hypoparthyroidism related to DiGeorge syndrome. It may also occur in patients receiving multiple transfusions because the preservative in blood products binds ionized calcium. Low levels of ionized calcium are treated with calcium chloride or calcium gluconate [3]. In addition to calcium, magnesium levels are monitored because hypomagnesemia may increase the risk of ventricular arrhythmias.

The most common electrolyte disturbance in the postoperative patient is hypokalemia, which usually manifests in rhythm disturbances. Hypokalemia is related to limited administration of potassium in the immediate postoperative period and early use of diuretics. Hyperkalemia may occur with severe postoperative renal dysfunction, with acidosis, or in patients receiving excessive potassium supplements. Elevated levels of potassium increase the risk of cardiac arrest. Treatments may include removal of all potassium from intravenous fluids, correction of acidosis, administration of potassium-binding substances, peritoneal dialysis, or hemodialysis.

Inadequate tissue perfusion resulting from decreased cardiac output often produces metabolic acidosis. Acidosis adversely affects myocardial function. Treatment involves correction of the underlying problem and administration of sodium bicarbonate [7]. The buffering action of bicarbonate increases systemic carbon dioxide concentration. Respiratory acidosis may result but is usually managed with adequate mechanical ventilation. Neonates are at risk for developing intraventricular hemorrhage from the concentrated sodium load; therefore, sodium bicarbonate is diluted to 0.5 mEq/mL and administered slowly in this population of patients.

Renal

Urine output is monitored as a gauge of renal perfusion and cardiac output. Minimal urine output is 0.5 to 1.0 mL/kg/h in pediatrics and 30 mL/h in adults. In the perioperative phase following CPB, urine output may be sufficient due to the stress response of surgery, intraoperative fluid administration, and an osmotic diuresis from elevated glucose levels in the CPB priming solution. Within several hours postoperatively, urine output usually diminishes in response to the effects of CPB and decreased perfusion. The use of hypothermia may further decrease renal perfusion. Inadequate intravascular volume stimulates the reticular activating system, increasing vasopressin production and the syndrome of inappropriate antidiuretic hormone secretion [3,4]. Diuretic therapy is usually initiated on the first postoperative day after the initial adverse effects of CPB diminish. Neonates require more time to diurese due to immature renal systems that have decreased glomerular filtration rates. Throughout the postoperative period, any decrease in cardiac output and tissue perfusion may impact renal function, resulting in decreased urine output. Excessive use of diuretics in an attempt to increase urine output and decrease edema may cause hyponatremia, hypokalemia, hypochloremia, and metabolic alkalosis [3].

Neurologic

Intraoperative or postoperative events associated with cardiac surgery have the potential to cause adverse neurologic sequelae. Among the risk factors are anesthesia, acidosis, electrolyte imbalance, hypoxia, embolic events, CPB, ischemia, and deep hypothermic cardiac arrest (DHCA). Although currently used judiciously and for short duration, DHCA allows for cessation of CPB to facilitate surgical repair of the aortic arch and intracardiac defects in infants [30]. Clancy and colleagues [31] reported that prolonged DHCA, aortic arch obstruction or the presence of genetic anomalies correlated with greater incidence of postoperative seizures in infants following cardiac surgery. Forbess and coworkers [32] found that DHCA greater than 39 minutes correlated with delayed visual-motor and fine motor skills and possibly decreased full-scale IQ scores in 5-year-old former cardiac surgical patients repaired in infancy.

The neurodevelopmental outcomes of infants who had transposition of great vessels and who underwent arterial switch operations using circulatory arrest (DHCA) or low-flow CPB strategies were studied in the Boston Circulatory Arrest Trial [33]. In this trial, longer periods of DHCA correlated with increased incidence of postoperative seizures and the release of brain creatinine kinase in the postoperative period [33]. Consecutive studies of the same group of patients at age 1 year [34], 4 years [35], and 8 years [36], demonstrated a greater likelihood of long-term delays in psychomotor function in patients assigned to primarily a DHCA strategy. In addition to lower motor function scores at age 4 years, the group assigned to DHCA was more likely to display delays in speech and oromotor control [35]. At age 8, the DHCA group performed worse on phonologic awareness, visual-motor tracking, and verbal fluency scores [36]. At this same age, the group assigned to a low-flow CPB strategy demonstrated worse scores on vigilance testing and received lower scores from their teachers on scales of appropriate behavior [36]. Overall, patients assigned to DHCA who had a ventricular septal defect in association with transposition of great vessels repeatedly demonstrated the worst neurodevelopmental outcomes of the entire cohort [33–36].

The development of seizure activity in the postoperative patient may be indicative of brain injury. Postoperative clinical or subclinical seizures in infants following cardiac surgery are associated with greater occurrence of neurobehavioral abnormalities in later development [37]. Hyperthermia and deficiencies in calcium, glucose, or magnesium levels predispose infants to seizure activity [7]. Measures to avoid and treat acidosis and hypoxia may assist in maintaining neurologic integrity. Neurologic assessment includes frequent evaluation of pupillary response and autonomic lability such as hypertension and tachycardia in the chemically paralyzed patient. After the effects of muscle relaxants no longer persist, clinical evaluation of neurologic integrity includes assessment of eye opening, motor, and verbal responses.

Analgesia and sedation

Although it may be difficult to assess anxiety and pain in the chemically paralyzed patient, physiologic parameters of hypertension, tachycardia, diaphoresis, and pupillary response are useful in assessing symptoms [10]. After the effects of muscle relaxants have dissipated, response to painful stimuli, fluctuations in respiratory movements, guarding, and facial grimacing provide additional information regarding patient comfort. Developmentally appropriate pain scales are effective in assessing levels of discomfort and the effects of pain treatments, especially in infants and younger pediatric patients [38]. Tools to measure sedation may be used to determine degree of agitation [39].

Combinations of opioid analgesics (such as morphine) and benzodiazepines (such as midazolam) provide efficacious postoperative analgesia and sedation [5,10]. Opioid analgesics may cause histamine release, with resultant vasodilation and elevations in PAP. Shorter-acting, synthetic opioids (like fentanyl citrate) may be effective analgesics that do not generally stimulate a histamine response [5]. Insufficient or excessive sedation, tachyphylaxis, dose dependence, and withdrawal associated with pain and sedative medications may be problematic. Acetaminophen and short-term nonsteroidal anti-inflammatory drugs (NSAIDs) such as ketorolac tromethamine may be effective adjuvants to other pain therapies and are not generally associated with the adverse effects of opioids and benzodiazepines. NSAIDs may cause nephrotoxicity and inhibition of platelet aggregation therefore may be contraindicated in the presence of existing renal insufficiency or postoperative bleeding [39].

Infection

Prophylactic antibiotics are used to reduce the risk of pneumonia and blood stream, urinary tract, and surgical site infections. A broad-spectrum antibiotic should be given before surgical incision and continued in the immediate postoperative period following cardiac surgery [40]. Data suggest that patients may benefit from antimicrobial therapy until all chest tubes have been removed [41]. Preventive strategies for the reduction of postoperative infections include strict adherence to sterile technique and prompt removal of invasive lines, catheters, and tubes. Fever in the immediate postoperative period is treated aggressively with antipyretic agents and cooling devices to reduce oxygen consumption. If fever persists, blood cultures are obtained to identify a specific organism.

Nutrition

Enteral nutrition in the postoperative period following congenital cardiac surgery provides essential nutrients and improves the immune response. Reduced splanchnic flow may alter the integrity of the gut and increase permeability to pathogenic organisms [42]. Protein-energy malnutrition reduces the number and function of T cells, phagocytic cells, and the release of IgA [43]. Stimulation of the gastrointestinal tract reduces the risk of bacterial overgrowth and translocation [44].

The nutritional goal for enteral feedings in infants who have congenital heart disease is 120 to 150 kcal/kg/d [45]. Enteral feedings should be initiated at 1 mL/kg/h for patients weighing less than 25 kg and 25 mL/h for children greater than 25 kg (N.J. Braudis and colleagues, Children's Hospital, Boston, unpublished data, 2001). Assessments should be made at 4-hour intervals and include abdominal girth, residual aspirate, and any episodes of gastrointestinal distress. If tolerated, feedings may be advanced to 2 mL/kg/h for children weighing less than 25 kg and 50 mL/h for those greater than 25 kg. This regimen may be repeated at 4-hour intervals until maintenance has been achieved or a fluid restriction has been attained (N.J. Braudis and colleagues, Children's Hospital, Boston, unpublished data, 2001).

If the patient is unable to tolerate enteral feedings, then total parenteral nutrition should be established to maximize caloric intake to 80 to 90 kcal/kg/d [46]. Pediatric patients are at risk for development of stress ulceration and gastritis. Histamine$_2$ blockers or antacids should be used prophylactically in patients requiring extended hemodynamic and respiratory support [5].

The risk of necrotizing enterocolitis in patients who have congenital heart disease was reported at 3.3% or 10 times the risk for normal-term infants [47]. Clinical symptoms of necrotizing enterocolitis vary but may include temperature instability, lethargy, acidosis, abdominal distention, vomiting, bloody stools, or pneumatosis intestinalis [48]. Initial treatment includes nasogastric suction, intravenous maintenance fluids, and broad-spectrum antibiotics.

Summary

Intraoperative and postoperative events have the potential to produce adverse multisystem sequelae. Comprehensive postoperative management focuses on a preemptive approach in preventing deleterious effects associated with CPB and intraoperative events. A disciplined approach to the assessment and integration of clinical, laboratory, and physical examination data is essential. Provision of optimal postoperative care of the pediatric cardiac surgery patient requires an interdisciplinary team of skilled clinicians.

References

[1] Flori HR, Johnson LD, Hanley FL, et al. Transthoracic intracardiac catheters in pediatric patients recovering from congenital heart defect surgery: associated complications and outcomes. Crit Care Med 2000; 28(8):2997–3001.

[2] Gold JP, Jonas RA, Lang P, et al. Transthoracic intracardiac monitoring lines in pediatric surgical patients: a ten-year experience. Ann Thorac Surg 1986;42:185–91.

[3] Roth SJ. Postoperative care. In: Chang AC, Hanley FL, Wernovsky G, et al, editors. Pediatric cardiac intensive care. Philadelphia: Lippincott, Williams, and Wilkins; 1998. p. 163–87.

[4] Craig J, Fineman LD, Moynihan P, et al. Cardiovascular critical care problems. In: Curley MAQ, Moloney-Harmon P, editors. Critical care nursing of infants and children. 2nd edition. Philadelphia: WB Saunders; 2001. p. 579–654.

[5] Laussen P. Pediatric cardiac intensive care unit. In: Jonas RA, editor. Comprehensive surgical management of congenital heart disease. London: Arnold; 2004. p. 65–115.

[6] Jaggers J, Ungerleider RM. Cardiopulmonary bypass in infants and children. In: Mavroudis C, Backer CL, editors. Pediatric cardiac surgery. 3rd edition. Philadelphia: Mosby; 2003. p. 171–91.

[7] Backer CL, Badden HP, Costello JM, et al. Perioperative care. In: Mavroudis C, Backer CL, editors. Pediatric cardiac surgery. 3rd edition. Philadelphia: Mosby; 2003. p. 119–42.

[8] Wessel DL. Managing low cardiac output syndrome after congenital heart surgery. Crit Care Med 2001; 29(10):S220–30.

[9] Hoffman TM, Wernovsky G, Atz AM, et al. Efficacy and safety of milrinone in preventing low cardiac output syndrome in infants and children after corrective surgery for congenital heart disease. Circulation 2003;February 25:996–1002.

[10] Odegard KC, Laussen PC. Pediatric anesthesia and critical care. In: Sellke FW, delNido PJ, Swanson SJ, editors. 7th edition. Sabiston and Spencer: surgery of the chest, vol. 2. Philadelphia: Elsevier; 2005. p. 1863–77.

[11] Wernovsky G, Wypij D, Jonas RA, et al. Postoperative course and hemodynamic profile after the arterial switch operation in neonates and infants: a comparison of low-flow cardiopulmonary bypass and circulatory arrest. Circulation 1995;92:2226–35.

[12] Bailey JM, Miller BE, Lu W, et al. The pharmacokinetics of milrinone in pediatric patients after cardiac surgery. Anesthesiology 1999;90(4):1012–8.

[13] Chang AC, Atz AM, Wernovsky G, et al. Milrinone: systemic and pulmonary hemodynamic effects in neonates after cardiac surgery. Crit Care Med 1995;23(11):1907–14.

[14] Laussen PC, Roth SJ. Mechanical circulatory support. In: Sellke FW, delNido PJ, Swanson SJ, editors. 7th edition. Sabiston and Spencer: surgery of the chest, vol. 2. Philadelphia: Elsevier; 2005. p. 1851–62.

[15] Wessel DL, Almodovar MC, Laussen PC. Intensive care management of cardiac patients on extracorporeal membrane oxygenation. In: Duncan B, editor. Mechanical circulatory support for cardiac and respiratory failure in pediatric patients. New York: Marcel Dekker; 2001. p. 75–111.

[16] Jaggers JJ, Forbess JM, Shah AS, et al. Extracorporeal membrane oxygenation for infant postcardiotomy support: significance of shunt management. Ann Thorac Surg 2000;69:1476–83.

[17] Leroy SS. Clinical dysrhythmias after surgical repair of congenital heart disease. AACN Clin Issues 2001; 12(1):87–99.

[18] Perry JC, Walsh EP. Diagnosis and management of cardiac arrhythmias. In: Chang AC, Hanley FL, Wernovsky G, et al, editors. Pediatric cardiac intensive care. Philadelphia: Lippincott, Williams, and Wilkins; 1998. p. 461–80.

[19] Hanisch D. Pediatric arrhythmias. J Pediatr Nurs 2001;16(5):351–62.

[20] Walsh EP, Saul P, Sholler GF, et al. Evaluation of a staged treatment protocol for rapid automatic junctional tachycardia after operation for congenital heart disease. J Am Coll Cardiol 1997;29(5):1046–53.

[21] Drifus LS, Fisch C, Griffin JC, et al. Guidelines for implantation of cardiac pacemakers and antiarrhythmia devices ACC/AHA task force report. J Am Coll Cardiol 1991;18:1.

[22] Castaneda AR, Jonas RA, Mayer JE, et al. Perioperative care. In: Castaneda AR, Jonas RA, Mayer JE, et al, editors. Cardiac surgery of the neonate and infant. Philadelphia: WB Saunders; 1994. p. 65–104.

[23] Bissonnette B, Holtby HM, Davis AJ, et al. Cerebral hyperthermia in children after cardiopulmonary bypass. Anesthesiology 2000;93(3):611–8.

[24] Beghetti M, Silkoff PE, Caramori M, et al. Decreased exhaled nitric oxide may be a marker of cardiopulmonary bypass-induced injury. Ann Thorac Surg 1998;66: 532–4.

[25] Adatia I, Wessel DL. Diagnostic and therapeutic uses of inhaled nitric oxide in congenital heart disease. In: Zapol WM, Bloch KD, editors. Nitric oxide and the lung. New York: Marcel Dekker; 1997. p. 365–92.

[26] Adatia I, Atz AM, Jonas RA, et al. Diagnostic use of inhaled nitric oxide after neonatal cardiac operations. J Thorac Cardiovasc Surg 1996;112(5):1403–5.

[27] Chang AC, Zucker HA, Hickey PR, et al. Pulmonary vascular resistance in infants after cardiac surgery: role of carbon dioxide and hydrogen. Crit Care Med 1995; 23(3):568–74.

[28] Russell IA, Zwass MS, Fineman JR, et al. The effects of inhaled nitric oxide on postoperative pulmonary hypertension in infants and children undergoing surgical repair of congenital heart disease. Anesth Analg 1998;87:46–51.

[29] Ghofrani HA, Pepke-Zaba J, Barbera JA, et al. Nitric oxide pathway and phosphodiesterase inhibitors in

pulmonary arterial hypertension. J Am Coll Cardiol 2004;43(12):68S–72S.

[30] DiNardo JA. Profound hypothermia and circulatory arrest. In: Lake CL, Booker PD, editors. Pediatric cardiac anesthesia. 4th edition. Philadelphia: Lippincott, Williams, and Wilkins; 2005. p. 253–65.

[31] Clancy RR, McGaurn SA, Wernovsky G, et al. Risk of seizures in survivors of newborn heart surgery using deep hypothermic circulatory arrest. Pediatrics 2003; 111(3):592–601.

[32] Forbess JM, Visconti KJ, Bellinger DC, et al. Neurodevelopmental outcomes after biventricular repair of congenital heart defects. J Thorac Cardiovasc Surg 2002;123(4):631–9.

[33] Newburger JW, Jonas RA, Wernovsky G, et al. A comparison of the perioperative neurologic effects of hypothermic circulatory arrest versus low-flow cardiopulmonary bypass in infant heart surgery. N Engl J Med 1993;329(15):1057–64.

[34] Bellinger DC, Jonas RA, Rappaport LA, et al. Developmental and neurologic status of children after heart surgery with hypothermic circulatory arrest or low-flow cardiopulmonary bypass. N Engl J Med 1995;332(9):449–55.

[35] Bellinger DC, Wypij D, Kuban KC, et al. Developmental and neurological status of children at 4 years of age after heart surgery with hypothermic circulatory arrest or low-flow cardiopulmonary bypass. Circulation 1999;100:526–32.

[36] Bellinger DC, Wypij D, duPlessis AJ, et al. Neurodevelopmental status at eight years in children with dextro-transposition of the great arteries: the Boston Circulatory Arrest Trial. J Thorac Cardiovasc Surg 2003;126(5):1385–96.

[37] Rappaport LA, Wypij D, Bellinger DC, et al. Relation of seizures after cardiac surgery in early infancy to neurodevelopmental outcome. Circulation 1998;97: 773–9.

[38] Merkel SI, Voepel-Lewis T, Shayevitz JR, et al. The FLACC: a behavioral scale for scoring postoperative pain in young children. Pediatr Nurs 1997;23(3): 293–7.

[39] Jacobi J, Fraser GL, Coursin DB, et al. Clinical practice guidelines for the sustained use of sedatives and analgesics in the critically ill adult. Crit Care Med 2002;30(1):119–41.

[40] Mangram A, Horan T, Pearson M, et al. Guideline for prevention of surgical site infection, 1999. Centers for Disease Control and Prevention (CDC) Hospital Infection Control Practices Advisory Committee. Am J Infect Control 1999;27:97–134.

[41] Maher KO, VanDerElzen K, Bove DL, et al. A retrospective review of three antibiotic prophylaxis regimens for pediatric cardiac surgical patients. Ann Thorac Surg 2002;74:1195–200.

[42] Stechmiller JK, Treloar D, Allen N. Gut dysfunction in critically ill patients: a review of the literature. Am J Crit Care 1997;6(3):204–8.

[43] Chandra RK. Nutrition and immunology: from the clinic to cellular biology and back again. Proc Nutr Soc 1999;58:681–3.

[44] Heyland DK, Cook DJ, Guyatt GH. Enteral nutrition in the critically ill patient: a critical review of the evidence. Intensive Care Med 1993;19:435–42.

[45] Norris MK, Hill CS. Nutritional issues in infants and children with congenital heart disease. Crit Care Nurs Clin North Am 1994;6(1):153–63.

[46] Jaksic T, Shew SB, Keshen TH, et al. Do critically ill surgical neonates have increased energy expenditure? J Pediatr Surg 2001;36(1):63–7.

[47] McElhinney DB, Hedrick HL, Bush DM, et al. Necrotizing enterocolitis in neonates with congenital heart disease: risk factors and outcomes. Pediatrics 2000;106(5):1080–7.

[48] Kalhan SC, Price PT. Nutrition and selected disorders of the gastrointestinal tract. In: Klaus MH, Fanaroff AA, editors. Care of the high-risk neonate. 5th edition. Philadelphia: WB Saunders; 2001. p. 147–94.

ELSEVIER
SAUNDERS

Crit Care Nurs Clin N Am 17 (2005) 417–429

CRITICAL CARE
NURSING CLINICS
OF NORTH AMERICA

Pediatric Sepsis: The Infection unto Death

Patricia A. Moloney-Harmon, RN, MS, CCNS, CCRN, FAAN

Children's Services, Sinai Hospital of Baltimore, 2401 W. Belvedere Avenue, Baltimore MD 21215, USA

A significant percentage of pediatric patients admitted to an ICU have an infectious disease process. Many of these infants and children go on to develop sepsis, still a major cause of death in the intensive care unit. Caring for these children presents a collaborative challenge because of the multifactorial etiology and the complicated pathophysiology.

Worldwide, sepsis is the most common cause of death in infants and children [1]. In 1995, there were more than 42,000 cases of severe sepsis in children ≤ 9 years of age [2]. Even though sepsis-related mortality in children has decreased [3], severe sepsis is still among the leading causes of death in children, and accounts for more than 4300 deaths annually [2].

The incidence of sepsis in children demonstrates a bimodal distribution. The first peak is in the neonate where the incidence is 4.3 per 1000 neonates. Sixty percent of cases occur in the first 5 days and have an overall mortality of approximately 20%. The second peak is at about 2 years of age. These two age periods are critical times in the development of the immune system [4].

Definitions

Sepsis represents a clinical syndrome and there have been a variety of definitions used to describe it. A consensus conference of the Society of Critical Care Medicine and American College of Chest Physicians developed a new set of definitions for sepsis and related conditions, such as septic shock, which made sepsis a more precise diagnosis [5]. However, the definitions were not pediatric specific. Although

there were some pediatric-specific diagnostic criteria for sepsis that were presented at a 2001 consensus conference, there was scant consensus in the literature of a definition for pediatric sepsis [6]. In 2002, the International Pediatric Sepsis Consensus Conference participants met and modified the adult systemic inflammatory response syndrome (SIRS) criteria for children, and revised the definitions of severe sepsis and septic shock for the pediatric population.

SIRS is defined as the presence of at least two of the following conditions, one of which must be abnormal temperature or leukocyte count. The conditions include:

- core temperature $> 38.5°C$ or $< 36°C$
- tachycardia, defined as a mean heart rate > 2 SD above normal for age in the absence of external stimulus, chronic drugs, or painful stimuli; or otherwise unexplained persistent elevation over a 30 minute to 4 hour time period; or for children less than 1 year of age, bradycardia, defined as a mean heart rate less than the 10th percentile for age in the absence of external vagal stimulus, β-blocker drugs, or congenital heart disease; or otherwise unexplained persistent depression over a 30 minute time period
- mean respiratory rate > 2 SD above normal for age or mechanical ventilation for an acute process not related to underlying neuromuscular disease or the receipt of general anesthesia
- leukocyte count elevated or depressed for age (not secondary to chemotherapy-induced leukopenia) or the presence of $> 10\%$ immature neutrophils [7].

An infection is defined as a suspected or proven (by positive culture, tissue stain, or polymerase chain

E-mail address: pmoloney@lifebridgehealth.org

0899-5885/05/$ – see front matter © 2005 Elsevier Inc. All rights reserved.
doi:10.1016/j.ccell.2005.08.004

Box 1. Organ dysfunction criteria

Cardiovascular dysfunction
Despite administration of isotonic intravenous fluid $\geq$ mL/kg in 1 hour

- Decrease in blood pressure (hypotension) $< 5^{th}$ percentile for age or systolic blood pressure < 2 SD below normal for age

OR

- Need for vasoactive drug to maintain blood pressure in normal range (dopamine > 5 μg/kg/min or dobutamine, epinephrine, or norepinephrine at any dose)

OR

- Two of the following:

Unexplained metabolic acidosis: base deficit > 5.0 mEq/L
Increased arterial lactate > 2 times upper limit of normal
Oliguric urine output < 0.5 mL/kg/hr
Prolonged capillary refill > 5 sec
Core to peripheral temperature gap $> 3°C$

Respiratory

- $PaO_2/FiO_2 < 300$ in absence of cyanotic heart disease or pre-existing lung disease

OR

- $PaCO_2 > 65$ torr or 20 mmHg over baseline $PaCO_2$

OR

- Proven need or $> 50\%$ FiO_2 to maintain saturation $\geq 92\%$

OR

- Need for nonelective invasive or non-invasive mechanical ventilation

Neurologic

- GCS ≤ 11

OR

- Acute change in mental status with a decrease in GCS ≥ 3 points from abnormal baseline

Hematologic

- Platelet count $< 80,000/mm^3$ or a decline of 50% in platelet count from highest value recorded over the past 3 days (for chronic hematology/oncology patients)

OR

- International normalized ratio > 2

Renal

- Serum creatinine > 2 times the upper limit of normal for age or 2-fold increase in baseline creatinine

Hepatic

- Total bilirubin ≥ 4 mg/dL (not applicable to newborn)

OR

- ALT 2 times upper limit of normal for age

From Goldstein B, Giroir B, Randolph A. International pediatric sepsis consensus conference: definitions for sepsis and organ dysfunction in pediatrics. Pediatric Crit Care Med 2005;6(1):2–8; with permission.

reaction test) infection caused by any pathogen or a clinical syndrome associated with a high probability of infection. Evidence of infection includes positive findings on clinical exam, imaging, or laboratory tests (eg, white blood cells in a normally sterile body fluid, perforated viscus, chest radiograph consistent with pneumonia, petechial or purpural rash, or purpura fulminans) [7].

Sepsis is defined as SIRS in the presence of or as a result of a suspected or proven infection [7]. Severe sepsis is defined as sepsis plus one of the following:

- cardiovascular organ dysfunction
- acute respiratory distress syndrome
- two or more other organ dysfunctions (respiratory, renal, neurologic, hematologic, or hepatic) [7].

Organ dysfunctions are described in Box 1. Septic shock is defined as sepsis plus cardiovascular organ dysfunction as described in Box 1.

Etiology

A child is an immunocompromised host for a variety of reasons. Developmental differences in the immune system alone place a child at risk for sepsis. In addition to host factors (eg, age), immunodeficiencies, surgery, anesthesia, nutritional factors, pharmacologic and immunosuppressive interventions, and stress predispose a child to sepsis.

Organisms that cause sepsis vary with age. In newborns, the most common pathogens are those isolated from the maternal gastrointestinal and genital tracts. Group B streptococcus is currently the most common etiologic agent of neonatal sepsis in the United States, although *Escherichia coli*, *Enterococcus* organisms, *Listeria* organisms, *Haemophilus influenzae, Staphlococcus aureus, Pseudomonas aeruginosa, Candida albicans*, and *Salmonella* may also be implicated. *H influenzae, Streptococcus pneumoniae*, and *Neisseria meningitidis* are the pathogens that most commonly cause sepsis in children 3 months to 5 years of age. These are also the pathogens often associated with meningitis. *Staphylococcus aureus*, gram negative bacilli, and *P aeruginosa* are often associated with sepsis in the immunocompromised host. Also, children with hypogammaglobulinemia, agammaglobulinemia, splenic dysfunction, and AIDS are at increased risk for developing overwhelming sepsis associated with encapsulated bacteria such as *S pneumoniae, H influenzae, N meningitidis*, and *E coli*. Cytomegalovirus should also be considered in the immunocompromised patient who presents with a clinical sepsis syndrome [4].

Pathophysiology

Current knowledge of sepsis demonstrates that the normal response of the immune system goes wildly out of control. When the immune system is working as it is supposed to, it functions like finely tuned choreography; however, in the child who has sepsis, this choreography turns into chaos.

Children stricken by sepsis lose the proper functioning of their immune system. The host's own immune system is responding to toxins released by microorganisms that mediate the tissue damage and other harmful effects associated with sepsis. The changes that occur in sepsis are directly related to the endothelial damage and the release of the circulating mediators. The event is initiated when a microorganism or its toxins trigger the inflammatory/immune response. Once in the circulation, the byproducts of the microorganism, such as endotoxin, stimulate the release of mediators. Mediators, along with procoagulant factors and agents that inhibit fibrinolysis, stimulate three responses: (1) initiation of inflammation, (2) commencement of coagulation, and (3) interference with fibrinolysis [8].

Inflammatory response

Inflammatory cytokines that are released in response to stimulation of the inflammatory/immune response include tumor necrosis factor-α (TNFα), interleukin-1 (IL-1), interleukin-6 (IL-6), and platelet activating factor. After the release of various mediators, arachidonic acid is metabolized to form leukotrienes, thromboxane A, and prostaglandins. IL-1 and IL-6 activate T-cells to produce interferon, interleukin-2 (IL-2), interleukin-4 (IL-4), and granulocyte-monocyte colony stimulating factor. In an effort to re-establish homeostasis, IL-4 and interleukin-10 (IL-10), both anti-inflammatory cytokines, are released [8]. Some initial studies propose that TNFα and IL-6 actually augment the actions on one another during inflammation and can actually overcome an anti-inflammatory process put in place by IL-10 [9,10]. As excessive inflammation results, impaired tissue function and tissue damage occur [8].

Coagulation

Activation of the complement cascade results in vascular abnormalities, including the formation of thrombin, which results in the conversion of fibrinogen to fibrin, and amplifies the pro-coagulant state [11]. Pervasive fibrin deposits impede blood flow, which then may interfere with tissue oxygenation in spite of adequate cardiac output [12]. Levels of anti-coagulant factors, such as antithrombin and protein C, are decreased in sepsis, which enhances the pro-coagulant state [8,13].

Fibrinolysis

Normally, when the coagulation pathway is initiated, fibrinolysis occurs to encourage breakdown of clots. However, with sepsis, the fibrinolysis system is subdued by the release of plasminogen activator inhibitor-1 and thrombin activatable fibrinolysis inhibitor [8]. Under normal circumstances, these inhibitors protect the body from excessive fibrinolysis, but with sepsis the process is suppressed and coagulopathy occurs.

Endothelium

The endothelium is the largest organ in the body and is known to play a key role in the processes of inflammation, prothrombosis, and impaired fibrinolysis associated with sepsis [8]. Mediators, such as TNFα, platelet activating factor, leukotrienes, thromboxane A, and prostaglandins cause endothelial damage. The continuous release of these mediators produces an increase in endothelial permeability. The endothelial cells release adhesion molecules, which encourages buildup of leukocytes and platelets at the site of injury. The consequence of platelet adhesion is microemboli formation. The damage to the endothelium promotes the movement of inflammatory cells

and fluid from the blood into the interstitial spaces, which further contributes to endothelial cell damage and inflammation [8]. Endothelial damage finally results in a severe capillary leak syndrome and increased vascular permeability, which leads to profound interstitial edema, diffuse parenchymal cell injury and persistent hypovolemia, followed by multiorgan dysfunction, multiorgan failure, or death. Fig. 1 illustrates the processes that occur with severe sepsis.

Hemodynamic response

The establishment of pediatric definitions for sepsis and related conditions is important because there are developmental differences in the hemodynamic response to sepsis in children when compared with adults. Adults with sepsis tend to have myocardial dysfunction, which shows as decreased ejection fraction while cardiac output is usually sustained by tachycardia and ventricular dilation. If these mechanisms are not in place to maintain cardiac output, the prognosis is poor [14].

In children, it is a decrease in cardiac output, not systemic vascular resistance that is associated with mortality in septic shock [15]. Based on this developmental difference, achieving a therapeutic goal of a $3.3-6.0$ L/min/m^2 cardiac index (CI) may result in better survival [15]. In addition, in children, oxygen delivery is the major determinant of oxygen consumption as opposed to oxygen extraction, so achieving oxygen consumption > 200 mL/min/m^2 may also be associated with a better outcome [16,17].

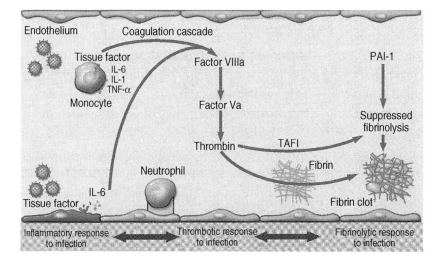

Fig. 1. Inflammation, coagulation, and impaired fibrinolysis in severe sepsis. (*From* Eli Lilly and Company, Indianapolis, IN; with permission.)

In 1998, Ceneviva and coworkers reported positive outcomes when aggressive fluid resuscitation was used (60 mL/kg in the first hour) and when therapy was directed toward a cardiac index of 3.3–6.0 L/min/m^2 and normal pulmonary capillary wedge pressures [15]. Fifty children who were in fluid refractory ($\geq$ 60 mL/kg in the first hour) experienced dopamine-resistant shock. Fifty-eight percent had a decreased cardiac output and an increased systemic vascular resistance; only 22% had a decreased cardiac output and a decreased systemic vascular resistance. Thirty-three percent of the patients experienced persistent shock. Cardiac function decreased significantly over time, necessitating the addition of inotropes and vasodilators. The achievement of a normal CI and systemic vascular resistance (SVR) was obtained through goal-directed therapy using inotropes, vasopressors, and vasodilators [18]. The results of this study demonstrated a significant decrease in mortality, which was different from the mortality results reported in a 1985 study by Pollack and colleagues, where aggressive fluid resuscitation was not used [15,17].

Clinical manifestations

Clinical manifestations may vary based on the age of the child. Children with an infection often present with a classic inflammatory triad of fever, tachycardia, and vasodilatation, which result from the release of IL-1 and other inflammatory mediators from polymorphonuclear leukocytes and the reticuloendothelial system. However, these children rarely have sepsis; sepsis is clinically suspected when children have accompanying signs of hypoperfusion, such as change in mental status (demonstrated by inconsolable irritability, lack of interaction with parents, or inability to be aroused) [18]. The clinical diagnosis of septic shock is made in children who have a suspected infection demonstrated by temperature change (hypo- or hyperthermia) and have clinical signs of diminished perfusion, including decreased level of consciousness, prolonged capillary refill time > 2 seconds, or rapid capillary refill, decreased or bounding peripheral pulses, mottled cool extremities, or a urine output < 1 mL/kg/hr [18]. Overall, in the early stages of sepsis, increased cardiac output and O$_2$ transport is seen along with a decrease in systemic vascular resistance and oxygen extraction ratio. During the warm phase, the child usually shows a widened pulse pressure with an increased cardiac index, a decreased SVR (secondary to increased levels of IL-1, catecholamines, and other vasoactive media-

tors), and increased pulmonary vascular resistance (PVR) (caused by thromboxane release). The changes brought about by a decrease in systemic vascular resistance are the result of increased blood flow to the skin. The child may be flushed with a normal or rapid capillary refill time. They often have a high fever, though hypothermia may be present. In the high cardiac output state, bounding pulses are present, the result of an increased stroke volume with a decreased systemic vascular resistance. If sepsis persists, the child moves into the late stage, which results in manifestations of low cardiac output [19]. These manifestations include a decreasing CI, normal or mildly elevated SVR, hypoxia, and metabolic acidosis. Hypotension is not an absolute for a clinical diagnosis of septic shock but its presence in a child with other signs of infection is confirmatory [18]. Hypotension results because the increase in vascular tone is not sufficient to maintain homeo-

---

Box 2. Definitions of shock

Cold or warm shock: Decreased perfusion including decreased mental status, capillary refill > 2 seconds (cold shock) or flash capillary refill (warm shock), diminished (cold shock) or bounding (warm shock) peripheral pulses, mottled cool extremities (cold shock), or decreased urine output < 1 mL/kg/hr

Fluid-refractory/dopamine-resistant shock: Shock persists despite $\geq$ 60 mL/kg fluid resuscitation in first hour and dopamine infusion to 10 µg/kg/min

Catecholamine resistant shock: Shock persists despite use of catecholamines-epinephrine or norepinephrine

Refractory shock: Shock persists despite goal-directed therapy use of inotropic agents, vasopressors, vasodilators, and maintenance of metabolic (glucose and calcium) and hormonal (thyroid and hydrocortisone) homeostasis.

From Carcillo JA, Fields AI. Clinical practice parameters for hemodynamic support of pediatric and neonatal patients in septic shock. Crit Care Med 2002;30:1370; with permission.

Table 1
Phases and associated symptoms of septic shock

Organ system	Sepsis	Septic shock	
		Early	Late
Central nervous system	Change in activity	Clouded sensorium	Disorientation
	Change in feeding	Irritability	Lethargy
	Change in response	Disorientation	Obtundation
		Lethargy	
Cardiovascular	Sinus tachycardia	Sinus tachycardia	Sinus tachycardia
	Bounding pulses	Bounding pulses	Weak, thready pulse
		Warm, dry, flushed skin	Dysrhythmias
		Widened pulse pressure	Narrowed pulse pressure
		± Diminished perfusion	Diminished perfusion
		± Mottled extremities	Mottled extremities ↓
		↑↓ Capillary refill	↓ Capillary refill
		Generalized edema	Generalized edema
		Relative hypovolemia	
		Progressive hypotension	Hypotension
Pulmonary	Tachypnea	Tachypnea	Pulmonary edema
		Progressive hypoxemia	
Metabolic	Fever or hypothermia	Fever or hypothermia	Fever or hypothermia
	Respiratory alkalosis	Hyperglycemia or hypoglycemia	Hyperglycemia or hypoglycemia
		Progressive metabolic acidosis	Severe metabolic acidosis
Hematology/immunology	Leukocytosis/leukopenia	Leukocytosis/leukopenia	Leukocytosis/leukopenia
	↑ Immature neutrophils (bands)	↑ Immature neutrophils (bands)	
Renal		↓ Urine output	↓ Urine output

Data from Carcillo JA. Management of pediatric septic shock. In: Holbrook PR, editor. Textbook of pediatric critical care. Philadelphia: WB Saunders; 1993. p. 114–42; Robbins EV. Maldistribution of circulating blood volume. In: Secor VH, editor. Multisystem organ failure: pathophysiology and clinical implications. St. Louis (MO): Mosby-Year Book; 1996. p. 107–34; Rosenthal-Dichter C. Septic shock. In: Slota MC, editor. Core curriculum for pediatric critical care nursing. Philadelphia: WB Saunders; 1998. p. 638.
From Dichter CH, Curley MAQ. Shock. In: Curley MAQ, Moloney-Harmon PA, editors. Critical care nursing of infants and children. 2nd edition. Philadelphia: WB Saunders; 2001. p. 921–45; with permission.

stasis. Box 2 provides the definitions of shock. Table 1 presents the phases and associated symptoms of septic shock. In newborns, the symptoms can be subtle and difficult to differentiate from other disorders. The infant may present with respiratory distress, apnea, temperature instability, abdominal distention, vomiting, diarrhea, jaundice, loss of muscle tone, lethargy, seizures and an altered body temperature, either hypo- or hyperthermia.

Monitoring and laboratory data

All children with sepsis receive routine monitoring in the pediatric intensive care unit (PICU). However, if sepsis is progressing to sepsis syndrome or septic shock and the child is not responding to therapies directed to perfusion, perfusion pressure, or oxygen saturation, a pulmonary artery catheter may be considered so that oxygen use and hemodynamic values can be monitored [18]. Ceneviva's study

showed that in children with fluid-refractory and dopamine-resistant shock, a pulmonary artery catheter identified inappropriate cardiovascular support based on an inaccurate assessment of the child's hemodynamic status [15]. Table 2 summarizes the hemodynamic and oxygenation profile changes that are associated with septic shock.

There are a variety of laboratory tests that are used to determine the presence of sepsis. Laboratory tests to determine microbiologic indicators of sepsis include bacterial cultures to distinguish specific etiologic agents, latex particle agglutination tests to detect bacterial antigens, gram stains, fungal cultures, and viral cultures. Indirect indicators include the white blood cell (WBC) count and differential, erythrocyte sedimentation rate (ESR), and C-reactive protein (CRP). Neutrophilia ($\geq 20,000$ WBC/mm^3) and neutropenia (≤ 5000 WBC/mm^3) with a shift to the left are more likely to be associated with infection. ESR (0–10 mm/hr) is a reflection of an acute-phase reaction in inflammation and infection. However, it is a

Table 2
Hemodynamic and oxygenation profile changes in septic shock

Parameter	Normal values	Septic shock	
		Early	Late
Heart rates (beats/minute)	Newborn–3 mo: 85–205 3 mo–2 yr: 100–190 2–10 yr: 60–140 >10 yr: 60–11	Increased	Increased
MAP	>60 mmHg	Normal$_{Compensated}$	Decreased$_{Decompensated}$
CI	2.5–5.5 L/min/M^2	Increased	Decreased
RAP/PAWP	2–6 mmHg/6–12 mmHg	Decreased	Increased
PVRI	PVRI = Mean PA-PCWP/CI × 80 Norm: 80–240 dyne-sec/cm^5/M^2	Normal or increased	Normal or increased
SVRI	SVRI = MAP – RAP/CI × 80 Norm: 800–1600 dyne-sec/cm^5/M^2	Decreased	Increased
DO$_2$	DO$_2$ = CaO$_2$ × CI × 10 Norm: 620 ± 50 mL/min/M^2	Increased	Decreased
VO$_2$	VO$_2$ = arterial DO$_2$ – venous DO$_2$ Norm: 120–200 mL/min/M^2	Increased	Decreased
OER	CaO$_2$ – CvO$_2$/CaO$_2$ × 100 Norm: 25% + 2%	Normal/increased	Decreased
SvO$_2$	Norm: 75% (60%–80%)	Normal/decreased	Increased

Abbreviations: CI, cardiac index; DO$_2$, oxygen delivery; MAP, mean arterial pressure; OER, O$_2$ extraction ratio; PAWP, pulmonary artery wedge pressure; PVRI, pulmonary vascular resistance index; RAP, right atrial pressure; SVRI, systemic vascular resistance index; VO$_2$, oxygen consumption.

Adapted from Dichter CH, Curley MAQ. Shock. In: Curley MAQ, Moloney-Harmon PA, editors. Critical care nursing of infants and children. 2nd edition. Philadelphia: WB Saunders; 2001. p. 921–45; with permission.

non-specific indicator. CRP is a nonspecific, acute-phase protein that rises in response to infectious and non-infectious inflammatory processes. Levels begin to rise within 4–6 hours of the onset of signs of infection or tissue injury and peak 24–48 hours later. They rapidly disappear as the infection or inflammatory process resolves. The degree of response may be dependent on the amount of tissue damage present.

The indirect indicators of sepsis were discussed during the International Pediatric Sepsis Consensus Conference. Conference participants considered whether biochemical markers of inflammation, such as ESR, CRP, base deficit, IL-6, and procalcitonin levels, may actually be more objective and reliable than physiologic variables. These indicators have been described as potential biochemical markers of SIRS; however, they lack specificity at this time, and so were not added to the general definition [7].

Collaborative management

The treatment for sepsis remains largely supportive. Newer broad-spectrum antibiotics have enhanced the ability to destroy the causative organisms; however, the root of therapy still focuses on sustaining oxygen delivery and maintaining homeostasis. The emphasis for newer therapies is to slow or stop the sepsis cascade.

Collaborative management begins with prevention. There needs to be close attention to preventing nosocomial infections. Attempts should be made to identify sources of infection before the infection occurs. For example, Persico and colleagues found that otitis media, detected with daily inspection, also identified organisms that were associated with those cultured during bacteremia and sepsis [20]. In addition, there are data that show the younger the child in the PICU, the higher the risk for nosocomial infection. Children under 2 years of age have the highest infection rates; up to 25% of this age group is affected [21]. This study also showed that primary bloodstream infections were the most common type, followed by pneumonia and urinary tract infections [21]. A survey of bacteremia and fungi in a PICU showed an incidence of 39.0 per 1000 admissions, or 10.6 per 1000 bed days. Of these, 64.1% were acquired in the ICU and 20.6% were community acquired. The remainder (15.3%), were acquired in other areas of the hospital [22].

Length of stay in the PICU is also a risk factor for nosocomial infection. One study identified that 90% of children with nosocomial infections developed the infection after the beginning of their second week of hospitalization [23].

Early recognition, prompt treatment, and removal of the source of infection are critical to a good outcome. A key component of early recognition is defining the infection itself. Failure of clinical sepsis trials of single therapeutic agents has been linked to the fact that the study populations have not been homogenous in their host characteristics or sites and types of infections [24]. The International Sepsis Forum on Sepsis in Infants and Children recently published definitions of the most common infections in neonates, infants, and children [25].

Initial resuscitation

Clinical practice guidelines for treatment of sepsis and septic shock recommend that goals for the first hour of resuscitation remain focused on airway, breathing, and circulation. The therapeutic endpoints include a capillary refill time < 2 seconds, normal pulses, no differential between peripheral and central pulses, warm extremities, a urine output > 1 mL/kg/hr, normal mental status, and normal blood pressure for age [18]. Monitoring includes heart rate, oxygen saturation, blood pressure, temperature, urine output, glucose, and ionized calcium. The decision to intubate the patient is based on manifestation of increased work of breathing, hypoventilation, and decreased level of consciousness. Vascular access is rapidly obtained and intravascular volume expansion is accomplished with fluid boluses of 20 mL/kg of isotonic saline or colloids. It may be necessary to administer as much as 200 mL/kg in the first hour, although the average is 40–60 mL/kg. The goal of fluid resuscitation is to attain normal perfusion and blood pressure [18]. Monitoring the response is critical because children with septic shock demonstrate a less consistent response to fluid replacement [26]. One study found that in children with septic shock after fluid resuscitation, only 20% had a high cardiac output and low SVR, whereas 80% had a low cardiac output with variations in SVR [27].

Vasoactive agents may be necessary during resuscitation. Dopamine is an effective first line agent; however, the development of dopamine resistant shock should be recognized rapidly if it does develop. In that case, epinephrine is used for cold shock or norepinephrine is used for warm shock to restore normal perfusion and blood pressure [18].

Hydrocortisone may be lifesaving in the child with catecholamine resistant shock. Dose recommendations for treatment of shock are 50 mg/kg followed by the same dose as a 24 hour infusion. [18]

Ongoing therapy

Once the initial resuscitation has taken place, vigilance is required to determine the effects of hypovolemia and cardiac and vascular dysfunction, and precise management become necessary. The goals of stabilization, according to the clinical practice guidelines, are normal perfusion, a perfusion pressure normal for age, superior vena cava or mixed venous oxygen saturation > 70%; and a CI > 3.3 L/min/m^2 and < 6.0 L/min/m^2 [18]. The therapeutic endpoints are a capillary refill time < 2 seconds, normal pulses with no difference between peripheral and central pulses, warm extremities, urine output > 1 mL/kg/hour, normal mental status, a CI > 3.3 L/min/m^2 and < 6.0 L/min/m^2 and superior vena cava or mixed venous oxygen saturation > 70%. Cardiac index is maximized by enhancing preload [18]. Monitoring includes heart rate, oxygen saturation, blood pressure, temperature, urine output, central venous pressure, pulmonary artery pressure, cardiac output, glucose, and calcium.

Because a diffuse capillary leak can contribute to ongoing fluid losses and persistent hypovolemia, fluid replacement should be directed toward perfusion, pulmonary capillary occlusion pressure, and cardiac output [18]. The use of inotropes, vasopressors, and vasodilators will vary. The child in septic shock with cardiac failure frequently requires the addition of vasodilators to decrease SVR and improve CO. In particular, reduction of PVR and right ventricular afterload may be necessary to decrease intracardiac shunting and to prevent right ventricular failure. Nitroprusside and nitroglycerin are first-line vasodilators in patients with epinephrine-resistant shock and a normal blood pressure. Children with predominant vascular failure often require the addition of an inotrope over time as cardiac dysfunction occurs. Occasionally, children shift their hemodynamic requirements from vasopressor to inotrope or vice versa [18]. Table 3 presents a summary of the pharmacologic therapy used in the treatment of septic shock.

In addition to improving tissue perfusion, oxygenation must be maximized. Increasing the hemoglobin concentration (> 10 g/dL), oxygenation, or cardiac output can increase oxygen delivery. However, increasing O_2 delivery is helpful only if it is associated with an accompanying increase in O_2 consumption. Pollack and coworkers reported that a CI between 3.6 and 6 L/min/m^2, an O_2 consumption > 200 mL/min/m^2, and an oxygen extraction ratio > 28% are associated with improved outcome. [17]

Table 3
Pharmacologic therapies used in septic shock

Drug	Site of action	Dose (μg/kg/min)	Primary effect*	Secondary effect
Dopamine	Dopaminergic	2–5	Increase renal perfusion	Dysrhythmia
	Dopaminergic and β_1	2–10	Inotropy	
			Chronotropy	
			Increase renal perfusion	
	α	10–20	Vasoconstriction	
Norepinephrine	$\alpha > \beta$	2–10	Vasoconstriction	>MVO$_2$
			Inotropy	Dysrhythmias
				<Renal BF
Epinephrine	α and β	0.05–1.5	Vasoconstriction	>MVO$_2$
			Inotropy	Dysrhythmisa
			Chronotropy	< Renal BF
Dobutamine	β_1	5–20	Inotropy	Tachycardia
				Dysrhythmia
				Vasodilatation
				Hypotension
Sodium nitroprusside	NA	0.5–10 (light sensitive)	Vasodilatation (balanced)	<PVR
				>V/Q mismatch
				Cyanide toxicity
Nitroglycerin	NA	0.2–20	Vasodilatation (venous)	<PVR
				>ICP
Amrinone	NA	5–10 (load with up to 3 mg/kg over 20 min)	Inotropy	Dysrhythmias
			Vasodilatation	<PVR
				Thrombocytopenia
Milrinone	NA	0.75–1.0 (load with 75 μg/kg over 20 min)	Inotropy	Dysrhythmias
			Vasodilatation	<PVR
			Improves diastolic function	

Abbreviations: BF, blood flow; ICP, intracranial pressure; MVO$_2$, myocardial oxygen consumption; PVR, pulmonary vascular resistance; V/Q, ventilation/perfusion.

* Difficult to predict the dose-response effect. Management requires individual titration at the bedside.

From Dichter CH, Curley MAQ. Shock. In: Curley MAQ, Moloney-Harmon PA, editors. Critical care nursing of infants and children. 2nd edition. Philadelphia: WB Saunders; 2001. p. 937.

Treatment of infection

When sepsis is suspected, empiric antibiotic therapy is begun once blood cultures are drawn without waiting for results. The initial antibiotic therapy will be based on the suspected organism, organisms typically found in a particular institution, whether the child is neutropenic, duration of the neutropenia, organisms associated with a particular patient population, central nervous system penetration, toxicity, and the child's hepatic and renal function [4,28]. Once the results of the cultures and susceptibility tests are available, antibiotics should be evaluated. If the clinical findings are normal and the cultures are negative, the antibiotics should be discontinued [4]. With continued antibiotic use, it is important to monitor for efficacy; an overall clinical improvement of infection should be evident within 24–48 hours of starting antibiotics. The length of therapy depends on

the initial response to the appropriate antibiotic but generally ranges from 10 to 14 days in the child with sepsis and minimal or localized infection [4]. The lack of a response may indicate an inappropriate antibiotic or incorrect dose, inability to achieve adequate levels at the site of infection, a fungal organism, continuing contamination or undrained purulent focus, resistance, poor absorption of oral antibiotics, or immunodeficiency [29,30].

Antibiotic therapy should continue to be assessed every few days and special attention given to therapy maintained for more than 10 days. This is to prevent the emergence of antibiotic resistant strains, which has produced a crisis in hospitals throughout the world. Some of the mechanisms involved in antibiotic resistance include enzymatic breakdown of the antibiotic, changes in the binding site of the antibiotic within the bacteria, changes in the cell wall structure of the organism that inhibit entry of the antibiotic, and efficient pumps that eliminate the antibiotic from the bacteria as quickly as they can enter the cell wall [31]. Antibiotic resistance has developed because of misuse and overuse of antibiotics; dissemination has occurred because of poor compliance with hand washing and isolation procedures [28].

Respiratory management

As many as 80% of critically ill children with septic shock are intubated and started on mechanical ventilation within 24 hours of admission. Forty percent of children have the criteria for acute respiratory distress syndrome (alveolar infiltrates, PaO_2 < 60 mmHg on room air, and a pulmonary capillary wedge pressure of ≤ 15 mm Hg) [4]. This is thought to be facilitated in part by white blood cell-induced autoinjury, macrophage-released mediators, complement, ischemia, and endotoxin. The result is increased capillary permeability with alveolar collapse, increased extravascular lung water, and decreased lung compliance. In the child with cardiac dysfunction, the work of breathing can require as much as 25% of O_2 consumption so early intubation and ventilation is recommended [4]. Determining an optimal level of positive end expiratory pressure (PEEP) is important to protect against volutrauma which has been shown to cause the release of cytokines [32]. Using the PaO_2/FiO_2 ratio or compliance can determine the optimal PEEP [33].

Preservation of renal function

Renal function is critical to maintaining cardiopulmonary and metabolic homeostasis in early and middle stages of septic shock. Renal function is maintained through the maintenance of renal blood flow; low dose dopamine may be indicated for this (Table 3). If the child develops oliguria or anuria, use of diuretics is the first line of therapy. Fluid restriction is not indicated because of the significant capillary leak, which leads to intravascular hypovolemia and decreased renal blood flow. Dialysis or hemofiltration is indicated for the child who has sepsis and capillary leak syndrome, oliguria or anuria unresponsive to diuretics, hyperkalemia, a blood urea nitrogen > 100 mg/dL, and refractory metabolic acidosis [4].

Management of metabolic dysfunction

Hypocalcemia, hypophosphatemia, and metabolic acidosis are common during septic shock. Hypocalcemia correlates with a decrease in CO, so the cor-

rection of low ionized calcium levels is important. Hypophosphatemia should also be corrected because phosphate is crucial to cardiac, diaphragmatic, and mitochondrial function. Metabolic acidosis has numerous negative effects on cardiac function; sodium bicarbonate is the treatment of choice. Hyper- or hypoglycemia may be present in children during early sepsis. Hyperglycemia is often accompanied by an insulin resistance, which may necessitate the use of glucose, insulin, and potassium infusion. Hypoglycemia is treated aggressively since it is associated with poor neurological outcomes [33].

Nutrition

Though there are few data to direct nutritional support in critically ill pediatric patients with sepsis, Curley and Castillo recommend beginning nutritional support as soon as possible [34]. Enteral nutrition is recommended and the transpyloric route is preferred over the gastric route because critical illness impedes gastric emptying. Total parenteral nutrition will be indicated for those children who cannot tolerate enteral feedings. One source recommends a feeding protocol during the acute period of sepsis, which includes a glucose infusion of 4 to 8 mg/kg/min, protein intake of 2 to 3 g/kg/day, and limited administration of fat except for essential fatty acids [4].

Management of coagulation abnormalities

Alteration of the coagulation cascade is common in children during septic shock. Alteration can result in disseminated intravascular coagulation (DIC). DIC is distinguished by extreme activation of coagulation factors that surpasses the ability to replace those factors, which results in the rapid production of thrombin and activated factor X, or disproportionate bleeding caused by the failure of clot formation. All of these mechanisms may contribute to organ failure. With sepsis, the bacterial processes induce activating factors that commence the intrinsic coagulation system [35]. The surface of the vascular endothelium favors coagulation activation and antifibrinolysis, which leads to enhanced vascular thrombosis, potential for decreased blood flow to the organs, and an increased risk of multiorgan system failure [36]. Fig. 2 illustrates the pathophysiology of DIC. Diagnosis is usually validated by combining factors known to predispose the child to DIC along with abnormal laboratory parameters (prolonged prothrombin time, activated partial thromboplastin time, and decreased platelet count and fibrinogen levels) [36]. The initial focus is

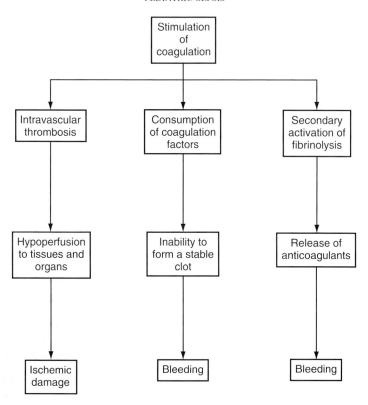

Fig. 2. Pathophysiology of disseminated intravascular coagulation. (*From* Dressler DK. Patients with coagulopathies. In: Clochesy JM, et al, editors. Critical care nursing. Philadelphia: WB Saunders; 1992; with permission.)

on treating the cause of the DIC but if the process is moving too rapidly, the child is supported with blood component therapy. Fresh frozen plasma and cryoprecipitate are used to treat prolonged prothrombin time, activated partial thromboplastin time, and abnormal fibrinogen levels [19].

Purpura fulminans may also occur in the child with septic shock and DIC. It often occurs in association with meningococcal and *Haemophilus influenzae* infection and results from alterations in coagulation [19]. Various treatments are under investigation.

Decreasing energy expenditure

Since O₂ supply is less than demand, it is critical to minimize the expenditure of energy. Fever, pain, shivering, tachycardia, and anxiety all cause energy expenditure and increase O₂ demand. Nurses play a key role in addressing these issues. Fever is identified and treated which is critical (for each degree Celsius, metabolic demands change 13%) [19], the child's comfort is addressed by providing analgesia and sedation, which decreases restlessness, tachycardia, the work of breathing, and shivering. All of these interventions help to preserve O₂ for use by major organs. Family needs are also addressed so that they can focus on supporting their critically ill child.

Alternative therapies and controversies

Alternative therapies in sepsis and septic shock have been aimed at interrupting the pathophysiologic process. One therapeutic intervention that has received much attention is activated drotrecogin alfa (Xigris). Drotrecogin alfa has been shown to effectively treat sepsis in adults through a number of mechanisms including, suppression of inflammation, prevention of microvascular coagulation, and the reversal of impaired fibrinolysis [37]. However, in April 2005, Eli Lilly announced that it was ending a clinical trial of drotrecogin alfa in children after an interim analysis demonstrated that the drug would unlikely show a benefit over placebo. According to a letter posted on the product's website, an independent safety panel also detected a higher rate of central nervous system bleeding among patients given drotrecogin alfa during the 6-day infusion period in the drotrecogin alfa group compared with placebo (4 versus 1). Three of the four intracranial hemorrhage events in the drotrecogin alfa group occurred in patients 2 months old or younger [38].

There are several other alternative therapies for sepsis currently under investigation. Further study is needed to find effective treatment for this devastating disorder.

Outcomes

Pediatric sepsis remains a major health issue with high mortality and morbidity worldwide [1]. More successful treatment of many diseases may actually increase the incidence of sepsis; however, advances in treatment may decrease mortality. As mortality decreases, it becomes necessary to examine other end points in clinical trials. Several that are proposed are organ dysfunction resolution, long-term outcomes, functional health assessment, quality of life assessment, intensive care unit costs, and biomarkers [39]. These alternative outcome measures will provide a better picture of the true impact of this disorder on the pediatric population.

Summary

It is obvious that sepsis in children provides a real challenge for the practitioner. However, astute assessment skills and collaboration among the entire health care team will promote the best possible outcome for the child. Outcomes have improved dramatically, but more work is still needed.

References

[1] Watson RS, Carcillo JA. Scope and epidemiology of pediatric sepsis. Pediatr Crit Care Med 2005; 6(3 suppl.):S3 – 5.

[2] Watson RR, Carcillo JA, Linde-Zwirble WT, et al. The epidemiology of severe sepsis in children in the United States. Am J Respir Crit Care Med 2003; 167(5):695 – 701.

[3] Stoll BJ, Holman RC, Schuchat A. Decline in sepsis-associated neonatal and infant deaths in the United States, 1979 through 1994. Pediatrics 1998;102(2):e18.

[4] von Rosentiel N, Von Rosentiel I, Adam D. Management of sepsis and septic shock in infants and children. Paediatr Drugs 2001;3:9 – 27.

[5] Bone RC, Balk RA, Cerra FB, et al. Definitions for sepsis and organ failure and guidelines for the use of innovative therapies in sepsis. The ACCP/SCCM Con-

sensus Conference Committee. American College of Chest Physicians/Society of Critical Care Medicine. Chest 1992;101(6):1644 – 55.

[6] Levy MM, Fink MP, Marshall JC, et al. 2001 SCCM/ESICM/ACCP/ATS/SIS international sepsis definitions conference. Intensive Care Med 2003;29(4):530 – 8.

[7] Goldstein B, Giroir B, Randolph A. International pediatric sepsis consensus conference: definitions for sepsis and organ dysfunction in pediatrics. Pediatr Crit Care Med 2005;6(1):2 – 8.

[8] Kleinpell R. Advances in treating patients with severe sepsis: role of Drotrecogin alfa (activated). Crit Care Nurse 2003;23(2):16 – 29.

[9] Cunneen J, Cartwright M. The puzzle of sepsis: fitting the pieces of the inflammatory response with treatment. AACN Clin Issues 2004;15(1):18 – 44.

[10] Okusawa S, Gelfand JA, Ikejima T, et al. Interleukin 1 induces a shock-like state in rabbits. Synergism with tumor necrosis factor and the effect of cyclooxygenase inhibition. J Clin Invest 1988;81(4):1162 – 72.

[11] Ahrens T, Tuggle D. Surviving severe sepsis: early recognition and treatment. Crit Care Nurse 2004; (suppl):2 – 15.

[12] Ahrens T, Vollman K. Severe sepsis management: are we doing enough? Crit Care Nurse 2003;23(5 Suppl): 2 – 17.

[13] Aird WC. Vascular bed-specific hemostasis: role of endothelium in sepsis pathogenesis. Crit Care Med 2001;29(7 Suppl):S28 – 34.

[14] Parker MM, Shelahmer JH, Bacharach SL, et al. Profound but reversible myocardial depression in patients with septic shock. Ann Intern Med 1984;100(4): 483 – 90.

[15] Ceneviva G, Paschall JA, Maffei F, et al. Hemodynamic support in fluid refractory pediatric septic shock. Pediatric 1998;102(2):e19.

[16] Pollack MM, Fields AI, Ruttimann UE. Distributions of cardiopulmonary variables in pediatric survivors and nonsurvivors of septic shock. Crit Care Med 1985; 13(6):454 – 9.

[17] Pollack MM, Fields AI, Ruttimann UE. Sequential cardiopulmonary variables of Infants and children in septic shock. Crit Care Med 1984;12(7):554 – 9.

[18] Carcillo JA, Fields AI. Clinical practice parameters for hemodynamic support of pediatric and neonatal patients in septic shock. Crit Care Med 2002;30:1365 – 78.

[19] Dichter CH, Curley MAQ. Shock. In: Curley MAQ, Moloney-Harmon PA, editors. Critical care nursing of infants and Children. 2nd edition. Philadelphia: WB Saunders; 2001. p. 921 – 45.

[20] Persico M, Barker GA, Mitchell DP. Purulent otitis media – a "silent" source of sepsis in the pediatric intensive care unit. Otolaryngol Head Neck Surg 1985; 93(3):330 – 4.

[21] Stover BH, Shulman ST, Brachter DF, et al. Nosocomial infection rates in US children's hospitals' neonatal and pediatric intensive care units. Am J Infection Control 2001;29(3):152 – 7.

[22] Gray J, Grossain S, Morris K. Three-year survey

of bacteremia and fungemia in a pediatric intensive care unit. Pediatr Infect Dis J 2001;20(4):416–21.

[23] Sarginson RE, Taylor N, Reilly N, et al. Infection in prolonged pediatric critical illness: a prospective four-year study based on knowledge of the carrier state. Crit Care Med 2004;32(3):839–47.

[24] Brilli RJ, Goldstein B. Pediatric sepsis definitions: past, present, and future. Pediatr Crit Care Med 2005; 6(3 suppl):S6–8.

[25] Randolph AG. International sepsis forum on sepsis in infants and children. Pediatr Crit Care Med 2005; 6(3 suppl):S1–164.

[26] Tabbutt S. Heart failure in pediatric septic shock: utilizing inotropic support. Crit Care Med 2001; 29(10 suppl.):S231–6.

[27] Ceneviva G, Paschall JA, Maffei F, et al. Hemodynamic support in fluid-refractory pediatric septic shock. An Pediatr (Barc) 1998;102(2):e19.

[28] Grant MJ. Host defenses. In: Curley MAQ, Moloney-Harmon PA, editors. Critical care nursing of infants and Children. 2nd edition. Philadelphia: WB Saunders; 2001. p. 461–509.

[29] Mollitt DL. Infection control: avoiding the inevitable. Surg Clin N Am 2002;365–78.

[30] Heath PT, Breathnach AS. Treatment of infections due to resistant organisms. Br Med Bull 2002;61:231–45.

[31] Bradley JS. Old and new antibiotics for pediatric pneumonia. Semin Respir Infect 2002;17(1):57–64.

[32] Plotz FB, Vreugendahl HA, Slutsky AS, et al. Mechanical ventilation alters immune response in children without lung pathology. Intensive Care Med 2002; 28(4):486–92.

[33] Carcillo JA. Pediatric septic shock and multiple organ failure. Crit Care Clin 2003;19(3):413–40.

[34] Curley MAQ, Castillo L. Nutrition and shock in pediatric patients. New Horiz 1998;6:212–25.

[35] Brinker D, Moloney-Harmon PA. Hematologic critical care problems. In: Curley MAQ, Moloney-Harmon PA, editors. Critical care nursing of infants and Children. 2nd edition. Philadelphia: WB Saunders; 2001. p. 821–50.

[36] Nimah M, Brilli RJ. Coagulation dysfunction in sepsis and multiple organ system failure. Crit Care Clin 2003; 19(3):441–58.

[37] Barton P, Kalil AC, Nadel S, et al. Safety, pharmacokinetics, and pharmacodynamics of drotrecogin alfa (activated) in children with severe sepsis. Pediatrics 2004;113(1):7–17.

[38] US Food and Drug Administration. Xigris drotrecogin alfa (activated). Available at: http://www.fda.gov/med watch/safety/2005/safety05.htm#xigirs2. Accessed July 5, 2005.

[39] Curley MAQ, Zimmerman JJ. Alternative outcome measures for pediatric clinical sepsis trials. Pediatr Crit Care Med 2005;6(3 suppl):S150–6.

ELSEVIER
SAUNDERS

Crit Care Nurs Clin N Am 17 (2005) 431 – 440

CRITICAL CARE
NURSING CLINICS
OF NORTH AMERICA

Safety in the Pediatric ICU: The Key to Quality Outcomes

Bonnie A. Rice, ARNP, MSN, CCNS*, Carla Nelson, MPH, CPHQ

Quality and Outcome Department, All Children's Hospital, 801 Sixth Street South, Saint Petersburg, FL 33701, USA

A bedside nurse fails to identify a patient before administering a medication intended for another. The pharmacist confuses milliequivalents per day with milliequivalents per liter, and a patient dies of potassium toxicity. Who is to blame for these mistakes? In each case, the health care provider did not mean to harm anyone. Instead of doing the right thing wrong, they did the wrong thing right. Does the doctor, the nurse, or the pharmacist deserve a reprimand? Or did the health care system fail to protect patients by not insisting that all health care providers standardize practice with national guidelines? Why have large health care firms failed to incorporate checklists, redundancy, and prompts throughout processes to eliminate error?

There are significant deficiencies in the ICUs' systems of care delivery, of which bedside practitioners are aware. The process, as it stands, relies on intellect, vigilance, memory, and a hierarchical communication system that has been a tradition since the professions of medical doctor and registered nurse were established. So why are health care systems not as safe as high reliability industries like nuclear power plants or aviation?

Safety within health care delivery is not unique. As James Reason stated in his chapter in the Institute of Medicine's Report *To Err is Human* in 1999 [1], "The users of health care technology (are like any other industry and) bring certain characteristics to a task such as the quality of their knowledge and training, level of fatigue, and careful or careless habits. They also bring characteristics that are common to everyone, including difficulty recalling material and making occasional errors." Human limits and potential for error should be considered during process design in health care. Specifically, at the bedside, systems should reduce reliance on memory, standardize processes as much as possible, and use redundancy (eg, double-checking and checklists) wherever appropriate. Forcing functions should be built into medical technology to assure that steps are not skipped in care delivery, such as patient identification, before care is delivered. Reliance on professional vigilance to prevent errors has not been successful in other industries, and it creates blame, which further divides the health care team.

Nurses often feel that they are in the position of being the last line of defense for all errors that potentially could harm the patient. Rather than a person, the design of standardized processes should guard the patient from medical error with all members of the health care team using evidence-based protocols for common care situations. Error reduction should be focused on process redesign validated by outcome measurement.

The organization has accountability for recognizing the effects of substandard working conditions on health care providers. According to Reason, heavy workloads, staffing ratios, sources of distraction, and inversion of assigned shifts (affecting a worker's circadian rhythm) may affect alertness on the job and jeopardize patient safety [1]. High turnover, downsizing, and temporary workers may all increase the potential for error. Organizational tracking of error rates in relation to staffing patterns and patient acuity enhances awareness of these influences.

* Corresponding author.
E-mail address: riceb@allkids.org (B.A. Rice).

Many invasive and complicated treatment modalities, such as continuous veno-venous hemofiltration (CVVH) and extracorporeal membrane oxygenation (ECMO), have been developed without programming in the redundancy prompts to ensure that the treatment is administered correctly. Until health care is delivered safely and all adverse events are avoided, the concept of quality care cannot be realized. Every stakeholder in the health care system, from insurance companies to hospitals, nursing organizations to pharmaceutical companies, has an obligation to redesign safety into the fragmented maze of health care settings. Without safety designed into every level of the system, human error always will be the source of needless deaths and a waste of resources aimed at palliating medical mistakes after the fact.

With the publication of *To Err is Human* and *Crossing the Quality Chasm*, the Institute of Medicine has put the issue of preventable medical errors foremost in the minds of most hospital administrators. In *Crossing the Quality Chasm*, the Committee on Quality of Health Care in America identified six dimensions of health care quality (Box 1) [2]. Safety is listed as the first dimension, and the other five dimensions cannot be achieved without first providing safe health care. In 1977, Forrest and colleagues [3] delineated four characteristics of childhood that distinguish it as a unique period of life—the four Ds. They are developmental change; dependency on parents and other adults for accessing and receiving health care; differential epidemiology; and demographic patterns [3]. These four Ds add a level of complexity to caring for pediatric patients. Children are dependent upon an adult to communicate signs and symptoms to health care providers and to determine which signs and symptoms merit communication. Children's differential epidemiology influences many aspects of care delivery. For instance, many prescription medications have not been tested

in pediatric populations. Merely adjusting a dosage for the child's size and weight (even a nearly adult-size adolescent) may not be adequate given that children may metabolize medication at a different rate. It is vital to keep this added complexity in mind when dealing with issues in the pediatric ICU (PICU). The dimensions of health care quality and the four Ds of childhood are clearly interrelated.

It is not necessary to redesign the entire care delivery process. It often is preferable not to undertake a project that is too large in scope. It is important to focus on changes that can be made that will result in a small improvement in quality. This strategy is particularly useful when initiating a culture of continual improvement in the unit. After experiencing success on a small scale, the size of projects can be increased slowly.

Health care has long been considered an amalgam of art and science; however, today's health care environment requires that organizations focus on reducing variation. Reduction of variation is a hallmark of quality improvement activities. The greater the number of methods used to complete any task on the unit, the more opportunity there is for variation in the outcome. Accomplishing a task with multiple methods adds difficulty in pinpointing the cause when an unexpected outcome occurs. Not all situations should be treated alike. Specification and standardization are appropriate when the levels of certainty and clinical agreement are high, and the science base is consistent [2].

Standardizing processes and eliminating random variation will allow for analysis of which changes in care result in improved outcomes for patients. It is helpful to use a tool, or model to help quantify the effects of small changes. The Model for Improvement is a useful tool in testing the effects of a change [4]. The improvement starts with building knowledge about the system or process that requires change. The Model starts with three questions:

What are we trying to accomplish?
How will we know that a change is an improvement?
What changes can we make that will result in improvement?

All change does not result in improvement. Without a standardized way to evaluate changes there is no way of knowing if improvement occurred. The Plan, Do, Study, Act (PDSA) cycle is an efficient method for "trial and learning." The three questions and the PDSA cycle form the basis for the Model for Improvement [4]. By applying this model to small changes made in the PICU, it is possible to document

---

Box 1. Institute of Medicine's dimensions of health care quality

Health care should be:

Safe
Effective
Patient-centered
Timely
Efficient
Equitable

how incremental changes in nursing care result in improved outcomes for patients.

Silence kills in the pediatric ICU

Communication begins with respect and creates a reality. As David Berwick points out, "Language does not just classify reality, it creates reality. The creation of a dysfunctional reality by the choice of bad language is a privilege that responsible leaders simply do not have"[5]. Administrators, physicians and nurses are all guilty of communicating poorly at times. As the caregivers at the bedside begin to feel unsafe, they may revert to unhealthy communication patterns. Patterson and colleagues described two common responses when communications become emotional or unsafe. Individuals may become silent and withhold information out of fear, or they may become violent by trying to force others to accept information without question [6]. The option to remain silent does avoid conflict, but it does not meet the advocacy needs of the patient if the plan of care does not address the patient's problems. Violence uses a verbal strategy to control or compel others to refrain from questioning a decision or plan of care. In the medical hierarchy, a superior to eliminate suggestions or opinions about the patient's care uses violence. If communication begins with the belief that everyone at the bedside has the patient's interests as the primary goal, caregivers can feel a sense of mutual purpose. Conversations become safer, and true meaning flows much easier.

An overlooked element when designing and delivering health care is how the patient and family perceive the process. Family-centered care mandates that care delivery processes are examined from the perspective of the patient. In the PICU, this perspective must include the parents or guardian, and possibly the extended family of the patient. Families observe the providers' interactions with the patient and the interactions that take place within the unit. They overhear tidbits of conversations that take place between providers. If a portion of conversation is taken out of context it may seem to be inappropriate, and it may affect the way the entire episode of care, and the manner in which health care organization is viewed.

Using respectful words that stick to the point rather than emotional words that distract from the goal are important when caregivers disagree. Once a caregiver has decided what they believe the patient needs are, staying focused on that goal in a matter-of-fact style is much more effective than silence or violence, according to Patterson and colleagues [7].

According to Silversin and Kornacki [6], one of the barriers to effective communication between physicians, nurses, and administrators is a shift in how effective leadership is viewed in the new health care market. Physicians have valued autonomy in decision-making in the past. Small physician groups essentially were small business owners competing in a marketplace of other small business owners. Physicians had the objectives of representing their own interests in the hospital, competing for resources, and possibly, rallying other physicians against a common enemy. In the current managed care climate, teamwork for physicians becomes even more important. Physicians will benefit from forming a cohesive workforce of administrators, physicians, and nurses in the acute care hospital, which is accomplished through physician leaders building collaborative relationships with all other health care providers in the system. Physicians, nurse leaders, and administrators are encouraged to examine the "old" leadership paradigm and consider if the current leadership model will result in the success of the overall health care system. As Kornacki and Silversin state, "It is not that the 'old' leadership styles are bad, it is simply that they do not work in a new environment" [6].

Communication with parents and patients in the PICU is undergoing change as well. Some suggest promoting the parent to the head of the health care team, because they will be managing the child's illness and medications after discharge. Parents should be encouraged to be present during rounds held at an hour when they can attend easily and interact with the health care team at their child's bedside. Dr. Daniel Sands [8], at Beth Israel Deaconess Hospital in Baltimore, has gone a step further. He has suggested that patients are put in charge of their own health care by providing access to a secure PatientSite website, where patients can view, and be educated on laboratory results and medications, track their own health data, schedule appointments with providers, and even replace office visits with e-mail consultations. In the PICU, parent kiosks can allow parents to view their child's electronic medical record, as well as communicate with family and friends by way of a website that they can set up for their child.

One method that is being used to improve team cohesiveness and assure that all caregivers' concerns regarding patient needs are being addressed is a daily goals worksheet initiated during multi-disciplinary rounds. A daily goals worksheet encourages everyone to "be on the same page" literally, sharing the same goals for each patient, and individualizing care daily to ensure that the team compensates for the variability of each patient's response to illness. Provonost and colleagues [9] developed a daily goal worksheet, and demonstrated a reduction in the ICU length of stay. In their study, which was conducted at Johns Hopkins University, the ICU length of stay decreased from 2.2 days to 1.1 days. The daily goals worksheet was signed by the physician every day on rounds, and all providers—including nursing, respiratory therapy, pharmacist, and consultants—sign the sheet daily to document that they have reviewed the goals. The team can update the sheet if the goals for the day change suddenly.

Another method for improving communication among caregivers is the SBAR method for transmitting data about patient problems. This method is particularly useful when obtaining telephone orders. The SBAR stands for: situation, background, assessment and recommendation. An example that was presented in a lecture by Maureen Bisognano at the 2004 Institute for Health Care Improvement Forum in 2004 [10] is presented in Box 2.

Using an organized communication matrix to relay patient information reduces omission of important data and promotes fully describing the current problem. It also gives the on-site caregiver a chance to recommend the needed level of involvement from the off-site physician.

Communication barriers are one of the biggest safety challenges that face the ICU team. Care provided to a child should be a team effort, goal-oriented, evidence-based, and transparent to the family. Effective communication requires education, self-control, and diplomacy. It is a skill that all individuals in a team must master to realize their full contribution to each patient and family.

Box 2. Situation, background, assessment, recommendation

Situation: "I am calling about John Smith, who is short of breath."

Background: "He is a patient with lung disease, and he has been headed downhill all day."

Assessment: "He has decreased breath sounds on the left, and I believe he has a punctured lung."

Recommendation: "I think he probably needs a chest tube, and I need you to see him now."

Mortality prediction as a quality indicator

The pediatric risk of mortality scores (PRISM) have been used for over 2 decades to predict the probability of mortality based on certain physiologic variables [11]. The scoring is based on the first 12 or 24 hours of data after PICU admission. Individual scores of predicted mortality are not useful; however, populations of patients can be studied and the actual rate of mortality in a PICU can be compared with the predicted rate of mortality based on PRISM scoring. The benefit is that the PICU health care team can assess whether more patients are living to discharge in their ICU over a predicted value based on the physiologic instability of the total population. An unsafe environment would result in a higher mortality than predicted because of deaths from medical error.

Some statistical concepts are necessary to use PRISM scoring appropriately. PRISM scoring is reliable and valid in classifying (at the first 12 hours after admission) whether a child is at high risk for death during a PICU stay. The PRISM score is not an interval level of measurement, but it is a sophisticated ordinal scale (ie, a patient with a PRISM score of 6 is not at twice the risk of mortality as a patient with a PRISM score of 3). The scores do discriminate successfully between children who probably will live or die, but the difference in illness between a child scoring 10 and a child scoring 11 would not be clearly evident at the bedside. Therefore, it is important to focus on the probability of mortality. The probability of mortality calculated from the PRISM score does help to describe how acutely ill a child is, and discriminates well whether a child is at high risk of dying. It is not intended as an indicator to caregivers about the futility of care, or a prediction of probable outcome for an individual set of parents.

Severity of illness adjusted length of stay for the pediatric ICU

Severity of illness as determined by a physiologic scoring system (PRISM) is a valid predictor of length of stay [12]. Comparison of expected length of stay with actual length of stay can highlight problems with discharge criteria or unintended PICU stay due to atypical complications or as a result of medical error.

In the past, it has been difficult to compare the practice patterns of physicians at the provider level [13]. If the comparison is looking at compliance with a guideline (eg, the number of children receiving oral steroids during an asthma exacerbation), a severity of illness measure is not needed. Some situations involving physician variation in practice can be ascertained by comparing higher length of stay with higher hospital charges. Health care providers who have high complication rates, who are not practicing cost-effective care, or who provide inappropriate care (eg, empiric antibiotics for long periods of time) can be identified through these measures. Unfortunately, there is no mechanism to ascertain if the provider's patient population is more critically or chronically ill, which in turn, may drive up the length of stay and hospital charges. Severity of illness risk-adjusted length of stay becomes important in provider groups with unusually sick populations.

Patient identification as a safety issue

"We know our patients." This is an oft-repeated phrase in response to inquiries into patient identification concerns. Another often heard lament is that there is not time to check the identification bracelet every time there is an interaction with the patient; however, improving the accuracy of patient identification remains the Joint Commission on Accreditation of Health care Organization's (JCAHO) number one patient safety goal for 2005 [14]. If health care is to become a high reliability industry, every single provider needs to take the time to follow all procedures regarding patient identification. No pilot ever leaves the ground without conducting a thorough preflight inspection of the plane, and a power check at the end of the runway. Pilots have a vested interest in the plane arriving at its destination, because they want to arrive safely. The same holds true for health care providers. The same sense of urgency is required regarding patients' safety. Reputations, individually and collectively, suffer whenever care is not delivered with the utmost of responsibility.

Patient identification does not need to be a time consuming process, especially with children who are verbal and oriented. At the beginning of each shift it is possible to enter the room and introduce yourself to the child in a manner that elicits a response from the child. "Good morning, how did I end up with Hillary Duff as my patient today?". To this the child will respond that is not their name, and provide their actual name. This type of interaction can provide one identifier—the patient name.

For preverbal patients, using a minimum of two identifiers, (eg, patient name, birth date, or medical record number) is crucial. Infants often are approximately the same size and age and are difficult to distinguish, especially in the case of multiple births. Always check at least two identifiers on every patient.

Patient identification does not stop at looking at the identification bracelet. Open-ended questions should be used to ascertain the correct patient. At admission or whenever the parent is present, questions such as "What is your child's name?" and "And her birthday is?" can determine patient identity. Whenever a patient is transferred to another caregiver within the organization, an identification check should occur. The individual who receives the patient should read the identification bracelet while the caregiver who is relinquishing possession of the patient provides the patient's full name and birth date.

Patient identification encompasses more than verifying interaction with the correct patient. It extends to performing the correct procedure, drawing the correct laboratory sample, treating the correct side or site, delivering the correct meal, and administering the correct medication. Laboratory samples should be labeled when taken, at the bedside. Leaving the patient care area without having the sample labeled increases the risk of error. Patient/parent education is another part of patient identification. Patients and their families should come to expect that every caregiver who approaches the patient checks the identification bracelet. Patients should be so accustomed to having their identification bracelet checked that they should present the bracelet any time a hospital employee enters their room.

Checking patient identification is not a time consuming process. Not taking care to double check patient identification is more costly. One patient who is harmed by an error; wrong medication, wrong sample drawn, or wrong procedure costs more than the time that is consumed in double-checking. Also, error investigations take the nurse's time and the resources of others who are examining the error.

Catheter-related bloodstream infections

Central venous lines have become an essential component of the care rendered to critically ill children. Unfortunately, there are significant risks of infection associated with use during insertion and maintenance.

There may be situations when line infection cannot be avoided. Children using highly invasive technologies, such as CVVH and ECMO, have a much higher risk of catheter-related bloodstream infection (CRBSI) [15]. Children in certain diagnostic categories, such as transplants and other immuno-suppressive illnesses, may be more prone to line infection than the standard PICU population. For most of the population, CRBSI is a preventable nosocomial infection that is financially costly and increases the PICU length of stay [15].

The Centers for Disease Control and Prevention issued Guidelines for the Prevention of Intravascular Devices in 2002 [16]. These guidelines have been controversial because there is a limited amount of research on the benefits of some recommendations in pediatrics. If a PICU discovers the CRBSI rate is running over the National Nosocomial Infection Surveillance benchmarks [17], standardizing the insertion and maintenance of central lines should be attempted. If adult medications can be used off label without a clear understanding of the risks involved [18], it seems prudent to suggest that practitioners within the PICU accept infection reduction strategies if the CRBSI rate is unacceptable, although the benefits have been documented only in the adult population.

Unplanned endotracheal extubations

The airway is the source of most pediatric emergencies. Establishing and maintaining an airway through endotracheal intubation is a fundamental part of critical care for children and infants. Loss of an airway by unplanned extubation can result in a longer length of ventilator dependence, a longer length of stay in the PICU, and increased risk of mortality [19].

Unplanned extubations should be expressed as a rate per 100 ventilator days. When a rate is used, it allows for comparison based on the total volume of ventilated patients. Unplanned extubations can be classified as deliberate self-extubations or accidental extubations that occur when the tube is dislodged as care is being rendered.

Standardization of care should be attempted whenever possible. A procedure for taping the endo-tracheal tube, or techniques for using a commercially available tube holder should be consistent throughout an institution.

Popernack and colleagues [20] performed a prospective, 10-year study that examined the use of a nurse-driven sedation protocol to decrease successfully the unplanned extubation rate. The sedation protocol reduced the number of unplanned extubations without increasing the length of stay in the ICU. This finding suggests that the nurse-driven sedation protocol did not result in oversedation leading to increased time on mechanical ventilation [20]. The infant and toddler population often can extubate the trachea by a sudden turn of the head. A nurse-driven sedation protocol would reduce this behavior until the patient is ready to wean to extubate.

Restraints

A restraining therapy, or restraint, is a treatment aimed at improving a medical condition or preventing complications by restricting a patient's movement or access to his or her body [21]. Historically, restraints have been used in health care to promote patient safety, while maintaining comfort and individual dignity to the extent possible [21]. Restraints may be physical or pharmacologic. A physical restraint is any mechanical device that restricts a patient's movements [21]. Common devices used in the PICU are net beds, arm restraints, freedom restraints, mitts, bubble top beds, and elbow restraints (no-no's). Many organizations use one or more of these devices to protect medical sites. However, the use of restraints has come under increased scrutiny from institutions, external regulatory bodies, and the public [22]. In 2001, the American Nurses Association adopted the position that restraints should be used only when no other viable option is available. When restraint, seclusion, or therapeutic holding is determined to be "clinically appropriate and adequately justified," registered nurses—who possess the necessary knowledge and skill to effectively manage the situation—must be involved actively in the assessment, implementation, and evaluation of the selected intervention [23]. The least restrictive restraint option should be used for the shortest duration necessary [21]. Box 3 lists the American College of Critical Care Medicine's Restraint Recommendations.

There are several alternatives to restraints that may be considered before their application. Diversionary tactics may be used to calm an agitated patient or to redirect a patient's attention. The local environment also might be altered to minimize sensory stimuli.. These may include limiting noise from alarms, avoiding unnecessary arousal of the patient, and scheduling activities during waking hours. Increased vigilance of the patient may allow for the elimination of restraints, and some organizations are using friends and family as "sitters." Other members of the hospital staff also can be used as sitters [21].

Once the decision has been made to use a restrictive device, its application should be completed by an RN or supervised by an RN if applied by another qualified staff member. The application always should be completed in a way that upholds the patient's rights and dignity as much as possible. The

Box 3. American College of Critical Care Medicine's Restraint Recommendations

1. Institutions should strive to create the least restrictive but safest environment for patients in regard to restraint use. This is in keeping with the goals of maintaining the dignity and comfort of our patients while providing excellence in medical care.
2. Restraining therapies should be used only in clinically appropriate situations and not as a routine component of therapy. When restraints are used, the risk of untoward treatment interference events must outweigh the physical, psychologic, and ethical risks of their use.
3. Patients must always be evaluated to determine whether treatment of an existing problem would obviate the need for restraint use. Alternatives to restraining therapies should be considered to minimize the need for extent of their use.
4. The choice of restraining therapy should be the least invasive option capable of optimizing patient safety, comfort, and dignity.
5. The rationale for restraint use must be documented in the medical record. Orders for restraining therapy should be limited to a 24-hour period.
6. Patients should be monitored for the development of complications from therapies at least every 4 hours, more frequently if the patient is agitated or if otherwise clinically indicated. Each assessment for complications should be documented in the medical record.
7. Patients and their significant others should receive ongoing education as to the need for, and nature of, restraining therapies.
8. Analgesics, sedatives, and neuroleptics used for the treatment of pain, anxiety, or psychiatric disturbance of the ICU patient should be used as agents to mitigate the need for restraining therapies and not overused as a method of chemical restraint.
9. Patients who receive neuromuscular blocking agents must have adequate sedation, amnesia, and analgesia. The use of neuromuscular blocking agents necessitates frequent neuromuscular blockade assessment to minimize the serious sequelae associated with long-term paralysis. Neuromuscular blocking agents should not be used as chemical restraints when not otherwise indicated by the patient's condition.

From Maccioli GA, et al. Clinical practice guidelines for the maintenance of patient physical safety in the intensive care unit: use of restraining therapies – American College of Critical Care Medicine Task Force 2001–2002. Crit Care Med 2003;31(11): 2665–76, with permission.

patient or their family should be provided information regarding the need for the restraint. The restraint should be removed easily in the event of an emergency [21].

The critical care team should assess patient readiness for reduction or removal of the restraint at least every 8 hours. This should not be considered a hard and fast rule. Reassessment may be conducted more frequently based upon the patient's clinical circumstances and existing plan of care [21].

The Center for Medicaid and Medicare Services (CMS) guidelines are silent as to the application of their guidelines to pediatric patients. During recent surveys, CMS has insisted to organizations that the same guidelines for adults be applied to children of all ages, in regard to protective measures and documentation. Organizations' policies should be specific regarding nursing responsibilities having to do with restraints.

Medication safety

Elimination of medication errors has proven to be a difficult problem with no simple solution. No single task within the acute care environment has been studied as intensively and standardized. Medication administration guidelines are a central part of any kind of medical training, and yet, it remains the source of significant morbidity and mortality in hospitalized children [24].

Medication administration in children is a complex process in comparison with adults. Many medications must be administered to children in intravenous or liquid form, because they are unable to swallow pills. The process necessitates an adult strength medication be withdrawn and diluted to the appropriate strength for the infant or child. The opportunity for 10-fold errors is high [25]. Most medication errors occur during drug ordering (79%), and involve incorrect dosing (34%), anti-infective drugs (28%), and intravenous medications (54%) [26].

It has been suggested that Computerized Physician Order Entry (CPOE) will reduce medication errors significantly in the pediatric inpatient setting [27]. Unfortunately, CPOE is not a panacea. The software for CPOE must include brand and generic names—with adult and pediatric dosing—and interact with other programs that hold allergies and laboratory information to truly be effective.

Bedside nurses should rethink any double-checking protocol before a medication is administered. All double-checks should be independent; without the presence of the patient's nurse, and take into consideration all pertinent factors about the effects of the medication (ie, instead of just checking a digoxin dose, the patient's identifiers, allergies, other medications, heart rate and last potassium level should be checked). This process is time consuming but could reduce the chance for catastrophe as effectively as having a pilot and copilot in an airplane.

One adjunct to bedside care that might aid nurses in the double-checking process is the personal digital assistant (PDA). PDAs can store readily accessible medication information at the point of care [28]. Some drawbacks of the PDAs are small size (making them easy to lose), small screen size, and a lack of security and compliance with Health Information Portability & Accountability Act guidelines if patient information is stored [29].

The case for transparency

In chapter 3 of *Crossing the Quality Chasm* [2], the Institute of Medicine delineates 10 rules for redesigning and improving patient care (Box 4). One of these rules is the need for transparency, which means that the health care system should make information available to patients and their families so that they can make informed choices regarding their provider or treatment options. Patients' care will remain confidential, but information regarding the performance of the health care system will be widely available. Some states are already posting informa-

> **Box 4. Institute of Medicine's 10 rules to redesign and improve care**
>
> Care based on continuous
>   healing relationships
> Customization based on patient needs
>   and preferences
> The patient is the source of control
> Shared knowledge and the free flow
>   of information
> Evidence-based decision making
> Safety as a system property
> The need for transparency
> Anticipation of needs
> Continuous decrease in waste
> Cooperation among clinicians

tion regarding health care providers and hospitals on web sites for health care consumers.

The idea of transparency may sound frightening to many health care providers, but it ultimately will result in improved outcomes for patients. Trust will be built through public disclosure of results, even of the system's own problems [2].

Atul Gawande notes an excellent example of transparency in his recent article in *The New Yorker*, "The Bell Curve" [30]. He reports on Cincinnati Children's Hospital's efforts at openness regarding their cystic fibrosis program and its efforts to improve. Their initial forays into transparency with their patients tested some patients' loyalty, but is paying off in improved systems and processes of patient care.

Pay for performance is fast becoming a reality. The government is leading the way, and some insurers (eg, Aetna and Blue Cross-Blue Shield), are instituting pay for performance in adult populations across the country [30]. CMS has tied increased Medicare reimbursement to quality data. At the request of CMS, the National Quality Forum (NQF) is planning a workshop in early 2005 on rewarding physicians and hospitals for improving the quality of care [31]. Many providers are uncomfortable with the notion of paying for performance. The flip side of pay for performance is docking pay for mediocrity [30]. When viewed from this vantage point, pay for performance may enhance health care performance. All health care providers want to provide high quality, safe care for their patients. Providers that strive to be the best will be compensated for their drive.

Measurement and analysis of safety and quality

Quality and safety are driving the market in health care. Efforts are accelerating by government, accrediting bodies, large purchasers, and employer coalitions, among others, to track quality at the national, statewide, and provider levels [32]. Multiple entities are influencing this focus on safe care. The Agency for Health care Research and Quality has developed two sets of indicators: quality indicators and patient safety indicators [32]. The Institute of Medicine has developed 20 priority areas for national action to improve the quality of health care. Leaders in the public and private sectors created the NQF as a mechanism to bring about national change by developing and implementing a national strategy for health care quality measurement and reporting [33]. The Leapfrog Group was formed in 2000, and is a growing consortium of Fortune 500 companies and other large private and public health care purchasers. The organization is working to initiate breakthrough improvements in the safety, quality, and affordability of health care for Americans by agreeing to base their purchase of health care on principles that encourage provider quality improvement and consumer involvement. The consortium is made up of health care purchasers that provide health benefits to more than 34 million Americans in all 50 states [34]. JCAHO releases its list of National Safety Goals and requirements annually. Organizations that wish to obtain or maintain accreditation must show that they are meeting these requirements.

Several private organizations also are driving the focus on health care quality and safety, specifically for children. The Child Health Corporation of America is one such organization. It is a network of 41 of North America's children's hospitals, and strives to be a catalyst for continuous performance improvement, through performance improvement and patient safety initiatives [35]. The National Association of Children's Hospitals and Related Institutions (NACHRI) is an organization of children's hospitals with 181 members in the United States, Canada, Mexico, and Puerto Rico. NACHRI promotes the health and well-being of all children and their families by helping children's hospitals measure, improve, and innovate in their service delivery [36].

The Institute for Health care Improvement (IHI) is a not-for-profit organization that is driving the improvement of health by advancing the quality and value of health care [37]. The IHI incubated the National Initiative for Children's Health care Quality, which was founded in 1999 and is an education and research organization dedicated solely to improving the quality of health care provided to children [38].

Summary

Many of the organizations mentioned above have initiatives and indicators that overlap in one or more areas, but the number of indicators of quality health care in children's hospitals has grown tremendously in the past 5 years. Management and use of outcomes data are beyond the scope of the daily activities of the bedside nurse. How does this affect the nurse at the bedside? It is important that nurses be aware of the emphasis that is being placed on health care quality and safety. Safety is the first dimension of health care quality delineated by the Institute of Medicine, and the other dimensions are reliant upon the delivery of safe care. Consumer awareness is becoming a national priority, and all health care providers should be prepared for changes in their day-to-day work. As providers of a service, it is important that health care providers anticipate the needs and demands of their customers (patients and their families). As some states and organizations lead the way in providing information to the public, patients and their families will come to expect information about the performance of hospitals and providers. By anticipating these new expectations, nurses can provide safer service to their patients.

An individual focus on health care safety and improvement also is vital for each nurse in performing his or her daily duties. Once nurses are aware of the safety indicators that are being used to improve children's health care, they can begin to integrate the tools and processes into their daily routines to improve continually the care they provide.

References

[1] Reason J. To err is human. Washington (DC): The Institute of Medicine; 1999.

[2] The Institute of Medicine. Committee on Quality of Health Care in America. Crossing the Quality Chasm: A New Health System for the 21st Century. Washington DC: National Academy Press; 2001.

[3] Forrest C, Simpson L, Clancy C. Child health services research challenges and opportunities. JAMA 1997; 277(22):1787–93.

[4] Langely GJ, Nolan K, Nolan TW, et al. The improvement guide: a practical approach to enhancing organizational performance. San Francisco (CA): Jossey-Bass; 1996.

[5] Berwick D. Introduction. In: Silversin J, Kornacki M, editors. Leading physicians through change. Tampa

(FL): American College of Physician Executives; 2000. p. ix–xi.

[6] Silversin J, Kornacki M. Leading physicians through change. Tampa (FL): American College of Physician Executives; 2000.

[7] Patterson K, Grenny J, Mcmillan R, et al. Crucial conversations: tools for talking when stakes are high. New York: McGraw-Hill; 2002.

[8] Sands D. New Information Technology Can Help Keep Patients Safer. Available online at: http://www.ihi.org. Accessed January 14, 2005.

[9] Provonost P, Berenholtz S, Dorman T, et al. Improving communication in the ICU using daily goals. J Crit Care 2003;18(2):71–5.

[10] Biscognano M, Plsek P. Top ten improvement ideas from 2004: emerging and promising approaches. Presented at the Institute for Healthcare Improvement Forum. Orlando, Florida; December 3–10, 2004.

[11] Pollack MM. PRISMIII: an updated pediatric risk of mortality score. Crit Care Med 1996;24:743–52.

[12] Ruttimanm UE, Patel KM, Pollack MM. Length of stay and efficiency in the pediatric intensive care units. J Pediatr 1998;133(1):79–85.

[13] Spath P. Creating valid profiles of physician hospital practices. Available online at http://www.brownspath. com/original_articles?validprofiles.htm. Accessed January 11, 2005.

[14] Joint Commission. 2005 Patient Safety Goals. Available at: http://www.jcaho.org/accredited+organizations/ patient+safety/npsg.htm. Accessed January 11, 2005.

[15] Odetola F, Moler F, Dechert R, et al. Nosocomial catheter-related bloodstream infections in a pedaitric intensive care unit: Risk and rates associated with various intravascular technologies. Pediatr Crit Care Med 2003;4(4):432–6.

[16] Centers For Disease Control. Guidelines for the prevention of intravascular catheter-related infections. MMWR 2002;51(RR10):1–26.

[17] Centers For Disease Control. National nosocomial infections surveillance system report. Am J Infect Control 2004;32:470–85.

[18] Groopman J. The pediatric gap. The New Yorker, January 10, 2004 [Available online at http://www. newyorker.com].

[19] Sadowski R, Dechert R, Bandy K, et al. Continuous quality improvement: reducing unplanned extubations in a pediatric intensive care unit. Pediatrics 2004; 114(3):628–63.

[20] Popernack M, Thomas N, Lucking S. Decreasing unplanned extubations: utilization of the penn state children's hospital sedation algorithm. Pediatr Crit Care Med 2004;5:58–62.

[21] Maccioli GA, Dorman T, Brown BR, et al. Clinical practice guidelines for the maintenance of patient physical safety in the intensive care unit - use of restraining therapies. American College of Critical Care Medicine Task Force 2001–2002. Crit Care Med 2003;31(11):2665–76.

[22] Kapp MB. Physical restraint use in critical care: legal issues. AACN Clin Issues 1996;7:579–84.

[23] ANA Board of Directors Position Statement, Congress on Nursing Practice and Economics, Reduction of Patient Restraint and Seclusion in Health Care Settings. October 17, 2001. Available at: www.nursingworld. org/readingroom/position/ethics/ctresrnt.htm.

[24] Koren G. Trends of medication errors in hospitalized children. J Clin Pharmacol 2002;42(7):707–10.

[25] Fortescue E. Prioritizing strategies for preventing medication errors and adverse drug events in pediatrics. Pediatrics 2003;111:722–9.

[26] Kaushal R, Bates D, Landrigan C, et al. Medication errors and adverse drug events in pediatric inpatients. JAMA 2001;285(16):2114–20.

[27] American Academy of Pediatrics. Prevention of medical errors in the pediatric inpatient setting. Pediatrics 2003;12(2):431–6.

[28] Rosenbloom M. Medical error reduction and PDAs. Int Pediatr 2003;18(2):69–77.

[29] Cascardo D. Mastering PDA: Small steps can yield big efficiency improvements. Available at: http://www. medscape.com. Accessed January 12, 2005.

[30] Gawande A. The bell curve. The New Yorker, December 6, 2004 [Available at: http://www.newyorker.com].

[31] Troop C. Pediatric measures: looking back at 2004... and ahead to 2005. Child Healthcare Corporation of America. Webcast December 15, 2004. Available at: www.chca.com.

[32] Remus D, Fraser I. Guidance for using the AHRQ quality indicators for hospital-level public reporting or payment. Rockville, MD: Department of Health and Human Services, Agency for Healthcare Research and Quality; 2004 [AHRQ Publication #04–0086-EF].

[33] National Quality Forum. Available at: http://www. qualityforum.org/about/home.htm. Accessed January 3, 2005.

[34] The Leapfrog Group. Available at: http://www.leapfrog group.org/about_us/leapfrog-factsheet. Accessed January 3, 2005.

[35] Child Health Corporation of America. Available at: http://chca.com/about.html. Accessed January 3, 2005.

[36] National Association of Children's Hospitals and Related Institutions. Available at: http://www.childrens hospitals.net/Template.cfm?Section=About_Us. Accessed January 5, 2005.

[37] The Institute for Healthcare Improvement. Available at: http://www.ihi.org/ihi/about. Accessed January 3, 2005.

[38] National Initiative for Children's Healthcare Quality. Available at: http://www.nichq.org/about/. Accessed January 5, 2005.

ELSEVIER
SAUNDERS

Crit Care Nurs Clin N Am 17 (2005) 441 – 450

CRITICAL CARE
NURSING CLINICS
OF NORTH AMERICA

Adverse Responses: Sedation, Analgesia and Neuromuscular Blocking Agents in Critically Ill Children

Lauren R. Sorce, RN, MSN, CCRN, CPNP-AC/PC

Pediatric Critical Care, Children's Memorial Hospital, 2300 Children's Plaza Box 246, Chicago, IL 60614, USA

Managing critically ill children produces many challenges for today's advanced practice nurse (APN). One small part of daily management of critically ill children includes the selection, prescription, and monitoring of sedation, analgesia, and neuromuscular blockade. No guidelines exist for the use of sedation, analgesics, and neuromuscular blocking agents (NMBA) in pediatric critical care (PCC). Although it is simple to memorize the pharmacodynamics and pharmacokinetics of these medications, the use of any one of them in an individual child may result in a new experience for the APN. Additionally, when used for prolonged periods of time, adverse responses that are not seen with time-limited use may present. This article focuses on the adverse responses of moderate- to long-term use of these medications.

Sedation and analgesia are used commonly in critically ill children to relieve pain, facilitate procedures, reduce stress of critical illness, promote ventilator synchrony, and to reduce oxygen consumption [1]. Before using sedation or analgesia, the APN must rule out physiologic causes of agitation, including hypoxemia, pain, hypercapnia, and cerebral hypoperfusion [1]. The clinical condition will guide appropriate medication selection because there is a variety of medications from which to choose. For example, if a child needs sedation for a short time, the APN would select a short-acting sedative. Table 1 shows categories, mechanism of action, and sample medications.

E-mail address: lsorce@childrensmemorial.org

NMBAs also are used in PCC, although less frequently. Indications for use include the following: facilitate mechanical ventilation, facilitate procedures, facilitate treatment of status epilepticus, decrease oxygen demands, assist with control of increased intracranial pressure, eliminate shivering, and maintain immobilization after surgery [2,3]. Two classes of NMBAs are available (see Table 1). Again, the clinical condition of the child will guide appropriate medication selection.

Adverse responses

Tolerance, dependence, and withdrawal

Inherent in the long-term use of benzodiazepines and opioids is the risk of tolerance, dependence, and withdrawal. Tolerance is a decrease in a drug's effect over time or the need to increase the dose delivered to obtain the same effect [4]. This is believed to be related to an alteration at the level or distal to the receptor at the cellular level [5]. Withdrawal is a constellation of symptoms that arise when a benzodiazepine or opioid is ceased abruptly in a patient who has developed tolerance [5]. Physiologic dependence is defined as the continued need for the medication to prevent withdrawal [5]. Psychologic dependency is beyond the scope of this article. With increasing technology and critical illness in children, the incidence of these phenomena is being seen with increased frequency and with other medications, including barbiturates.

Table 1
Medication table

Medication	Activity	Sedative properties	Analgesic properties	Examples
Benzodiazepines	↓ CNS (limbic & reticular formation) by binding to GABA receptor	Yes	No	Midazolam Diazepam Lorazepam
Barbiturates	↓ CNS (reticular activating system) by binding to GABA receptor	Yes	No	Pentobarbital Methohexital Thiopental
Anesthetics	Variable; dependent on the medication	Variable	Variable	Ketamine Propofol Etomidate
Opioids	Inhibits ascending pain pathways, CNS depressant	Some	Yes	Morphine Fentanyl Sufentanyl Hydromorphone
Alpha adrenergic agonist	Stimulates alpha$_2$ adrenoreceptors in the brain stem	Yes	No	Clonidine Dexmedetomidine
NSAIDs	Prevents prostaglandin synthesis	No	Yes	Ketorolac Naproxen
Depolarizing neuromuscular blocking agents	Depolarizes the motor endplate to cause muscle paralysis	No	No	Succinylcholine
Non-depolarizing neuromuscular blocking agents	Binds with cholinergic receptors to block acetylcholine transmission at the neuromuscular junction	No	No	Pancuronium Vecuronium Rocuronium Atracurium Cisatracurium

Abbreviations: CNS, central nervous system; GABA, γ-aminobutyric acid; NSAID, nonsteroidal anti-inflammatory drug.
Data from: http://online.lexi.com/crlsql/servlet/crlonline.

Because critically ill children frequently are on a plethora of medications which may be linked to withdrawal syndromes, determining which medication is contributing to the symptoms may be onerous. Tobias [5] identified signs and symptoms of sedation/analgesic withdrawal to include gastrointestinal disturbances, sympathetic hyperactivity, and central nervous system activation (see Table 2 for specific listing). Dominguez and colleagues [6] studied neonates who had fentanyl withdrawal. Higher total doses of fentanyl and longer duration of use were associated with increased risk of withdrawal. The most frequent symptoms of withdrawal were sleep within 3 hours of feeding and increased muscle tone. Lugo and colleagues [7] studied children and fentanyl withdrawal. Of the children studied, 50% had symptoms of withdrawal; the most frequent symptoms were hyperreflexia, tremors, and diaphoresis. Fonsmark and colleagues [8] studied the incidence of withdrawal in critically ill children who were sedated with midazolam. In this retrospective study, 35% of the children had withdrawal symptoms. A total dose of midazolam of more than 60 mg/kg was statistically significant for the incidence of withdrawal, but length of therapy was not significant. Other investigators have studied opioid and benzodiazepine withdrawal; the incidence was greater than originally considered before the study, and was associated with length of therapy [9,10]. Using the aforementioned information, one may be able to identify children who are at risk for the development of withdrawal and potentially decrease the risk.

Reducing the length of therapy may reduce the risk of withdrawal. In the adult literature, there is evidence that nurse-managed protocols not only decrease length of sedation, but also decrease time on the ventilator, need for tracheotomy, and decrease ICU and hospital length of stay [11]. Additional research showed that performing a daily wake-up from sedation also decreases the amount of sedation used, time on the ventilator, and ICU length of stay [12]. If studied, nurse-managed protocols and daily wake-up from sedation may also demonstrate decreased risk of withdrawal.

Table 2
Withdrawal symptoms

Gastrointestinal symptoms	Sympathetic hyperactivity	CNS activation
Feeding intolerance	Tachycardia	Irritability
Diarrhea	Tachypnea	Hypertonicity
Vomiting	Hypertension	Hyperreflexia
Uncoordinated suck/swallow		Increased wakefulness
Decreased gastric emptying		Tremors
		Sneezing
		Delirium
		Frequent yawning
		Clonus
		Fever
		Inability to concentrate
		Seizures
		High-pitched cry and exaggerated Moro reflex in infants

Data from: Tobias JD. Tolerance, withdrawal and physical dependency after long-term sedation and analgesia of children in the pediatric intensive care unit. Crit Care Med 2000;28(6):2122–32.

Withdrawal therapy

Therapy for withdrawal may be as simple as increasing the offending agent back to the dose that the child was receiving when there was no evidence of withdrawal; however, if the goal is to stop the medication, this approach is not feasible. In weaning medications that have an inherent risk for withdrawal, monitoring for and measuring withdrawal is desirable. A frequently used scoring system was developed in 1975 by Finnegan and colleagues [13] to measure withdrawal in neonates who were born to opioid addicted mothers. It has been used by other researchers to identify withdrawal in children although it was not developed for this purpose and has not been validated in this population. There are other scales that primarily measure withdrawal in neonates and have not been validated in children [4]. Unfortunately, there is not a widely accepted withdrawal scale for children.

With this in mind, it is important to delineate the goal of medication weaning before initiating a modification in care. If the child is receiving sedation and analgesia and will continue to require hospitalization, the goal of therapy will be different from the child who is being prepared for discharge. Collaborating with the team allows for easy identification of goals of therapy. A variety of methods for weaning exists throughout PCC. For example, one method is to wean over the same period of time that the child has been receiving the medication. Another method is to wean by 10% to 20% each day. The weaning process will vary depending on the length of therapy, medication dosages, and goals of treatment. When intravenous (IV) access is being used only for sedation and analgesia, to allow for removal of the catheter and reduce the need for continued IV access, weaning may be done enterally or subcutaneously.

Tobias [14] described nine children who were receiving IV fentanyl and midazolam. A subcutaneous (SQ) catheter was placed, and the children were weaned by way of the SQ route using their standard protocol of weaning fentanyl by 1 μg/kg/h every 12 to 24 hours and weaning midazolam by 0.05 mg/kg/h every 12 to 24 hours. No children exhibited evidence of withdrawal using the Finnegan score. Hydromorphone, morphine, and meperidine also have been delivered safely by way of the SQ route [1,14,15]. Methadone may cause considerable tissue reaction, and thus, is not recommended for SQ delivery [14]. To use this method of delivery intermittently or continuously, increased medication concentration is needed to limit maximum infusion rates [4,15].

Another method of weaning is to substitute longer-acting medications or alternate routes of delivery to simplify care. For example, morphine or fentanyl may be converted to methadone and midazolam may be converted to lorazepam. Conversions from one opioid to another may seem to be the same; however, to the child, it may represent a decremented decrease. To reduce the risk of withdrawal with conversions of opioids, Anand and Arnold [4] recommended converting to an equianalgesic dose for the first 24 hours before decreasing the dose to reduce the risk of withdrawal. Dexmedetomidine has been used in a couple of cases of withdrawal from opioids, benzodiazepines, and illicit drugs [16,17].

The most important element of weaning these medications is vigilance for withdrawal. Withdrawal may occur at any time during the weaning process, and may not develop until several half lives of the medication have passed because of slow decrements in plasma concentration [4]. Identifying the agent associated with the withdrawal symptoms may be possible if medications are being weaned individually instead of at the same time, and if the medications have different pharmacodynamics. For example, withdrawal from a medication with a short half-life likely will become obvious sooner than a medication with a long half-life. To begin to treat withdrawal, identify the contributing agent and provide an additional dose of this medication. Next, adjustments need to be made to the weaning method which may include increasing the dosage or decreasing the interval of delivery.

Specific methods for weaning children from these medications need to be developed individually to account for the child's illness, therapies, and goals for care. Weaning a child from these medications should not complicate the care of the child, but rather, should simplify it by reducing invasive lines and frequency of medication delivery. Regardless of the method selected, it must accommodate the goal of therapy.

Muscle weakness

Muscle weakness is a significant adverse response to NMBAs because it may account for increased mechanical ventilation and the subsequent need for tracheotomy, increased length of intensive care hospitalization, increased length of overall hospitalization, and interim inpatient rehabilitation [18–20], which all result in increased health care costs. Therefore, it is imperative to identify muscle weakness in the critically ill population.

Muscle weakness acquired during critical illness has been well-described in the adult population over the past 20 years [21–23]. A variety of terms has been used to describe this condition, depending upon its features. Critical illness polyneuropathy (CIP) is a commonly used phrase to identify a primarily "distal, axonal degeneration of the motor and sensory fibers" [21] without evidence of inflammation, occurring as a complication of sepsis or systemic inflammatory response syndrome [21,24]. The incidence of CIP among adults who have sepsis is approximately 70%, although an indeterminate link exists [25]. In one study of 830 children who were admitted to the pediatric ICU for at least 24 hours, the incidence of muscle weakness was 1.7%; 57% of these children were transplant recipients [20]. Although the incidence in children seems to be low, this likely is reflective of limited research.

CIP is characterized by normal or prolonged nerve conduction tests, reduced motor and sensory potential amplitudes, fibrillation potentials on the electromyelogram with normal creatine kinase levels, and the demonstration of demyelination on muscle biopsy [26,27]. Clinically, patients who have CIP have flaccid tetraplegia, reduced or absent deep tendon reflexes, and difficulty weaning from ventilatory support [26].

Critical illness myopathy (CIM) is used to refer to the syndrome of muscle weakness that encompasses a variety of conditions, each with its own major pathologic feature [28]. The use of NMBAs and steroids has been associated with the development of myopathy in critical illness [18,19,29].

Thick filament myopathy (TFM) is the type of CIM that specifically is related to the use of NMBAs. This syndrome is described as motor weakness with elevated creatine kinase levels, normal nerve stimulation tests, low amplitude of compound muscle action potentials, low amplitude of motor unit potentials, and loss of myosin of the muscle fiber on biopsy [24,30]. TFM also may be referred to as acute quadriplegic myopathy syndrome in the literature [31]. Clinically, patients who have TFM have weakness which is diffuse and flaccid—including all muscle groups—and they may have altered reflexes [29].

CIP and CIM are described in the pediatric population, but less frequently. Benzig and colleagues [32] described a 28-month-old boy who had a history of reactive airways disease who developed desquamative interstitial pneumonia and required intubation, mechanical ventilation, NMBAs, steroids, and sedation. He developed severe paresis in his extremities that lasted for 6 weeks. His muscle biopsy demonstrated areas of atrophy and terminal axon degeneration. His electromyelogram demonstrated changes that were consistent with neuromuscular junction disorder. The investigators attributed this condition to neurotoxicity secondary to the use of NMBAs. Petersen and colleagues [26] described a 6.5-year-old child who suffered a head injury secondary to a motor vehicle accident. He required therapies for respiratory failure, intracranial hypertension, and subsequent multi-organ system failure that was due to sepsis, including sedation, analgesia, NMBAs, and antibiotics. He developed loss of his deep tendon reflexes which was especially marked in his lower extremities. He underwent electrophysiologic studies which demonstrated reduced amplitudes of the nerves and ongoing denervation of his extremities which were consistent with CIP. Other investigators have described cases of CIP and CIM [20,27]. Although muscle and nerve impairment are evident in children who have been exposed to NMBAs during critical illness, the data remain controversial of direct effect.

Disuse atrophy is another form of muscle weakness, and is defined as atrophic changes in the muscles due to lack of use [33]. It is associated with excessive doses and prolonged administration of NMBAs [34,35]. Typically, disuse atrophy results from immobilization and has no abnormal electrophysiologic findings or elevation in creatine kinase levels [26,27]. Limiting the duration and excessive dosing of these medications may decrease the incidence and severity of disuse atrophy.

Lastly, prolonged muscle weakness is associated with the use of NMBAs. This may result from prolonged use, accumulation of active metabolites of the parent medication, drug–drug interaction, or interactions between the medication and the patient's clinical condition [31]. For example, in a patient who develops hepatic failure, NMBAs that are reliant on hepatic metabolism may build up in the body. In patients who receive NMBAs that are reliant on the hepatic and renal systems for metabolism and excretion, alternate medications should be used if hepatic or renal insufficiency/failure occurs. See Table 3 for medications/conditions that interact with NMBAs.

Identifying muscle weakness is the first step for the APN. Other forms of muscle impairment diseases (eg, myasthenia gravis, Guillain-Barré syndrome, mitochondrial myopathy, etc.) must be ruled out before making the diagnosis of CIM. Unfortunately, there is no therapy aimed at CIP, CIM, or TFM. Treatment is supportive and should be geared toward rehabilitation [36]. Because of the limited amount of information on this topic in children, it is difficult to determine the long-term outcomes. Banwell and colleagues [20] described nine pediatric survivors of critical illness at 3 month after discharge; one child was normal and eight had persistent proximal weakness in the arms and legs. Of these eight, two were unable to walk without assistance; one child was normal by 8 months and one child regained strength but not endurance by 18 months after hospital discharge. In an adult study, of patients who were diagnosed with CIP and CIM, 44% and 48% were ambulatory at 4 months, respectively [37]. Other studies demonstrate an increased risk of mortality in adults who have CIP and severely prolonged weakness up to 5 years after discharge; some patients received NMBAs and some did not [38,39]. Overall, much research needs to be done to determine the relationship between muscle weakness and NMBAs.

Monitoring neuromuscular blocking agents

When using NMBAs, it is necessary to monitor their use to maximize therapy with the lowest dose infusion to minimize potential adverse responses to the medication. The guidelines for sustained NMBAs in adult critical care, which were created by the American College of Critical Care, Society of Critical Care Medicine in concert with the American Society of Health-System Pharmacists, and the American College of Chest Physicians, recommend clinical assessment and the use of peripheral nerve stimulation (PNS) by using train of four (TOF) testing

Table 3
Medications and conditions interacting with neuromuscular blocking agents

Potentiate effects	Antagonize effects
Acidosis	Alkalosis
Antibiotics	Chronic use of
Aminoglycosides (gentamicin,	steroids
amikacin, tobramycin);	Carbamazepine
polypeptides (polymyxin B)	Phenytoin
Other antibiotics (clindamycin,	Theophylline
streptomycin, tetracyclines,	Sympathomimetic
amphotericin B)	agents
Beta adrenergic blockers	Chronic exposure to
Calcium channel blockers	neuromuscular
Antiarrhythmics (quinidine,	blocking agents
procainamide, lidocaine,	Hyperkalemia
magnesium)	Hypercalcemia
Chemotherapy	Hyperthermia
(cyclophosphamide)	
Dantrolene	
Inhalational anesthetics	
(isoflurane)	
Diuretics (furosemide, thiazides)	
Lithuim	
Cyclosporine	
Hypokalemia	
Hypocalcemia	
Hyponatremia	
Hypothermia	
Neuromuscular diseases	

Data from: Grehn LS. Adverse responses to analgesia, sedation, and neuromuscular blocking agents in infants and children. AACN Clin Isssues 1998;9(1):36–48.

in adults [31]. Unfortunately, there is no guideline for pediatrics.

TOF is the simulation of a nerve with four burst stimuli in rapid sequence [3]. The ulnar nerve is stimulated most commonly; however, one also may use the facial, posterior tibial, or peroneal nerves [33]. The response to the TOF is graded according to the number of twitches. Twitch absence indicates 100% blockade, one twitch indicates 90% blockade, two twitches indicate 80% blockade, three twitches indicate 75% blockade, and four twitches indicates less than 75% blockade [3]. In adults, NMBAs should be titrated to effect of one or two twitches [31]; again, a guideline does not exist for pediatrics. This procedure may be done intermittently throughout the day to titrate NMBAs to the desired effect.

Foster and colleagues [40] elucidated potential problems with this method secondary to patient, operator, or equipment issues. Difficulties arise in patients who have edema, the presence of devices (eg, dressings, casts, lines) that impede proper electrode placement, or moist skin which may interfere with impulse conduction. Operators may hamper accurate use of the PNS with improper training, incorrect electrode placement, variability of twitch assessment, and reliability of twitch assessment. Furthermore, the PNS may allow for errors in measurement, including worn wires, low batteries, or dry electrode pads.

Clinical assessment is another way to monitor NMBAs simply by watching for dysynchrony with the ventilator or patient movement. If the patient does not move or breathe over the ventilator, it may be unclear if the patient is 100% blocked or maximally sedated. Performing a once daily drug holiday is another evaluation method whereby the medication is held and the patient is monitored for movement. When the patient demonstrates any sign of movement, an assessment of the length of time to first movement is compared with the known medication duration; an adjustment in medication infusion is made if needed. For example, if a child is receiving pancuronium with a duration of action of 60 to 100 minutes, one should expect the child to move within this time frame if he is blocked appropriately and has no evidence of hepatic or renal dysfunction. If it takes less than 60 minutes for the child to move, he is likely to be less blocked. If it takes more than 100 minutes for the child to move, he is likely to be overblocked. The medication should stay the same if the time frame is shorter or appropriate and the goals of NMBAs are being met. The medication should be decreased if the time frame is substantially greater than the outer limits of medication duration because it is likely that the child is receiving too much medication. Again, the goal is to titrate the medication to the desired effect and minimize the risk of adverse responses.

Decreased gastrointestinal motility

Opioids work centrally and directly on the gastrointestinal tract (GI) mu and delta opioid receptor sites and inhibit smooth muscle motility [41]. Therefore, gastric emptying time is reduced and peristalsis decreases with use [42]. Over time, this may result in constipation. Because tolerance to the GI effects of opioids does not occur, action must be taken to minimize constipation associated with opioid use in PCC.

Common therapies for constipation may be implemented in children who are receiving continuous infusions of opioids in addition to enteral feedings. For example, adequate fiber and water intake is necessary to reduce constipation. In children who are not receiving NMBAs, mobility and encouraging defecation are therapies that may be used. Additionally, stool softeners, laxatives, and enemas may be used to promote defecation. When all of the standard measures have been tried without success, additional therapies may be warranted.

Naloxone, an opioid antagonist, has been studied in adults who have constipation secondary to opioid use. Meissner and colleagues [43] studied adult patients on fentanyl who received naloxone or placebo, and evaluated the amount of gastric tube reflux, incidence of pneumonia, and time to first stool. The subjects who received naloxone had less gastric reflux and lower prevalences of pneumonia; however, there were no differences in time to first stool, ventilation time, length of ICU stay, or fentanyl dosing requirements when compared with those who did not receive naloxone. This study demonstrated that enteral naloxone may be given enterally and not affect the analgesic effects of the opioid. This is believed to work due to the extensive first pass metabolism of enteral naloxone therefore reducing the amount of circulating medication and thus limiting the impact on reversal of analgesia [44]. Lee and colleagues [45] studied the use of epidural naloxone in combination with morphine and their effect on GI hypomotility. Their study demonstrated that time to first flatus and first stool was decreased in adults who received naloxone in addition to morphine in the epidural space; there was equal pain relief in both groups. Some investigators report that the therapeutic window for naloxone is small and limits its use (ie, too much naloxone will reverse the analgesic effect of the opioid and potentially trigger withdrawal symptoms, whereas not enough is ineffective).

Methylnaltrexone is an opioid antagonist that does not cross the blood–brain barrier, and thus, does not alter the analgesic effects of opioids [44]. Multiple studies in adults have demonstrated its effectiveness. Yuan and colleagues [46] evaluated the effectiveness of SQ methylnaltrexone in adults. This study demonstrated a reduction in oral-cecal transit time with SQ methylnaltrexone in subjects who received morphine. Another study done using IV methylnaltrexone demonstrated similar findings and decreased time to laxative response [47]. Yuan and Foss [48] also demonstrated the effective use of oral methylnaltrexone.

Although both of these medications are promising to decrease constipation associated with opioid use, the pediatric data are significantly lacking; however, the information from the adult literature has been extrapolated to pediatrics. There are centers that use naloxone enterally to decrease constipation in dosages from 10 to 20 μg enterally every 8 hours to 20 to 30 μg/kg of weight enterally every 8 hours (S. Suresh, MD, personal communication, 2005). Given the lack of evidence and the wide dose range, it is prudent to start with low dosing and monitor the child for responsiveness. If the child does not respond in 1 to 2 days, increasing the dose may be required. During this time, it is imperative to observe the child vigilantly for withdrawal symptomatology and evidence of pain.

Corneal abrasions

When patients are not able to blink or maintain eye closure secondary to sedation, analgesia, or NMBAs, there is a risk for the development of a corneal abrasion [49]. Therefore, the patient's corneas are at risk for drying, infection, ulceration, perforation, scarring, and possibly the subsequent loss of visual acuity. The incidence of corneal abrasions ranges from 8% to 60% in adult studies [50–53]; however, there are no pediatric data.

In the literature, studies have evaluated protective strategies to reduce the prevalence of corneal abrasion. Cortese and colleagues [53] evaluated the effectiveness of two therapies: lubricating drops in one eye and creating a moisture chamber with plastic wrap over the other eye. The moisture chamber was associated with less corneal epithelial breakdown. Lenart and Garrity [50] compared the application of lubricating ointment with passive eyelid closure. The application of lubricating ointment was superior to passive eyelid closure in the prevention of exposure keratitis and corneal abrasions. Both of these studies were done in adults.

A multi-centered research trial is being done to evaluate the incidence of corneal abrasions and two therapies in critically ill children. Until the results of this study are available, the most important intervention is to maintain eye closure and moisture to reduce the potential risk of corneal abrasions. Monitoring for abrasions and consulting with ophthalmology to intervene upon suspicion of an abrasion is imperative to reduce this potential morbidity.

Cost

Overall, the cost for PCC is expensive. In a study by Chalom and colleagues [54], they determined that the year (1993) cost for children in their pediatric ICU was approximately $17,000,000 with an average cost per day of more than $5000 for a 3-day

length of stay and an average cost per day of more than $2000. Fifty-two percent of these costs were for the room fee, which included personnel and benefits; approximately 18% were for laboratory fees; and 6% to 8% each were for radiology, pharmacy, and respiratory therapies. The highest expenses were associated with the primary organ failure and diagnosis. As one can see here, there is a variety of ways to reduce costs.

The development of adverse effects also contributes to the cost of care. If a patient develops a corneal abrasion, costs will be incurred for an ophthalmology consult, medications, and follow-up care. Reduction of adverse responses can help to reduce costs. Rudis and colleagues [55] demonstrated muscle weakness secondary to prolonged NMBAs in adults resulted in a cost of $66,000 per subject for prolonged mechanical ventilation and increased length of stay. By using TOF testing, one might decrease the amount of NMBAs used (decreased cost of medication), improve neuromuscular recovery time, and improve time to spontaneous ventilation [56].

When it comes to medications, there is a variety of ways to determine cost of sedation, analgesia, and NMBAs. Economic considerations include the cost of the medication, access to administer it (eg, IV versus oral, tubing changes, line placement), cost of side effects (eg, prolonged weakness, withdrawal), and medication preparation [57]. Swart and colleagues [58] found that lorazepam was easier to use for sedation in adults than midazolam. They also found a lower average cost per day of $6.6 per subject for the lorazepam compared with $73.3 per subject for the midazolam. Lugo and colleagues [59] demonstrated an average cost savings of $42,904 for 30 children who were changed from parenteral midazolam to enteral lorazepam. When evaluating medication cost, it is necessary to identify the dosage to be used to achieve the therapeutic goal before determining a change to be fiscally sound. For example, drug A costs $2/mg and drug B costs $20/mg. For the same pharmacological impact, 30 mg of drug A is needed with a cost of $60 ($2/mg × 30), whereas only 2 mg of drug B is needed with a cost of $40 ($20/mg × 2). Thus, calculating cost savings with medications may be complex.

Nurse-managed protocols decrease the length of sedation, ventilator time, and length of stay as well as the need for tracheotomy; these translate into cost savings [11]. Daily wake-up tests also decrease sedation amount and time, and lead to decreased ventilator time and length of ICU stay; these also contribute to cost savings [12]. Decreasing the use of continuous infusion sedation also decreases ventilation time [60]. Randolph and colleagues [61] demonstrated an increased risk of extubation failure when children were more sedated; this increased ventilatory time. Mascia and colleagues [62] studied the institution of guidelines for sedation, analgesia, and NMBAs and the impact on cost and outcomes. They found a decrease in the use of NMBAs, no prolonged weakness, decreased ventilator time and ICU length of stay, decreased mean cost per day for medications, and an apparent improvement in functional outcomes after the institution of the guidelines.

Summary

APNs in PCC have specific challenges to reduce morbidity associated with sedation, analgesia, and NMBA therapies. Critically ill children who require sedation, analgesia, and NMBAs are at risk for a variety of adverse events. The APN as a part of a multidisciplinary team, can establish specific goals of therapy, implement research-based guidelines, perform vigilant monitoring, and implement changes as the critically ill child responds to therapy; this may provide a reduction in the incidents of these adverse responses.

References

[1] Tobias JD. Sedation and analgesia in pediatric intensive care units a guide to drug selection and use. Paediatr Drugs 1999;1(2):109–26.

[2] Tobias JD. The use of neuromuscular-blocking agents in children. Pediatr Ann 1997;26(8):482–9.

[3] Martin LD, Bratton SL, O'Rourke PP. Clinical uses and controversies of neuromuscular blocking agents in infants and children. Crit Care Med 1999;27(7): 1358–68.

[4] Anand KJ, Arnold JH. Opioid tolerance and dependence in infants and children. Crit Care Med 1994; 22(2):334–42.

[5] Tobias JD. Tolerance, withdrawal and physical dependency after long-term sedation and analgesia of children in the pediatric intensive care unit. Crit Care Med 2000;28(6):2122–32.

[6] Dominguez KD, Lomako DM, Katz RW, et al. Opioid withdrawal in critically ill neonates. Ann Pharmacother 2003;37(4):473–7.

[7] Lugo RA, Lee WE, Cash J, et al. Opioid abstinence syndrome in the PICU: frequency of signs [abstract]. J Pediatr Pharmacol Ther 2003;8(3):232.

[8] Fonsmark L, Rasmussen YH, Peder C. Occurrence of withdrawal in critically ill sedated children. Crit Care Med 1999;27(1):196–9.

[9] Carnevale FA, Ducharme C. Adverse reactions to withdrawal of opioids and benzodiazepines in paediatric intensive care. Intensive Crit Care Nurs 2003; 13(4):181–8.

[10] Franck LS, Vilardi J, Durand D, et al. Opioid withdrawal in neonates after continuous infusions of morphine or fentanyl during extracorporeal membrane oxygenation. Am J Crit Care 1998;7(5):364–9.

[11] Brook AD, Ahrens TS, Schaiff R, et al. Effect of a nursing-implemented sedation protocol on the duration of mechanical ventilation. Crit Care Med 1999;27(12): 2609–15.

[12] Kress JP, Pohlman AS, O'Connor MF, et al. Daily interruption of sedative infusions in critically ill patients undergoing mechanical ventilation. N Engl J Med 2000;342(20):1471–7.

[13] Finnegan LP, Kron RE, Connaughton JF, et al. A scoring system for evaluation and treatment of the neonatal abstinence syndrome: a new clinical and research tool. In: Morselli PL, Garattini S, Sereni F, editors. Basic and therapeutic aspects of perinatal pharmacology. New York: Raven Press; 1975. p. 139–52.

[14] Tobias JD. Subcutaneous administration of fentanyl and midazolam to prevent withdrawal after prolong sedation in children. Crit Care Med 1999;27(10): 2262–5.

[15] Dietrich CC, Tobias JD. Pediatric pain. American Journal of Pain Management 2003;13(4):146–50.

[16] Finkel JC, Elrefai A. The use of dexmedetomidine to facility opioid and benzodiazepine detoxification in an infant. Anesth Analg 2004;98(6):1658–9.

[17] Tobias JD, Berkenbosch JW, Russo P. Additional experience with dexmedetomidine in pediatric patients. South Med J 2003;96(9):871–5.

[18] Behbehani NA, Al-Mane F, D'yachkova Y, et al. Myopathy following mechanical ventilation for acute severe asthma. Chest 1999;115(6):1627–31.

[19] David WS, Roehr CL, Leatherman JW. EMG findings in acute myopathy with status asthmaticus, steroids and paralytics clinical and electrophysiologic correlations. Electromyogr Clin Neurophysiol 1998;38(6):371–6.

[20] Banwell BL, Mildner RJ, Hassall AC, et al. Muscle weakness in children. Neurology 2003;61(12): 1779–82.

[21] Bolton CF, Gilbert JJ, Hahn AF, et al. Polyneuropathy in critically ill patients. J Neurol Neurosurg Psychiatry 1984;47(11):1223–31.

[22] Heckmatt JZ, Pitt MC, Kirkham F. Peripheral neuropathy and neuromuscular blockade presenting as prolonged respiratory paralysis following critical illness. Neuropediatrics 1993;24(3):123–5.

[23] Bolton CF. Sepsis and the systemic inflammatory response syndrome: neuromuscular manifestations. Crit Care Med 1996;24(8):1408–16.

[24] Bolton CF. Critical illness polyneuropathy a useful concept. Muscle Nerve 1999;23(2):206–10.

[25] Sheth RD, Bolton CF. Neuromuscular complications of sepsis in children. J Child Neurol 1995;10(5):346–52.

[26] Petersen B, Schneider C, Strassburg H, et al. Critical illness neuropathy in pediatric intensive care patients. Pediatr Neurol 1999;21(4):749–53.

[27] Tabarki B, Coffinieres A, Van den Bergh P, et al. Critical illness neuromuscular disease: clinical, electrophysiological and prognostic aspects. Arch Dis Child 2002;86(2):103–7.

[28] Lacomis D, Zochodne DW, Bird SJ. Critical illness myopathy. Muscle Nerve 2000;23(12):1785–8.

[29] Lacomis D, Giuliani MJ, Van Cott A, et al. Acute myopathy of intensive care: clinical, electromyographic and pathological aspects. Ann Neurol 1996;4(40):645–54.

[30] Danon MJ, Carpenter S. Myopathy with thick filament (myosin) loss following prolonged paralysis with vecuronium during steroid treatment. Muscle Nerve 1991;14(11):1131–9.

[31] Murray MJ, Cowen J, DeBlock H, et al. Clinical practice guidelines for sustained neuromuscular blockade in the adult critically ill patient. Crit Care Med 2002;30(1):142–56.

[32] Benzig G, Iannaccone ST, Bove KE, et al. Prolonged myasthenic syndrome after one week of muscle relaxant. Pediatr Neurol 1990;6(3):190–6.

[33] Grehn LS. Adverse responses to analgesia, sedation and neuromuscular blocking agents in infants and children. AACN Clin Issues 1998;9(1):36–48.

[34] Rossiter A, Souney PF, McGowan S, et al. Pancuronium-induced neuromuscular blockade. Crit Care Med 1991;19(12):1583–7.

[35] Kupfer Y, Okrent DG, Twersky RN, et al. Disuse atrophy in ventilated patient with status asthmaticus receiving neuromuscular blockade. Crit Care Med 1987;15(8):795–6.

[36] Hund E. Myopathy in critically patients. Crit Care Med 1999;27(11):2544–7.

[37] Lacomis D, Petrella JT, Giuliani MJ. Causes of neuromuscular weakness in the intensive care unit: a study of ninety-two patients. Muscle Nerve 1998;21(5):610–7.

[38] Leijten FS, Harinck-deWeerd JE, Poortvliet DCJ, et al. The role of polyneuropathy in motor convalescence after prolonged mechanical ventilation. JAMA 1995;274(15):1221–5.

[39] Fletcher SN, Kennedy DD, Ghosh IR, et al. Persistent neuromuscular and neurophysiologic abnormalities in long-term survivors of prolonged critical illness. Crit Care Med 2003;31(4):1012–6.

[40] Foster JG, Kish SS, Keenan CH. National practice with assessment and monitoring of neuromuscular blockade. Crit Care Nurs Q 2002;25(2):27–40.

[41] Yaster M, Kost-Byerlye S, Maxwell LG. Opioid agonists and antagonists. In: Schechter NL, Berde CB, Yaster M, editors. Pain in infants, children and adolescents. 2nd edition. Philadelphia: Lippincott Williams and Williams; 2003. p. 181–224.

[42] Yuan CS, Foss JF. Antagonism of gastrointestinal opioid effects. Reg Anesth Pain Med 2000;25(6):639–42.

[43] Meissner W, Dohrn B, Reinhart K. Enteral naloxone reduces gastric tube reflux and frequency of pneumonia in critical care patients during opioid analgesia. Crit Care Med 2003;31(3):776–80.

[44] Holzer P. Opioids and opioid receptors in the enteric nervous system: from a problem in opioid analgesia to a possible new prokinetic therapy in humans. Neurosci Lett 2004;361(1–3):192–5.

[45] Lee J, Shim JY, Choi JH, et al. Epidural naloxone reduces intestinal hypomotility but not analgesia of epidural morphine. Can J Anesth 2001;48(1):54–8.

[46] Yuan CD, Wei G, Foss JF, et al. Effects of subcutaneous methylnaltrexone on morphine-induced peripherally mediate side effects: a double-blind randomized placebo-controlled trial. Clin Pharmacol Ther 2002;300(1):118–23.

[47] Yuan CS, Foss JF, O'Connor M, et al. Methylnaltrexone for reversal of constipation due to chronic methadone use: a randomized controlled trial. JAMA 2000;283(3):367–72.

[48] Yuan CS, Foss JF. Oral methylnaltrexone for opioid-induced constipation. JAMA 2000;284(11):1383–4.

[49] Wincek J, Ruttum MS. Exposure keratitis in comatose children. J Neurosci Nurs 1989;21(40):241–4.

[50] Lenart SB, Garrity JA. Eye care for patients receiving neuromuscular blocking agents or propofol during mechanical ventilation. Am J Crit Care 2000;9(3):188–91.

[51] Imanaka H, Taenaka N, Nakamura J, et al. Ocular surface disorders in the critically ill. Anesth Analg 1997;85(2):343–6.

[52] Hernandez EV, Mannis MJ. Superficial keratopathy in intensive care unit patients. Am J Ophthalmol 1997;124(2):212–6.

[53] Cortese D, Capp L, McKinley S. Moisture chamber versus lubrication for the prevention of corneal epithelial breakdown. Am J Crit Care 1995;4(6):425–8.

[54] Chalom R, Raphaely RC, Costarino AT. Hospital costs of pediatric intensive care. Crit Care Med 1999;27(10):2079–85.

[55] Rudis MI, Guslits BJ, Peterson EL, et al. Economic impact of prolonged motor weakness complicating neuromuscular blockade in the intensive care unit. Crit Care Med 1996;24(10):1749–56.

[56] Rudis MI, Sikora CA, Angus E, et al. A prospective, randomized, controlled evaluation of peripheral nerve stimulation versus standard clinical dosing of neuromuscular blocking agents in critically ill patients. Crit Care Med 1997;25(4):575–83.

[57] Jacobi J, Fraser GL, Coursin DB, et al. Clinical practice guidelines of the sustained use of sedatives and analgesics in the critically ill adult. Crit Care Med 2002;30(1):119–41.

[58] Swart EL, van Schijndel RJ, Strack M, et al. Continuous infusion of lorazepam versus midazolam in patients in the intensive care unit: sedation with lorazepam is easier to manage and is more cost effective. Crit Care Med 1999;27(8):1464–5.

[59] Lugo RA, Chester EA, Cash J, et al. A cost analysis of

enterally administered lorazepam in the pediatric intensive care unit. Crit Care Med 1999;27(2):417–21.

[60] Kollef MH, Levy NT, Ahrens TS, et al. The use of continuous IV sedation is associated with prolongation of mechanical ventilation. Chest 1998;14(2):541–8.

[61] Randolph AG, Wypij D, Venkataraman ST, et al. Effect of mechanical ventilator weaning protocols on respi-

ratory outcomes in infants and children. JAMA 2002; 288(20):2561–8.

[62] Mascia MF, Koch M, Midicis JJ. Pharmacoeconomic impact of rational use guidelines on the provision of analgesia, sedation and neuromuscular blockade in critical care. Crit Care Med 2000;28(7):2300–6.

ELSEVIER
SAUNDERS

Crit Care Nurs Clin N Am 17 (2005) 451 – 461

CRITICAL CARE
NURSING CLINICS
OF NORTH AMERICA

Enhancing Sibling Presence in Pediatric ICU

Janlyn R. Rozdilsky, RN, MN, CNCCP(C)

*Clinical Nurse Educator, Pediatric Intensive Care Unit, Royal University Hospital, 103 Hospital Drive, Saskatoon,
Saskatchewan, Canada S7N 0W8*

Four-year-old Jamie stands transfixed and rigid at the foot of his infant sister's crib. She has required intubation and ventilation for an acute viral respiratory illness. Jamie's eyes are wide. His mother strokes his hair, rumpled from a night of sleeping in the family waiting room. You ask if he has any questions. He shakes his head " no" but wants to leave immediately. Before you can reassure him, he is at the door. His mother escorts him back to the waiting area. He does not return for the remainder of your shift.

Samantha, 16 years old, rushes frantically over to her sister's bedside. Her 14-year-old sister, Sibyl, remains unresponsive, still under the effects of anesthesia from surgery to repair internal and orthopedic injuries sustained in a car crash last night. Sibyl's face is puffy and pale, with a few superficial abrasions and bruises. Samantha grabs her mother and cries, "Her face, her face—just look at her face. You said she was going to be okay." You explain the temporary nature of her sister's appearance, and Samantha becomes more upset. Sibyl begins to move and her monitor alarms. Samantha becomes even more distressed and is requested to return to the family waiting area.

Sam has cerebral palsy and yesterday had spinal surgery to correct severe scoliosis of the spine. Sam is intubated and asleep with the help of analgesics and sedatives. His 10-year-old brother, Jason, saunters into the room. He looks at his sleeping brother, then asks if Sam has had any seizures since his operation. The nurse answers that he has not had any. Jason then wants to know why his brother is not awake, and if Sam will be able to have dinner tonight.

Hospitalization of a child dramatically affects the entire family, including well siblings. A critically ill child demands highly technical and patient-focused nursing; how we respond to their well siblings influences the view, the response, and the coping of well brothers and sisters. Although family-centered care is integral to the pediatric settings, the focus often is on the critically ill child and parents. The needs of parents are widely identified [1–8]; however, little has been written regarding the brothers and sisters of the critically ill child. Nurses may overlook siblings and assume parents and other family members are supporting them; however, distraught parents may not have the insight to identify the needs of their well children [9], not know how to explain the situation [10], or even realize that well siblings benefit from being with their ill sister or brother. Siblings frequently remain invisible, are relegated to the waiting room, are rushed in and out, or are sent home with relatives.

Although most pediatric ICUs (PICUs) permit sibling visits [9,11], few have developed sibling policies or educational resources. This results in little staff or parental education regarding well sibling needs and little support for the sibling when present. Integrating knowledge of child development and well sibling stressors, along with understanding of illness and family adaptation, creates a sibling policy that enables PICU nurses to use their expertise and situation to provide holistic care to critically ill children and their family support systems.

Family: the changing center of children's lives

Family-centered care seeks to understand experiences from the perspective of the child and their

E-mail address:
janlyn.rozdilsky@saskatoonhealthregion.ca

family [12]. While families work toward maintaining integrity by supporting each other, each member's actions and reactions have a dynamic influence on roles and relationships within the family [1]. Because parental reactions strongly determine the family's abilities to cope and rebuild after critical illness of a child [1], assessing the impact of parental reactions, along with changes in routine and relationships within the family, is important in facilitating well sibling care.

Changes in parenting behaviors

Admissions to PICU cause a great deal of parental guilt associated with not recognizing symptoms, not seeking care quickly enough, or not preventing the occurrence. Parents are on a " roller coaster" of emotion during this time [1], and often must adjust to an outcome involving some form of loss [1,5]. Not surprisingly, the critically ill child becomes the focus of the parents' lives [1,2,5,13]. Everything else is put aside to protect, to comfort, and to make decisions related to the critically ill child [1–3,6,14] How this obvious stress, grief, preoccupation, and fatigue specifically influence parenting and interactions with well children has been explored only partially.

Changes in parent behavior are a significant source of stress [15–17]. Well siblings perceiving parenting changes of less supervision, less emotional availability, and greater anger showed higher stress compared with those not reporting these changes [10,15]. Greater parental behavior changes were reported by well siblings than by the parents themselves [18]; this indicated that parents are unaware of their own responses when immersed within the crisis of a critically ill child.

Because understanding of illness results from a interplay of educational, social, and cultural influences, parents with limited formal education or who are socially disadvantaged may have less understanding of the complexities of the situation, fewer problem-solving strategies, and fewer resources to cope with their ill child's situation. Therefore, they are less able to support well siblings [8,15]. Lower socioeconomic status of the mother correlates with increased well sibling anxiety [15,19], possibly related to less maternal attention toward well siblings and less ability to assist them through the event [15]. How specific cultural understanding of illness influences parental reactions has not been explored [8]. However, if language barriers, religious beliefs, and ethnic health care practices limit understanding or acceptance of the science and technology inherent in the intensive care setting, ensuing parental stress

and conflict is perceived by well siblings and adds to their stress.

Substitute caregivers

The extra demands of a critically ill child necessitate reframing and reassigning parenting and other family roles and duties [7], especially if the PICU is located some distance from the family home or hospitalization is of long duration. Although substitute parenting is undertaken in an effort to normalize the lives of well siblings [7], these arrangements can produce feelings of vulnerability, uncertainty, and emotional abandonment [15]. Research is unclear on what care arrangements minimize sibling stress. Knafl [20] found that siblings cared for outside their home or by rotating caregivers had increased stress as compared with well siblings who were cared for in their homes by a consistent caregiver. Simon [16] found that siblings who were cared for outside their home by neighbors had less stress than did siblings who were at home with relatives; differences were attributed to the relatives being more upset. Sibling stress also was greater if parents expected well siblings to adjust easily to these changes [20]. Clearly, changes from the usual living situation or routine [15–17] coupled with parental absence can create stress for the siblings.

Sibling relationships

Siblings play an important role in each other's emotional and psychologic development—and aside from parents—form the most long and enduring relationship within a child's life [21]. Sibling bonds before hospitalization influence well sibling reactions. Siblings describing themselves as "best friends" show increased stress levels as compared with those who rated their relationship as less close [16].

Pediatric intensive care hospitalization creates changes within sibling bonds. Carnevale [1] described the parental attachment to the injured child as immediately increasing, and bonds between the other well children strengthened to support each other through the initial crisis and parent's divided attention. At the same time, sibling bonds with the injured child weakened slightly, related to absence from the family unit and fear of losing the ill sibling. Siblings bonds often must be reworked following the critical illness, and may change permanently to protect or distance the ill or injured child.

Given changes in family social structure that produce more one-parent, two working-parent, and blended families, the impact of siblings on one another may be even greater [17,22]. Older siblings provide substitute parenting during hospitalization [2]. How this change in relationship alters future sibling relationships requires further study.

Siblings' perspectives of critical illness

Because there are no studies that explore responses of well siblings to the critical illness of their sister or brother, responses of children with siblings in other acute care settings, and children's general concepts of illness provide the framework for nursing and parental interventions.

Influence of maturation and experiences

Knowledge of growth and development is crucial in understanding well siblings' reactions and planning interventions [9,23–25]. Piaget [26] described understanding as constructed through increasingly sophisticated processes involving biologic maturation, assimilation of experiences, and social interactions. Children's understanding of illness follows a similar maturational pattern of prelogical, concrete logical, and formal logical sequencing [27].

In the prelogical stage, the young child is unable to see self as separate from others, and so react similarly to those around them. Thus, sensing their parents' emotional distress and physical reactions, the child reacts in like manner. Because object permanence has not developed, separation from parents and siblings produces distress; what is out of sight ceases to exist in the world of the toddler. This egocentric perspective places themselves central to world happenings with illness resulting from something immediate in their lives. For the toddler, cause and effect are unclear, and creates "magical thinking" where thoughts influence happenings (eg, not sharing a toy with a sibling can be seen as causing their sibling's illness). Likewise, not thinking about an event can prevent its happening. Jamie, the 4-year-old who was described earlier, wants to leave his infant sister's bedside and refuses subsequent visits as a way of coping with a situation that he does not understand. Unfortunately, hospitalization also may be seen as punishment, especially if parents have used this threat as disciplinary measure [23].

During the stage of concrete logical explanation, the preschooler to early school-aged child begins to distinguish self from surroundings and realize cause and effect. Illness, although not always visible, is something internal with an external cause, such as germs. Wellness is dependent upon conformity to rules, so children may become extremely diligent at routines, such as hand washing. Children understand more than they can articulate, so they need to be provided with information rather than having to ask questions. Although multiple points of view are understood, experience is lacking to determine the validity of each perspective; this results in misconceptions about illness if varying explanations are used.

The formal logical explanation of illness in the older child and adolescent, as in the adult, is grounded in the understanding of physiologic processes. Formal education, and social and cultural factors strongly influence the development of this abstract form of reasoning [23,28]; however, experientially acquired knowledge creates a novice-to-expert progression in conceptualizing illness, and increases perception and problem solving related to illness experiences [27]. Therefore, well siblings with previous illness experiences often have a greater understanding of their ill sibling's situation [27], especially if many of the circumstances are similar [28]. In the third vignette at the beginning this article, Justin, at 10 years of age, demonstrates a mixture of concrete and formal logic. He asks about Sam's seizures, something familiar, but he does not understand the other unfamiliar aspects of Sam's intensive care. Because most well siblings have no previous experience with the PICU environment, information provided by nursing staff and parents influences their interpretation and coping with critical illness.

A mixture of emotions and behaviors

Children are acutely aware of changes in their environment. When well-meaning adults try to shield them from unpleasant situations by providing little or no information, their stress is accentuated [5,15, 29–31]. Because children's imaginations are their strength and weakness, gaps in information are filled with vivid and imaginative pictures that often are more distressing than reality [5,21,29]. The situation—imagined or real—can produce emotional, psychologic, and physical disruptions [24] if coping resources are exceeded. Feelings of isolation and loneliness can be severe [32,33], fueled by diminished attention from parents, substitute caretaker arrangements, and lack of information about what is happening. Physical or emotional separation from parents also can be interpreted as withdrawal of love, abandonment, punishment, or rejection. Diminished attention from parents can lead to jealousy. This can be expressed in statements such as, "My parents pay less attention to me because they love me less" [1].

Feelings of resentment may surface in the form of angry outburst, acting out, and attention-seeking behaviors. Guilt surrounding these new feelings and behaviors only adds to the well siblings' stress and may precipitate regression or reversion to previous coping behaviors. Young siblings may require their favorite blanket or toy, seek more attention, or become withdrawn and cling to parents. Older children may disconnect from friends, depend excessively on parents, and need detailed instructions on previously mastered tasks. Other manifestations of stress in well siblings may include physical symptoms, such as inability to sleep, bad dreams, refusing to eat, overeating, or bedwetting [24,34]. Whether siblings are provided with information is not the question, but when and how this information is shared can add to sibling stress or enable growth within the crisis situation [24].

Sibling presence benefits family adaptation

Family members, including siblings, are not mere visitors but are an essential component of the ill child's life [1]. Sibling presence helps to facilitate family adaptation to hospitalization [15], can help to retain the feeling of "family" [7,33], and helps children integrate a stressful situation into their lives [9,16]. Presence at the bedside helps siblings cope with the intense emotions, stress, and change that are brought about by this event [1,10,11,16,21,31,34,35]. Siblings have an opportunity to see, feel, and touch their sibling, so they can reassure themselves that they really exist [15]; this helps them to dispel fantasies in young children, such as Jamie [5,33]. Being with their ill sibling may assist older well siblings in understanding the changes in their lives, why parents need to be with the ill child, and why parents are acting differently. Understanding can bring increased feelings of control that potentate adaptation and growth in the situation. Shared experiences, even if stressful and unpleasant, can unite a family and produce growth and adaptation within the family [36]. Support and interventions that are aimed at maintaining a functioning family unit will assist with the hospitalized child's recovery and integration back into their family [1].

Nurses caring for critically ill children are situated ideally to lessen the detrimental effects of intensive care hospitalization on well siblings through direct interventions that are aimed at preparing siblings for the PICU environment, and through indirect interventions that are aimed at parental education and support. Development of a sibling policy is instrumental in optimizing the well sibling's presence in the PICU; however, barriers to implementation need to be identified and eliminated for successful integration of siblings.

Sibling presence: a good idea but not on my shift

Despite evidence that supports the importance of including children in any family member's hospitalization, there has been resistance to children's presence in ICUs expressed as concerns of increased nursing time, increased risk of infections, effects on the patient, and psychologic trauma to the child. Whatever the underlying reason, children virtually have been unseen in many intensive care settings.

Children take nursing time

When children's hospitals were established, restricting visitors was a way of protecting them from the undesirable influence of their impoverished environments. With advances in medicine and professionally trained nurses, hospitals became militarily regimented institutions with "doctor knows best" paternalism. Families were relegated to short Sunday visits, least they upset their children and hospital routine [23].

Even now, despite more family-centered initiatives, nursing and medical staff still question the effect of children's presence on workflow [9,10,33] and nursing time [29], and worry about supervision [33,37]. Although there has been little investigation of staff concerns, several studies indicate increased staff acceptance following the experience of facilitated sibling visits; this suggests that reluctance is of habit, rather than necessity [37–39].

Children have infections

Transmission of infection from well siblings to brothers and sisters within the PICU has not been investigated; previous studies within neonatal intensive care settings have not validated these concerns [39–42]. Because most problematic organisms are hospital-acquired or of endogenous origin, the risk of infection from the well sibling should be no greater than from any other visitor, as long as infection-control measures (eg, hand washing) are adhered to (Sharon Cronk, RN, BSN, Infection Control Practitioner, personal communication, 2004).

There is no documentation of the reverse situation of well siblings contacting infection from the ill sibling or hospital setting. Although adherence to isolation precautions decreases the risk of infection, the development of antibiotic-resistant strains of bacteria and pandemics of little understood illnesses (eg, Severe Acute Respiratory Syndrome) raise the question of risk to well siblings. McIvor [43] acknowledged increased risk to infants younger than 9 months of age because of immature humoral immunity. Personal colleagues suggest that siblings who are younger than 2 years of age have little concrete understanding of the situation and immature immune responses, and should be restricted from bedside visitation. Although actual infection risks to well siblings needs further investigation, parents need to be informed of the infection risks to well children that are inherent in any hospital setting, not only the PICU.

It is upsetting to my patient

Studies done in adult intensive care concluded that family presence does not produce any greater physiologic stress, as reflected in vital signs, than other care interventions [44]. It is essential that PICU nurses assess the effects of any interactions—parental, sibling or health care staff—on their patient and implement alternatives if detrimental changes result. For the awake and aware child, sibling visitations help to maintain a feeling of normalcy and routine and foster a sense of caring and family integrity.

There is only one mention of a poorly supervised toddler pulling out a medication line. The resulting consequence was a stricter limitation on visiting by young siblings, rather than an increase in preparation and supervision of the sibling [35].

Children will have nightmares

The main reason cited by parents for limiting children's visits is the desire to protect the well siblings from the sights and sounds of the PICU [9–11,31]. Parents often feel unprepared or incapable of supporting the well sibling because of their own distress or believe that the child is too young to understand or cope [31]. However, this lack of information and the lack of bedside presence leaves well siblings formulating their own interpretations; they often imagine that the situation is worse than reality [21,29].

Simply permitting well siblings to visit without preparation and support may have unintended consequences. Well siblings who visited daily demonstrated greater stress than those who visited every other day or weekly; this suggests that intense contact may be more anxiety producing than reducing [16]. There are few anecdotal reports of children experiencing nightmares after a nonfacilitated visit to an adult ICU [25]; however, children who were prepared for what they saw before visiting a critically ill parent were not frightened but did desire more information [34]. Nicholson and colleagues [35] reported fewer negative behaviors in children who visited an adult ICU following a facilitated visitation program; this suggests the importance of nurse-based interventions.

The desire to protect is echoed by nursing staff that limit or deny sibling presence [9–11,31]. Nurses need to examine honestly whether this is used as a way to protect siblings or a way to shield themselves from the demands and emotions that are generated by children visiting because sibling presence humanizes the critically ill patient [9]. However difficult, providing emotional care for the siblings can provide rewards that are not gleaned from other aspects of intensive care nursing, and provide a way of knowing the ill child though his or her siblings [45]. This points to the importance of providing parents and nurses with education that alleviates their concerns and policies that provide strategies to support siblings at the bedside.

A sibling policy makes presence possible

A sibling policy indicates to families that they are valued and that thought is given to all members of the family. A sibling policy enables the nurse to make sound clinical decisions based on knowledge of growth and development; family systems theory; and current literature applied in a skilled, caring, consistent, and individualized manner—not just bending the rules whenever it seems to be justified [10].

Structured visitation programs have been introduced and advocated by adult and neonatal intensive care areas as a way of increasing staff comfort levels in dealing with children and diminishing resistance to child visitation [11,25,35,37–39]. These programs include a screening for infection, facilitated visits, and a debriefing session after the visit. Although evaluation of these programs is limited, no reports of such programs within PICU were found. This may be due to the PICU nurses' comfort in working with children and broad acceptance of family-centered care within these units. Help from the clinical nurse specialists, child life workers, and social workers may be valuable. Because not all PICUs have these supports and many situations occur during off hours, education of the bedside nurse is essential for ensuring sibling support is available night and day. Sibling policy should be reviewed with

Table 1
A parent's guide to helping children visit in the PICU

Age	How child sees world	Things to consider
Infant Up to 18 months	Afraid of separation from caregivers May be afraid of strangers Upset by changes in sleeping or eating times Watch parents and others around them to see how to react to new situations	Will not remember places or what happens but sense how those around them feel and will react in like manner Try to keep to child's usual schedule Visit when child not tired or hungry
Toddler 1.5 to 3 years	See themselves as center of their world May have magical thinking about why things happen Don't understand much about being sick or hurt Watch parents or others around them to see how to react to new situations Needs usual routines (nap time, snack time) to feel in control May have tantrums, more crying and clinging when stressed Needs space to run and play away from hospital	Keep explanations simple like "your brother has a sick tummy" or "your sister has a hurt head" Tell them nothing they did or thought about caused illness Keep favorite toys or blankets close by to help them feel safe Help them use words to tell about how they feel or ask questions. Give them lots of time to find words. Get them to draw a picture or tell a story about how they feel or what they see Keep time at hospital short
Preschool 3 to 5 years old	May ask many "why?" questions Take words to mean what they know from everyday life. For example, may think a "broken leg" is broken right off as with a broken doll May think that their thoughts or actions caused things to happen (eg, brother is sick because thought they didn't like him or sister is hurt because they bumped them with toy) May have trouble sleeping, eat less, or be active after visiting Only understand a bit of the situation	Keep explanations simple Try not to use scary words like "cut" Ask them about what they are feeling and give them lots of time to get their feelings and thoughts out Drawing pictures or telling stories with dolls or puppets may help Tell the child it is not their fault their brother or sister is sick even if it does not seem possible that they might think that May choose not to visit and use other ways to keep in touch (eg, pictures or videos) Child may respond in matter-of-fact way and want to leave soon Point out familiar things like toys, blanket, book
School age 6 to 12 years	Listens well and beginning to understand more complexity May say they understand to look more grown up May not want to ask questions because they are embarrassed Like to feel in control of situation May be embarrassed if express emotion such as crying Beginning to understand body injury and may have questions about death May remember details but in an exaggerated form May be afraid they will get sick as well	Ask what they know about the situation Provide more information even if don't ask Illustrations may help them to understand May feel guilty about brother or sister being sick or injured because can't help them May want 1 or 2 days to think about visiting and prepare themselves Keep visits short (5 to 10 minutes) in case embarrassed by emotions that are not controlled May benefit from concrete task (hold hand, put on lotion, read story) Point out familiar things like pictures, toys, blanket Let them know it is okay to cry and okay not to visit Let them know that the chance of them getting sick as well is small Keep answers honest. Tell them what you know and don't know.
Adolescent 12 to 17 years	Like to be in control Like to be with friends (peer group) Understand situation as whole and what it means in longer term May look physically grown-up but still need lots of support and understanding	Give them time to prepare for visiting Try to help them keep in touch with their friends if possible Carefully explore what they know and don't know, because they may worry about what others think and don't want to be embarrassed

(continued on next page)

Table 1 (*continued*)

Age	How child sees world	Things to consider
	May have many questions, some with no easy answer Have clear understanding of body injury and may have questions about death	Reactions may be out of proportion with event– may be upset or crying, or not talk at all Encourage them to talk about feelings instead of acting out feelings Try not to give them too many adult responsibilities during this time. They may not want to help with family decisions. Ask them about this. Keep answers honest. Tell them what you know and don't know. Have support persons (social worker, teacher, spiritual leaders) speak with them if appropriate

all parents, even those not asking about well sibling presence, because it introduces the possibility of sibling presence. It also provides time for parents to share concerns about sibling coping and care arrangements, and offers the nurse insight into family dynamics, adaptation, and understanding of the situation. It also may identify financial, travel, and accommodation concerns that require interventions through other resources and agencies.

Helping parents prepare

Preparation for the well sibling should begin with a discussion with the parents because they know their children the best. Although parental perspectives need to be respected, parents often express reservations about how to explain the situation to their children. The nurse can support the parents to do this or provide the previsit preparation for the sibling. Whoever is speaking with the child needs to be honest, even if this is painful. Children, who believe that they are lied to—even as a protective strategy— may develop distrust of the people they love and depend upon the most [24]. It is not necessary to tell everything, but rather to share the seriousness of the illness and understandings of what may happen, including the changes that may result in the well sibling's life. Reassure the sibling that they did nothing to cause the illness, and provide accurate information about the risk of themselves or others becoming ill with the same thing and measures that are taken to minimize the risk [5,24].

Helping parents to prepare for their well child's reactions and questions enables confidence in their parental role. Providing verbal or written information about common reactions of siblings provides examples of how to explain illness and deal with reactions in a developmentally appropriate manner (Table 1). Alerting parents to extreme reactions, such as per-

vasive feelings of guilt, persistent regressive behavior, use of alcohol or drugs, or threats of self-harm, needs to be included so parents recognize maladaptive behaviors and seek early professional interventions. It is essential that verbal explanations reinforce any written material to ensure comprehension where literacy and language difficulties exist.

Health screening

Previsit discussion should include a health screening that focuses on current health, immunization status, and contact with infectious disease. A structured approach using a checklist as a guide ensures that no important information is missed (Box 1). A brief visual check of the sibling can validate there are no "cold" symptoms, rashes, or other obvious exclusionary conditions. Rather than repeating the health screen with each sibling visit, educate parents to monitor the entire family's health, including adult visitors, and inform the staff of any changes before entering the PICU.

If the sibling does not meet the health screening criteria, it is essential that he or she receives an explanation of why he or she cannot visit. Siblings need to be assured that they have done nothing wrong, can visit in the future, and strategies should be undertaken to maintain sibling contact (eg, sending pictures, stories, or videos to be shared).

Offering alternative strategies and a tentative time as to when visiting may be feasible should be provided. Visiting with precautions may be warranted if opportunity for sibling presence is limited, as in end-of-life situations.

Guiding the visit

Parents often may feel hesitant about their abilities to represent the situation accurately and appreciate

---

Box 1. Sibling health screening tool

In an effort to protect the child in PICU from infection, please ensure that the following are asked:

Does the sibling have any of the following conditions or symptoms?

Sore throat
Cough
Runny nose
Fever
Stomach flu (vomiting, diarrhea)
Rash
Cold sore or herpes infection
Impetigo
Open wound or sore

Has the sibling been in contact with any of the following within the past 4 weeks?

Chickenpox or shingles
Mumps
German measles
Measles (rubella or rubeola)
Roseola
Fifth's disease (parainfluenza)
Strep throat
Pneumonia
Whooping cough (pertussis)
Tuberculosis
Hepatitis
Croup
Respiratory syncytial virus
''Colds''

If yes to any, check with physician or Infection Control Practitioner before permitting visit.

---

opmental level and urgency of the situation. For young children like Jamie, presenting information as close to the time of the visit as possible increases understanding and retention. Older children, like Samantha, may benefit from time to think about, ask questions, and psychologically prepare for the visit, which may lessen the emotional outbursts at the bedside. Provision of a handout tailored especially to the older sibling may help them to feel more included in the information process. Sibling decisions not to visit need to be respected but explored for misunderstandings that are leading to fears. The choice of visiting later should be left open to accommodate changing needs and desires (Box 2).

Whenever possible, arrange the first visit when the nurse can give the sibling some attention, guidance, and be available for questions. With 4-year-old Jamie, for example, pointing out familiar and normal behaviors (eg, opening eyes) and familiar objects (eg, a mobile for his infant sister) can help him to feel more secure in a strange environment. Simple explanations of ECG leads as "special stickers" and intravenous lines as a way of getting water when someone cannot drink can reduce fear of equipment. Blood transfusions can be referred to as "special red medicine" for preschoolers who often equate blood with experiences of trauma. Although the most alarming sights (eg, wounds, external fixation de-

---

Box 2. Alternatives to visiting

Children may not want to visit their brother or sister. They should not be forced to visit. Ask them again in a few days because they may change their minds.

Here are some other ways that they can keep in contact with their sick brother or sister:

Choose pictures of family, themselves, or family pet or home to be in brother's or sister's room
Draw pictures of family, pets, and favorite activities to hang in room
Write a letter, story, or poem that describes how they feel about their brother or sister or about what they did today
Tape record stories, songs, or messages to be played for the brother or sister

---

the nurse's assistance. Preparation of the sibling should focus on what they will see, hear, and smell during the visit, including a brief general description as to their brother or sister's level of consciousness, obvious injuries, and invasive tubes and lines. Mentioning that their brother or sister is unclothed may help to alleviate discomfort for older school-aged children or adolescents who are struggling with body image and modesty.

Time should be given time for the well sibling to process this information, appropriate to their devel-

vices, drains) should be covered for young siblings who may not understand their necessity, the fascination of the school-aged sibling with technology may trigger questions about where tubes disappear to, what is under the covers, or the purpose of various equipment. Although answering questions does take up nursing time, how questions are answered is important. Words used with youngsters, such as Jamie, need to be chosen carefully because they can be interpreted in their literal sense. Avoid words with mixed meanings or synonyms, such as "dye" and "die." Death and anesthetized states should not be described as "going to sleep" because the young child then may fear going to sleep.

Keep initial visits brief, usually 5 to 10 minutes. Younger children have limited attention spans. As with 4-year-old Jamie, their concepts of permanence may have them wanting only a quick look to assure themselves that their sibling still exists and then wanting to leave. Older children and teenagers have concerns about how others see them, and may struggle to maintain composure. For them, an initial short visit provides a graceful way out of a difficult situation. Older children also want to appear grown up and knowledgeable so they may not ask any questions and say that they understand when they do not. Encouraging questions can provide the nurse with insight into what meaning the situation has for them and their family. The nurse also needs to anticipate overreaction by adolescents that may be out of proportion and border on hysterics. With Samantha, the nurse's calm demeanor and explanations of why her sister looks the way that she does and how this is expected to improve may dispel fears. Helping her focus on what she can do for her sister (eg, holding a hand or putting on lotion) may provide a channel for her emotions and a moment for her to regain composure.

It is important to address siblings directly—rather than through a parent—to help decrease their feelings of invisibility. During times of stress, sibling's normal feelings of jealousy, rivalry, and hostility may become more pronounced. An adolescent's angry, "You know he isn't the saint everyone is making him out to be" [1] illustrates the need for discussion of overwhelming and conflicting emotions. Acknowledgments of "You must have many feelings and questions about your brother/sister" can diffuse the situation, minimize parental reprimands, and focus attention away from the remark while still acknowledging sibling needs. Encourage parents to respond to the feelings behind the outbursts rather than what was said. Help parents reassure siblings that it is common to have a mixture of feelings during times of stress.

Although structured preparation is ideal, it should not limit the frequency and timing of sibling visits. A few minutes of briefing at the doorway or at the bedside to discuss the predominant sights, sounds, and smells may help the well sibling prepare if formalized preparation is not feasible, such as in a life-threatening situation. Children, like adults, may remember how they were treated more than what they actually were told or saw during stressful times. The nurse must also be able to accept silence—situations where words cannot express the emotional burden that is weighing on all members of the family.

Addressing concerns about death

Obviously, admission to a PICU signifies a life-threatening illness. Well siblings often ask the nurse, sometimes unexpectedly, if their brother or sister will die. Although the nurse needs to be respectful of the parent's decisions regarding how poor prognosis is explained, it is essential that the sibling receive honest answers. The nurse can assist the parents to share with them what is known and not known about the situation. When death is imminent, the nurse can share with parents what is known about children's understanding of death at different developmental levels. Remind parents that school-aged and older siblings probably already know the gravity of the situation having gleaned their own interpretations from overheard conversations, parents' demeanor, previous experiences, and their own observations.

Just as parents need time to say goodbye, so too do siblings. If possible, specific time for brothers and sisters with their parents should be provided, keeping in mind that older siblings may need privacy to express emotions. Give siblings the same opportunities that are offered to parents—the chance to hold infant siblings, or share a last snuggle in bed with an older sibling. Children should never be forced into behaviors. Giving a goodbye kiss may be awkward for the adolescent sibling, so suggesting giving a hand a squeeze or whispering a private message into the dying child's ear may be more accepted by this age group.

Siblings may remember little else but being included in this life event. Understanding of children's concepts of health, illness and death, developmental expressions, and coping strategies may better prepare the nurse for the emotional expressions of grief by the well siblings. Without this, strong emotional reactions of the sibling may be a source of extreme stress for the nurse who already is struggling with not being able to sustain the child's life. Being able to provide effective support by being attentive, calm, and honest during the ill child's death may assist the family bereavement process [46] as well as bring a sense of closure for the nurse.

Creating a child-friendly atmosphere

The hospital can be a frightening place for children. Efforts aimed at creating a child-friendly atmosphere need not be elaborate or costly. If the child is in a private room, inclusion of siblings' names on a family name board gives siblings feeling of inclusion and importance while assisting busy, often changing nurses in caring for the family. The physical atmosphere of the family area should be inviting to siblings. Inclusion of child-sized tables and chairs, movies, books, toys, and drawing materials at different developmental levels can make siblings feel welcome and help pass the time. Families should be encouraged to stay at child-friendly facilities with resources especially for siblings (eg, playrooms, outside play equipment, and communal family areas). This encourages interaction with siblings from other families, and provides much needed opportunities for play and interaction.

If isolation precautions are needed, the use of child-sized pajama gowns as isolation gowns can make the sibling feel more comfortable and provide better protection than a gapping adult gown. If time permits, the sibling can be given isolation masks to decorate. The use of various nose and whisker combinations can lighten the atmosphere; having the parents and health care team wear these creations give the sibling a sense of accomplishment and pride.

Summary

Although nurses provide many types of support to the ill child they cannot overlook the needs of well siblings. Nurses cannot and should not serve as surrogate parents; however, the support and education that they offer can diminish well sibling feelings of loneliness and isolation. Direct interventions that are aimed at helping the sibling prepare for sights and sounds of the setting help them to maintain a sense of control and help them feel included and useful.

Providing parents with research-based insights into the impact of hospitalization on the well siblings helps them to understand the effects of hospitalization, maintain a parenting role, and anticipate stress produced by altered routines. A sibling policy ensures that parents are aware of the possibility of sibling presence, helps them approach discussions with well siblings in a developmentally based way, and provides them with proactive strategies to assist well siblings to cope. For nurses, an understanding of well sibling stressors enhances preparation and guidance given to siblings, and diminishes nurse anxiety associated with sibling presence. A sibling policy provides nurses with a framework upon which to base assessments and ensures that interventions to support siblings are provided at the bedside; these enhance family-centered care.

Although the PICU setting is only a portion of a child's hospitalization, much of the family's adaptation to the illness and the future begins here. Although more research is required to strengthen the evidence to support the effectiveness of such interventions and demonstrate which interventions are most effective, helping to strengthen and maintain the ties that bind children to parents and siblings to each other can only enhance the family's abilities to care for each of its members.

References

[1] Carnevale FA. Striving to recapture our previous life: the experience of families with critically ill children. The Official Journal of the Canadian Association of Critical Care Nurses 1999;10(1):16–22.

[2] Chow SM. Parental stress in critical care [master's thesis]. Saskatoon, Saskatchewan, Canada: University of Saskatchewan; 2003.

[3] Fisher MD. Identified need of parents in a pediatric critical care unit. Crit Care Nurs 1994;82–90.

[4] Giganti AW. Families in pediatric critical care: the best option. Pediatr Nurs 1998;24(3):261–5.

[5] Hazinski MF. Psychosocial aspects of pediatric critical care. In: Nursing care of the critically ill child. 2nd edition. Philadelphia: Mosby; 1992. p. 19–77.

[6] Kirschbaum M. Needs of parents of critically ill children. Dimens Crit Care Nurs 1990;9:344–52.

[7] Mu PF, Tomlinson P. Parental experiences and meaning construction during a pediatric health crisis. West J Nurs Res 1997;19(5):608–36.

[8] Noyes J. A critique of studies exploring the experiences and needs of parents of children admitted to pediatric intensive care units. J Adv Nurs 1998;28(1): 134–42.

[9] Clarke C, Harrison D. The needs of children visiting on adult intensive care units: a review of the literature and recommendations for practice. J Adv Nurs 2001; 34(1):61–8.

[10] Clark M. Children visiting family and friends on adult intensive care units: the nurse's perspective. J Adv Nurs 2000;31:330–8.

[11] Johnson DL. Preparing children for visiting parents in the adult ICU. Dimens Crit Care Nurs 1994;13(3): 153–62.

[12] Saunders RP, Abraham MR, Crosby MJ, et al. Evaluation and development of potentially better practices for improvement of family centered care. Pediatrics 2003;11(4):437–49.

[13] Rennick JE. The needs of parents with a child in a pediatric intensive care unit [master's thesis]. Toronto, Ontario, Canada: University of Toronto; 1987.

[14] Kasper JW, Nyamthi AM. Parents of children in the pediatric intensive care unit: what are their needs. Heart Lung 1988;15:574–81.

[15] Craft MJ. Siblings of hospitalized children: assessment and intervention. J Pediatr Nurs 1993;8(5): 289–97.

[16] Simon K. Perceived stress of nonhospitalized children during the hospitalization of a sibling. J Pediatr Nurs 1993;8(5):298–304.

[17] Small L. Early predictors of poor coping outcomes in children following intensive care hospitalization and stressful medical encounters. Pediatr Nurs 2002;28(4): 393–401.

[18] Craft MJ, Craft JL. Perceived changes in siblings of hospitalized children: a comparison of sibling and parent reports. Child Health Care 1989;18:42–8.

[19] Craft MJ, Wyatt N. Effect of visitation upon siblings of hospitalized children. Matern Child Nurs J 1986;15: 47–58.

[20] Knafl KA. Parent's views of the responses of siblings to pediatric hospitalization. Res Nurs Health 1982;5: 13–20.

[21] Lewandowski LA. Needs of children during critical illness of a parent or sibling. Nurs Clin North Am 1992;4(4):573–85.

[22] Nelms BC. Sibling relationships: more important now than ever. J Pediatr Health Care 1990;4:57–8.

[23] Manworren RC, Woodring B. Evaluating children's literature as a source of patient education. Pediatr Nurs 1998;24(6):548–51.

[24] McCue K, Bonn R. Helping children through an adult's serious illness: roles of the pediatric nurse. Peds Nurs 2003;29(1):47–51.

[25] Pierce B. Children visiting in the adult ICU: a facilitated approach. Crit Care Nurs 1998;18(2):85–90.

[26] Piaget J. Psychology of the child. New York: Basic Books; 1969.

[27] Yoos HL. Children's illness concepts: old and new paradigms. Pediatr Nurs 1994;20(2):134–40.

[28] Kurt SP, Rodrigue JR. Concepts of illness causality in a pediatric sample: relation to illness duration, frequency of hospitalization and degree of life threat. Clin Pediatr (Phila) 1995;34(4):178–83.

[29] Wincek JM. Promoting a family-centered visitation makes a difference. AACN Clin Issues Crit Care Nurs 1991;2(2):293–8.

[30] Klieber C, Mongomery LA, Craft-Rosenburg M. Information needs of siblings of critically ill children. Child Health Care 1995;24:47–60.

[31] Titler MG, Cohen MZ, Craft MJ. Impact of adult critical care hospitalization: perceptions of patients, spouses, children, and nurses. Heart Lung 1991;20: 174–82.

[32] Hopper C. Perceptions of isolation: the impact of critically ill siblings on well children [master's thesis]. Montreal, Quebec, Canada: McGill University; 1994.

[33] Andrade TM. Sibling visitation: research implications for pediatric and neonatal patients. Online J Knowl Synth Nurs 1998;5(6). Available at: http://gort.ucsd. edu/newjour/o/msg/02454.html. Accessed January 30, 2004.

[34] Craft MJ, Cohen MZ, Titler M, et al. Experience in children of critical ill parents: a time of emotional disruption and need for support. Crit Care Nurs Q 1993; 16(3):64–71.

[35] Nicholson AC, Titler M, Montgomery LA, et al. Effects of child visitation in adult critical care units: a pilot study. Heart Lung 1993;22(1):36–45.

[36] Walker CL. Sibling bereavement and grief responses. J Pediatr Nurs 1993;8(5):325–34.

[37] Meyer EC, Kennally KF, Zika-Beres E, et al. Attitudes about sibling visitation in the Neonatal Intensive Care Unit. Arch Pediatr Adolesc Med 1996;150:1021–6.

[38] Montgomery LA, Klieber C, Nichols S, et al. A research-based sibling visitation program for the neonatal ICU. Crit Care Nurs 1997;17(2):29–40.

[39] Moore KS, Coker K, DuBusson AB, et al. Implementing potentially better practices for improving family centered care in the neonatal intensive care unit: successes and challenges. Pediatrics 2003;111(4):450–60.

[40] Hamrick WB, Reilly L. A comparison of infection rates in a newborn intensive care unit before and after adoption of open visitation. Neonat Net 1992;11: 15–8.

[41] Omphenour JK. Bacterial colonization in neonates with sibling visitation. J Obstet Gynecol Neonatal Nurs 1980;9:73–5.

[42] Solhiem K, Spellacy C. Sibling visitation: effects on newborn infection rates. J Obstet Gynecol Neonat Nurs 1988;17(1):43–8.

[43] McIvor D. Should children be restricted from visiting a relative in intensive care? Nurs Crit Care 1998; 3:36–40.

[44] Simpson T, Shaver J. Cardiovascular responses to family visits in coronary care unit patients. Heart Lung 1990;19:344–51.

[45] Benner P, Hooper-Kyriakidis P, Stannard D. Caring for patient's families. In: Clinical wisdom and interventions in critical care: thinking in action approach. Philadelphia: W. B. Saunders; 1999. p. 293–332.

[46] Meert KL, Thurson MA, Thomas R. Parental coping and bereavement outcome after the death of a child in the pediatric intensive care unit. Pediatr Crit Care Med 2001;2(4):324–32.

ELSEVIER
SAUNDERS

Crit Care Nurs Clin N Am 17 (2005) 463–479

CRITICAL CARE
NURSING CLINICS
OF NORTH AMERICA

Current Management of Status Asthmaticus in the Pediatric ICU

Kelly Keefe Marcoux, MSN, CPNP-AC, APRN-BC, CCRN[a,b,*]

[a]Department of Pediatrics, UMDNJ/Robert Wood Johnson Medical School, USA
[b]Bristol-Myer's Squibb Children's Hospital, New Brunswick, NJ, USA

In the past 2 decades, significant progress has occurred in understanding the pathophysiology of asthma. This has led to treatment modalities aimed at the underlying pathology. Guidelines for the diagnosis and management of asthma also have been developed. Despite these advances, asthma continues to be a significant health burden individually, nationally, and globally. Children who present to the pediatric ICU (PICU) in status asthmaticus (SA) are acutely ill and require prompt attention and management to prevent worsening respiratory distress and respiratory failure. This article reviews the pathophysiology, assessment, and management of the child with SA in the PICU to provide the critical care nurse with current information to facilitate optimal care.

Epidemiology

Pediatric asthma is the most common chronic condition in the United States and affects 9 million children who are younger than 18 years of age [1]. In 2002, it accounted for almost 200,000 hospitalizations for children younger than 18 years of age. The loss in productivity related to having a child hospitalized or home sick with asthma is estimated at $1.5 billion per year and has increased steadily in

the past decade [1]. The prevalence of children who have asthma also has increased steadily in the past 2 decades; from 1980 to 1994, it increased 160% in children younger than the age of 5 years, and 74% in children aged 5 to 14 years [2]. In 1994, for children 5 to 14 years old there was an average of 74.4 cases of asthma per 1000 children, and in 1980, there were only 42.8 per 1000 [3]. Children aged 0 to 4 years had the highest rate of emergency department visits, with a prevalence of 100 cases per 10,000 [2].

Despite the high morbidity rate of asthma, mortality is low; however, over the past 15 years, mortality has increased annually to a high of 3.3 deaths per 1 million children [4]. For children who received mechanical ventilation for acute asthma, recent data demonstrate an even higher mortality of 2% to 3% [5]. Pediatric asthma deaths have been attributed to an acute unexpected death in mild or newly diagnosed asthma or the progression of an asthma exacerbation in the child with poor asthma control [6,7]. Rarely, children who are cared for in the hospital die of acute asthma. Disproportionately, there has been a higher rate of African American children who die of asthma, are hospitalized with asthma, and who are afflicted with the disease. In 2000, African American children were almost twice as likely to have asthma than white children and had a mortality that was four times greater [4].

Pathophysiology

Asthma is "a chronic inflammatory disorder of the airways in which many cells and cellular elements

* Department of Pediatrics, Division of Critical Care Medicine, 100 Bayard Street, 3rd Floor, New Brunswick, NJ 08903.
  E-mail address: marcoukk@umdnj.edu

play a role, in particular, mast cells, eosinophils, T lymphocytes, neutrophils, and epithelial cells. An acute asthma exacerbation is an episode of progressive wheezing, cough, chest tightness, shortness of breath, or combinations of these symptoms…" [8]. SA is a progressively worsening asthma attack that is unresponsive to the usual appropriate therapy with β2-adrenergic agents and steroids leading to pulmonary insufficiency.

Historically, asthma has been identified as a disease with a triad of pathophysiologic processes: airway inflammation, edema, and airway hyperresponsiveness. Smooth muscle contraction was believed to be the primary mechanism of pathology in asthma; however, in the past decade or so, inflammation was recognized as the primary underlying pathogenesis, and management is aimed at decreasing and preventing this inflammation [9]. The airway hyperresponsiveness, airway limitation, and respiratory symptomatology that are seen in asthmatic patients can be attributed to this inflammation [9]. Recently, there also has been an appreciation for airway remodeling that occurs in asthmatic patients [10].

Cellular manifestations

The pathophysiology of asthma primarily involves a complex inflammatory cascade that occurs immediately or as a delayed response. Universal features of the inflammatory response in asthmatics include activation and infiltration of the airway by inflammatory cells. The initial or early phase reaction is caused by a stimulus that varies for each individual and each circumstance. Common stimuli include smoke, pollens, house dust mites, chemicals, cockroaches, stress, and infections, particularly viral infections. The immediate response to this stimulus is bronchospasm and smooth muscle contraction caused by the recruitment of various inflammatory mediators within the airway, such as mast cells, basophils, eosinophils, lymphocytes, and epithelial cells. Activation of mast cells releases histamine and leukotrienes, which along with the other mediators, lead to recruitment of eosinophils, neutrophils, lymphocytes, macrophages, and activated mononuclear cells into the airway. Eosinophils, once activated, possess leukotrienes, granular proteins, and oxygen-derived free radicals that can destroy the epithelium [11]. This damage results in decreased secretions and protective barrier dysfunction of the epithelium, and leads to the production of chemotactic cytokines which further increase inflammation [11]. The activated lymphocytes (T helper

cells) secrete cytokines, including interleukins (IL-2, IL-4, IL-5, IL-13), tumor necrosis factor–α, and interferon [10], which further promote migration and differentiation of eosinophils and mast cells into the airways [12]. Other inflammatory mediators which are responsible for bronchoconstriction are prostaglandin, thromboxane, platelet-activating factor, substance P, bradykinin, adenosine, neurokinin, and serotonin (Fig. 1) [13].

If the early phase is not responsive to β2 agonists, then the late phase reaction occurs 6 to 9 hours after the initial allergen exposure, and involves the continued release of these inflammatory mediators and movement of neutrophils, lymphocytes, eosinophils, and macrophages into the airway. This leads to cellular infiltration, airway edema, mucus secretions, subepithelial fibrosis, further airway hyperresponsiveness, bronchospasm, and smooth muscle contraction [14,15]. Without intervention, this results in atelectasis and mucus plugging. The airway is also narrowed as a result of leakage of plasma proteins which leads to an edematous airway wall [15].

The inflammatory changes that occur in asthma—epithelial alterations, thickening of the basement membrane, and submucosal infiltration with activated eosinophils, lymphocytes, and mast cells—occur along a continuum from mild to severe. In fatal asthma, progression of the inflammation is usually present and demonstrated by mucus plugging, hyperplasia of goblet cells, and hypertrophied smooth muscle [4,10]. Airway remodeling, recently appreciated as significant in the pathology of asthma, may be an irreversible process, and the degree of subepithelial thickening may affect disease severity significantly. The pathologic findings of increased basement membrane thickness and eosinophilia found on bronchial biopsy of children who have asthma are consistent with airway remodeling and the results of adult studies [16]. These findings further suggest that airway remodeling may occur simultaneously with chronic inflammation, rather than subsequent to it as is hypothesized generally [16]. These changes may be permanent and occur early in life [17] and lead to persistent airflow limitation that is not responsive to therapy. Based on adult studies, one of the cytokines that is involved in airway remodeling and chronic inflammation is transforming growth factor (TGF)-β type 1 receptor [16]. In a recent pediatric study, the decreased expression of TGFβ type 2 receptor was different for children who had asthma compared with children who had atopy without asthma, although basement membrane thickness and eosinophilia were similar [16]. This suggests that TGFβ may be an important cytokine in differ-

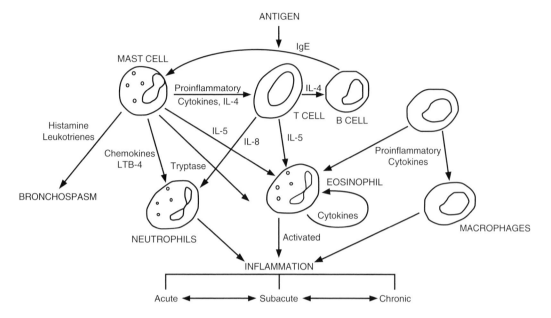

IL = interleukin, Ig = immunoglobulin, LTB = leukotriene

Fig. 1. Cellular mechanisms involved in airway inflammation. *Courtesy of* National Heart, Lung and Blood Institute. Guidelines for the diagnosis and management of asthma, expert panel report 2. NIH Publication No. 97-4051, 1997.

entiating the clinical manifestations of children who have asthma.

Clinical manifestations

The child who has SA has severe airway obstruction that is caused by bronchospasm, airway edema, mucus plugging, and airway hyperresponsiveness that leads to the use of accessory muscles to overcome airflow resistance. This results in increased work of breathing and the signs and symptoms that are associated with it (eg, retractions, tachypnea, shortness of breath, dyspnea). Because of impaired expiratory airflow, there is premature closure of the airway leading to increased functional residual capacity. In an attempt to overcome the "early" expiratory airway closure, the child must generate more inspiratory force to offset the resistance. Inspiratory muscle activity continues throughout expiration to try to increase the forces maintaining an open airway. Inspiration continues at higher, and subsequently higher, lung volumes resulting in hyperinflation and gas trapping. Initially, this increase in lung volume maintains, albeit temporarily, constricted bronchi open. As expiratory time increases,

expiration becomes an active, instead of passive, process that leads to respiratory muscle fatigue.

In the asthmatic, airflow obstruction is not uniform. Inspired air flows to the path of least resistance, so that obstructed alveoli remain so, and the open alveoli continue to receive the airflow resulting in maldistribution of ventilation. This leads to ventilation-perfusion mismatch and resultant hypoxemia. As the child continues to increase work of breathing to overcome airflow resistance, fatigue and respiratory failure ensue. Continued resistance to expiratory airflow will result in positive alveolar pressures at end-expiration, also known as auto-positive end-expiratory pressure (PEEP) or intrinsic PEEP.

Cardiac decompensation also may be evident as a result of changes in pulmonary vascular resistance, intrapleural pressure, and lung volumes during a severe asthma exacerbation. Intrapleural pressures remain significantly negative in spontaneously breathing asthmatic children throughout the respiratory cycle. This can lead to increased left ventricular afterload and increased alveolar/capillary permeability increasing the risk of pulmonary edema [18]. In addition, hypoxia can lead to pulmonary vasoconstriction, which coupled with acidosis and hyperinflation, may lead to increased right ventricular afterload [18]. Hyperinflation can compress the heart, decrease ventricular preload, decrease stroke volume, and result in hypotension (Fig. 2).

Clinically, the cardiopulmonary interaction of a severe asthma attack is evidenced by the presence of pulsus paradoxus. Pulsus paradoxus occurs when increased left ventricular afterload and decreased left atrial preload (caused by a shift to the left of the interventricular septum from right ventricular overload during inspiration) leads to decreased cardiac

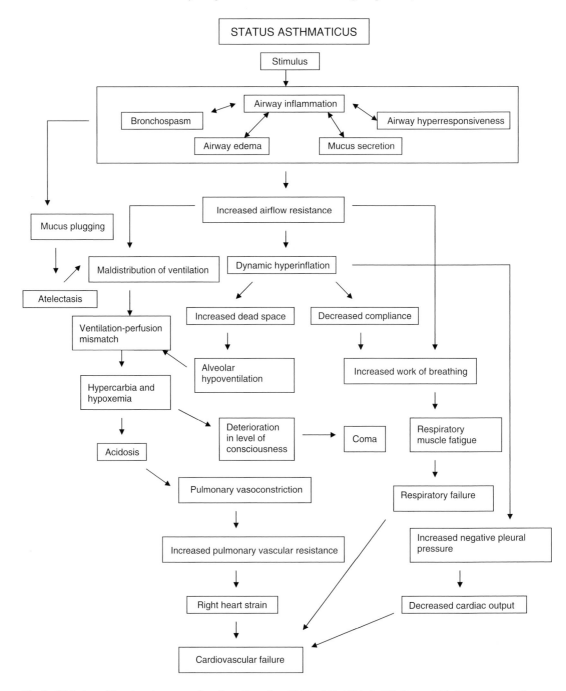

Fig. 2. Clinical manifestations in status asthmaticus. *Data from* Helfaer MA, Nichols DG, Rogers MC. Lower airway disease. In: Rogers MC, editor. Textbook of Pediatric Intensive Care. 3rd edition. Baltimore MD: Williams and Wilkins; 1996.

output with inspiration, followed by increased cardiac output with expiration. In the child who has SA, this is manifested by a decrease in systolic blood pressure with inspiration. An increased pulsus paradoxus is correlated clinically with the severity of the asthma exacerbation [19].

Derangements in acid–base balance and oxygenation also appear in the child who has SA. Initially, hypocarbia ($PaCO_2$ <35 mm Hg) may be present because of hyperventilation; however, as airway obstruction increases, hypercarbia ensues indicating respiratory decompensation due to muscle fatigue and impending respiratory failure. Hypoxemia also may be present; however, it may be masked by the administration of supplemental oxygen. Hypoxemia usually is indicative of impending respiratory failure, pneumothorax, or significant mucus plugging causing lung collapse [12]. The average PaO_2 is 69 mm Hg, and in most asthma exacerbations, hypoxemia is not profound [11]. Initially, respiratory alkalosis may be present, but as fatigue develops, respiratory acidosis occurs. With severe airflow obstruction, metabolic acidosis may be appreciated because of the development of lactic acidosis secondary to tissue hypoxia and lactate production because of muscle fatigue [11]. The combination of hypoxemia, hypercarbia, and acidosis may lead to cardiovascular compromise requiring prompt intervention.

Assessment: clinical scoring, patient history, clinical diagnostics, and physical examination

Clinical scoring

The implementation of asthma scoring systems has improved the assessment of asthma by providing an objective measure of disease severity. Wood and colleagues [20] described the Clinical Asthma Evaluation Score more than 30 years ago as an adjunct to assessment of arterial blood gases in children who have SA to predict respiratory failure. The clinical indicators scored by Wood and colleagues included cyanosis, inspiratory breath sounds, use of accessory muscles, expiratory wheezing, and cerebral function. At the time that this scoring system was developed, PaO_2 was the primary method of ascertaining hypoxemia; however, oxygen saturation measurement (SpO_2) often is substituted for the presence of cyanosis or PaO_2. (Table 1). The Wood scoring system correlates well with $PaCO_2$ and PaO_2 in children who have severe asthma [21]. Since this score was developed, it and other asthma scores have been used to provide an objective measurement of asthma severity, evaluate response to treatment, and predict outcome. Until recently, interrater reliability had not been determined [21–23]. One score recently developed, the Pediatric Asthma Severity Score, is based on three clinical assessments: wheezing, prolonged expiration, and work of breathing. It correlated with objective measurements of pulse oximetry readings and peak expiratory flow rate (PEFR) in children who had acute asthma with good to excellent interrater reliability [24].

Patient history

Information pertaining to the patient's medical history is particularly important in caring for children who have SA. The following information should be elicited from the child or guardian: time of onset; severity of symptoms; precipitating factor; recent increase in medications, particularly β-agonists and corticosteroids; current medication regimen; time of

Table 1
Clinical asthma score

Variables	0 Points	1 Point	2 Points
Oxygenation			
PaO_2 (mm Hg)	70 to 100 in air, or	70 in air, or	70 in 40% FIO_2, or
SpO_2 (%)	95 to 100 in air, or	94 in air, or	94 in 40% FIO_2, or
Cyanosis	None	In air	In 40% FIO_2
Inspiratory breath sounds	Normal	Unequal	Decreased or absent
Accessory muscles	None	Moderate	Maximal
Expiratory wheezing	None	Moderate	Marked
Cerebral function	Normal	Depressed/agitated	Coma

Scores may range from 0 to 10.
A score ≥5 indicates impending respiratory failure. A score ≥7 is consistent with respiratory failure.
Data from Ream RS, Loftis LL, Albers GM, et al. Efficacy of IV theophylline in children with severe status asthmaticus. Chest 2001;119(5);1480–8; and Wood DW, Downes JJ, Lecks HI. A clinical scoring system for the diagnosis of respiratory failure. Amer J Dis Child 1972;123:227–8.

last dose; medication compliance and plan of care; coexisting conditions; and presence of risk factors. Some of the factors that increase the risk of near-fatal or fatal asthma are previous hospitalizations, intubations, rapid progression of asthma exacerbations, severe nighttime wheezing, lack of perception of severity of disease, recent increase in use of β-adrenergic agonists, previous ICU admission, mechanical ventilation, poor access to health care, and exposure to smoke [7,11].

Children who have asthma may have difficulty associating their symptoms with disease severity, and thereby, delay medical treatment and increase their risk of a fatal asthma attack. A study in children who had life-threatening asthma found that by simulating the symptoms of an asthma exacerbation, particularly the increased amount of extrinsic resistive loads, children underestimate the severity of their asthma exacerbation which renders them more likely to have a near-fatal or fatal asthma attack [25].

Clinical diagnostics

Bedside pulmonary function testing

Bedside pulmonary function testing (PFT) should be performed if possible in children who are admitted who have SA. Bedside PFTs should include measurements of forced exhalation—peak expiratory flow rate (PEFR) and the forced expiratory volume in 1 second (FEV1)—on admission and at least daily [8]. Accurate PFTs can provide vital information regarding degree of airway obstruction; however, these tests require patient cooperation, which may limit their use in young children, mentally impaired children, and those in respiratory distress. A PEFR of less than 30% to 50% of predicted is associated with severe airway obstruction [10,12,26].

Pulse oximetry and arterial blood gas

Oxygenation status should be assessed frequently by way of pulse oximetry and possibly arterial blood gas (ABG) measurement. Continuous pulse oximetry is a noninvasive method of measuring oxygen saturation. An SpO_2 of less than 91% indicates significant ventilation-perfusion mismatch. ABGs are not indicated in the child who has SA unless there is significant respiratory compromise or the child fails to respond to escalating therapy. Possible ABG aberrations include hypoxemia due to air trapping, hypocarbia due to hyperventilation, hypercarbia due to respiratory fatigue, respiratory alkalosis, and metabolic acidosis. A normal $PaCO_2$ of 40 mm Hg is abnormal in a child with tachypnea and respiratory distress and indicates a severe attack. Routine ABG

monitoring may be indicated if the child is mechanically ventilated to guide ventilatory management and assess improvement or deterioration.

Pulsus paradoxus

Determination of pulsus paradoxus is an objective, quantifiable, often noninvasive measurement that is used to assess disease severity and should be performed in all critically ill children who have asthma. It is assessed noninvasively by way of auscultation of Korotkoff sounds or by plethysmography waveform analysis from pulse oximetry, or invasively by way of an arterial catheter. Recently, the plethysmography method has proven to be reliable, and at times, a more practical measurement of pulsus paradoxus in children who have acute asthma [19]. A pulsus paradoxus of more than 20 mm Hg usually is indicative of a severe asthma exacerbation.

Laboratory tests

Electrolytes should be obtained at baseline and repeated if indicated. If the child is receiving β-agonist therapy, potassium, phosphate, and magnesium should be followed because decreases may occur that necessitate replacement. Serum glucose should be monitored because the administration of steroids and concomitant use of β-agonists may cause hyperglycemia. A complete blood cell (CBC) count usually is not indicated for SA, but may be obtained if the child is febrile to differentiate bacterial from viral etiology. The CBC count may demonstrate leukocytosis that is due to stress or secondary to the administration of corticosteroids or β-agonists causing a demargination and increase in white blood cells. Measurement of cardiac troponin, creatine kinase (CK), and isoenzyme CK-MB fractions to assess for myocardial injury should be considered in the child who receives continuous β-agonists.

ECG

An ECG may be indicated in the critically ill child who has SA. Possible findings include right axis deviation, "p" pulmonale, and a right ventricular strain pattern.

Chest radiographs

Chest radiographs may be indicated for the child who has SA who requires intensive care monitoring or in the presence of a clinical examination that is suspicious for infection, air leak syndrome, foreign body, or other cause of wheezing. The chest radiograph in an asthmatic without any other etiology may be normal or demonstrate hyperinflation (Fig. 3). Typically, it reveals hyperexpanded lungs as evi-

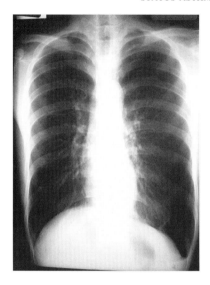

Fig. 3. Radiograph of child with status asthmaticus.

denced by flattened diaphragms and narrowed cardiac silhouette and mediastinum. There also may be areas of segmental or subsegmental atelectasis due to mucus plugging or smooth muscle hypertrophy, as well as thickening of the central bronchial wall. It is important to assess the radiograph to exclude other acute abnormalities, particularly if the child is not responding to escalating therapies.

Physical examination

Presentation

The clinical manifestations of a child presenting with an acute severe asthma exacerbation include wheezing, coughing, increased work of breathing, anxiety, tachypnea, tachycardia, pulsus paradoxus, and dyspnea. As respiratory failure ensues, diaphoresis, cyanosis, decreased level of consciousness, and markedly decreased or absent breath sounds will become apparent. Although audible wheezing is an integral symptom of an acute asthmatic event indicating sufficient airflow to cause turbulence and vibration, it is not a sensitive indicator of airway narrowing; its absence is a far more ominous sign which indicates impending respiratory failure. If the child becomes hypoxic or hypercarbic, he may become agitated, confused, and eventually obtunded.

Physical examination

The initial approach to any critically ill child includes an assessment of general appearance. For an asthmatic, this includes their mentation, use of accessory muscles, skin color, fatigue, ability to speak and

breathe simultaneously, body position, and presence of diaphoresis. Assessment of the asthmatic includes frequent monitoring of vital signs, particularly respiratory rate and heart rate; breath sounds, including presence, type, and quality of aeration; and symmetry of chest wall movement. It is important to reassess these parameters to monitor response to treatment on an ongoing basis. Further measurements should include pulse oximetry, PFTs, and the presence of pulsus paradoxus.

Management: pharmacologic and clinical management

The National Asthma Education and Prevention Program (NAEPP) established guidelines for asthma management in 1991, which were updated most recently in 2002 [10]. These guidelines provide a classification of asthma based on disease severity determined by patient symptomatology, measurement of pulmonary function, and outline recommended management. Asthma can be viewed as a disease on a continuum ranging from an acute exacerbation in which symptoms are reversed rapidly with bronchodilators, to a chronic condition that is characterized by inflammation and treated with anti-inflammatory medications, and finally to a disease of airway remodeling for which there is no defined treatment [10]. Its severity and sequence of symptoms can vary greatly among and between patients. For this article, acute management is focused on the child who has been treated in the emergency department (ED) and presents to the PICU with continued or worsening respiratory distress. Indications for admitting a child who has SA to a PICU include: history of mechanical ventilation, near-fatal asthma attack, inability to speak in full sentences, decreased level of consciousness, inaudible breath sounds, supplemental oxygen to maintain SpO_2 greater than 95%, $PaCO_2$ of greater than 40 mmHg, metabolic acidosis, lactic acidosis, air leak syndromes, ECG abnormalities, or if there is no improvement after β-agonist therapy (intermittent or continuous) and systemic steroids [12,27].

There has been an increase in the development and implementation of algorithms and critical care pathways for the management of asthma. These are helpful in identifying those patients who require hospitalization, particularly intensive care, and can streamline medical management and provide a cost savings [28]; however, they are no substitute for clinical judgment. Every child who is admitted to the PICU with SA should receive standard treatment, including oxygen, β-adrenergic therapy, corticosteroids, and anticholinergic medication as indicated. If the child does not improve with these initial therapies, management may escalate to include additional β-adrenergic medications, magnesium sulfate, methylxanthines, a mixture of helium and oxygen, invasive or noninvasive mechanical ventilation, anesthetic gases, and finally, extracorporeal support (Table 2).

Oxygen

Supplemental humidified oxygen should be administered to children who have SA to treat the ventilation-perfusion mismatch and maintain oxygen saturation at greater than 90% [10]. Oxygen is effective in improving the delivery of oxygen to peripheral tissues, promoting bronchodilation, and decreasing pulmonary vasoconstriction.

β-Adrenergic agonists

β-Adrenergic agonists are the first-line agent in the management of SA. Common β−agonists include epinephrine, albuterol, levalbuterol, isoproterenol, and terbutaline. β-Agonists that are selective for $β_2$ receptors (eg, albuterol, levalbuterol, terbutaline) are preferred to avoid the stimulation of the $β_1$ cardiac receptors. Stimulation of $β_2$ receptors on airway smooth muscle leads to smooth muscle relaxation and bronchodilation, reduces airway edema, and improves mucociliary clearance. Although these medications are selective for $β_2$ receptors, they may stimulate $β_1$ receptors and cause cardiac side effects, such as tachycardia, palpitations, arrhythmias, and myocardial ischemia.

In the United States, albuterol is the most commonly administered $β_2$ agonist in SA. It is administered by way of nebulization, either intermittently or continuously. Studies have found continuous or high-dose frequently administered albuterol, to be more efficacious [29] and superior to intermittent dosing. It decreases the rate of hospitalization and improves pulmonary function [6,30] without increasing the risk of cardiotoxicity [31]. Other advantages of continuous administration include more consistent medication delivery and a reduction in labor time and costs [30,32]. Continuous albuterol usually starts at 0.5 mg/kg/h [10] with a total dose range of 5 mg/h to 20 mg/h [33]. Alternative nebulized β-agonists include isoproterenol or terbutaline.

Albuterol is a racemic mixture of equal parts of R-isomer and S-isomer. The R-isomer, or the racemic isomer, is responsible for bronchodilation, whereas the S-isomer, once believed to be inert, may exaggerate airway hyperresponsiveness and possess proinflammatory properties [12,18]. S-albuterol metabolizes more slowly than R-albuterol, and may accumulate with frequent and repeated use of albuterol; this may increase the side effects. Recently, levalbuterol, which is the R-isomer, has been investigated as an alternative to albuterol. It decreased the rate of hospital admissions in children who presented to the ED with asthma, although it did not alter the length of inpatient stay or differ in adverse effects when compared with racemic albuterol [34]. It is approximately four times more expensive than racemic albuterol for equipotent doses [26]. It is not used routinely in the PICU pending further research on its advantages over albuterol in this setting.

Factors that affect medication delivery by way of nebulization include the patient's tidal volume, breathing pattern, and the gas flow of the nebulizer. To ensure optimal distribution to the alveoli, the flow rate of the nebulizer should be driven by oxygen and set to at least 10 to 12 L/min to decrease aerosol particle size [18]. Some patients may not improve with nebulized β-agonist therapy because of significant airway obstruction and mucus plugging which prevent the aerosol from reaching the distal airways. An alternative method of administration should be considered. Although intravenous (IV) albuterol is available in other countries, terbutaline is the most commonly administered IV β-agonist agent in the United States. Terbutaline is administered IV with a loading dose of 10 μg/kg over 10 minutes, followed by a continuous infusion of 0.4 μg/kg/min increasing in increments of 0.2 μg/kg/min to effect or to the appearance of adverse effects. Tachycardia, arrhythmias, and ST segment changes may be noted with the use of β-adrenergic agonists so prudent monitoring of ECG is warranted. Recent studies have not demonstrated any significant cardiac toxicity, as evidenced by cardiac troponin levels, ECG, or cardiac enzymes, in critically ill asthmatic children who received IV terbutaline [35,36]. IV isoproterenol has limited use in SA because of significant side effects, including myocardial ischemia, myocardial necrosis, cardiac toxicity, dysrhythmias, and death. In addition, epinephrine is no longer recommended in the management of SA because of its significant cardiac effects compared with equally efficacious nebulized agents [10].

Major side effects of β-agonists are primarily cardiovascular and include tachycardia, arrhythmias, hypertension, hypotension, and increased QTc interval. Other side effects include tremor, hypokalemia, nausea, headache, and worsened ventilation-perfusion mismatch [7,12]. Ventilation-perfusion mismatch may worsen initially as a result of the vasodilating effects of β−agonists, including perfusion to low ven-

Table 2
Medications for treating SA in the pediatric ICU

Medications	Dosage	Comments
Standard medications		
β-adrenergic agonists		
Albuterol Nebulizer solution 0.5% (5 mg/mL)	Intermittent: 0.15 mg/kg/dose (minimum 2.5 mg, maximum 5 mg) every 20 min × 3 doses; then 0.15–0.3 mg/kg (maximum 10 mg) every 1–4 hours. Continuous: 0.5 mg/kg/h, range 5–20 mg/kg.	Continuous nebulization is often preferred in the PICU, although frequent intermittent dosing is also effective.
MDI (90 μg/puff)	4–8 puffs every 20 min × 3 doses; then every 1–4 hours as needed.	MDI is as effective as nebulization, but not usually practical in the PICU.
Terbutaline 0.1% (1 mg/mL)	Nebulizer: 0.3 mg/kg (maximum 5 mg) every 20 min × 3 doses; continuous 2–4 mg/h. SC: 0.01 mg/kg (maximum 0.3 mg) every 20 min × 3. IV: loading dose 10 μg/kg, followed by infusion 0.4 μg/kg/min; increase by 0.2 μg/kg/min up to 3–6 μg/kg/min.	Titrate IV dose to effect or the appearance of adverse side effects.
Levalbuterol (R-albuterol) Nebulizer 0.63 mg/3 mL or 1.25 mg/3 mL	0.075 mg/kg (minimum dose 1.25 mg) every 20 min × 3 doses, then 0.075–0.15 mg/kg up to 5 mg every 1–4 hours as needed, continuous nebulization 0.25 mg/kg/h.	0.63 mg of levalbuterol is equivalent to 1.25 mg of racemic albuterol.
Anticholinergics		
Ipratropium bromide Nebulizer 0.25 mg/mL	0.25 mg every 20 min × 3 doses, then every 2–4 hours.	Can mix in same nebulizer with albuterol; not used as first line therapy, adjunct to β-agonist therapy.
Corticosteroids		
Methylprednisolone	Initial loading dose: 2 mg/kg (maximum 125 mg); followed by 1 mg/kg (maximum 40 mg) IV every 6 hours.	Enteral and parental steroids are equally efficacious. Parenteral is usually preferred in the PICU because of impaired respiratory status.
Prednisone/prednisolone	1–2 mg/kg/d divided every 12 hours for 3–5 days.	
Adjunctive medications		
Magnesium sulfate	25–100 mg/kg IV over 20 minutes.	Monitor serum magnesium level; optimal level not established, range of 3–5 mg/dL has not been associated with adverse effects.
Methylxanthines		
Aminophylline (aminophylline = 80% theophylline)	Loading dose: 6 mg/kg; infusion based on age: 2–6 mo 0.5 mg/kg/h 6 mo–1 y 1.0 mg/kg/h 1–9 y 1.5 mg/kg/h 10–16 y 1.2 mg/kg/h	Maintain serum theophylline levels at 10–15 mcg/mL.
Ketamine	Loading dose: 1–2 mg/kg IV Infusion: 0.5–2 mg/kg/h.	Often used for sedation for intubation and mechanical ventilation because of its bronchodilatory properties.

Abbreviations: MDI, metered dose inhaler; SC, subcutaneous.

Data from National Asthma Education and Prevention Program. Expert panel report: Guidelines for the diagnosis and management of asthma: update on selected topics 2002; 2003 Bethesda, US Department of Health and Human Services; National Institutes of Health; National Heart, Lung, and Blood Institute, Publication #02-5074; and Qureshi F. Management of children with acute asthma in the emergency department. Pediatr Emerg Care 1999;15(3):206–14.

tilation segments, but should improve as airway obstruction resolves.

Anticholinergics

Anticholinergic medications in conjunction with β-agonists improved pulmonary function in children [32,37–39], particularly school-aged children [38], and children who experienced a severe asthma attack [37]. Acetylcholine simulates the muscarinic receptors of the parasympathetic nervous system and results in bronchoconstriction and mucus secretion from the submucosal glands. Anticholinergic medications are acetylcholine antagonists that block these receptors and cause decreases in bronchomotor tone and secretions. The most commonly administered inhaled anticholinergic is ipratropium bromide, which is a quaternary derivative of atropine. It is a weak bronchodilator but works synergistically with β-agonists to improve and prolong bronchodilation [38].

The NAEPP guidelines include the recommendation for the use of ipratropium bromide as a component of the initial management strategy in an acute asthma exacerbation [10]. Most recent studies that investigated ipratropium bromide in asthma focused on children who had SA in the ED; few included hospitalized children—but not critically ill children—and these did not appreciate any added clinical benefit from the coadministration of ipratropium bromide with a β-agonist and steroid treatment regimen [40,41]. In one study, ipratropium bromide decreased the length of stay and improved asthma scores in older children; however, the results were not statistically significant [41]. Studies are needed on the efficacy and benefits of this medication in children who have SA and are cared for in the PICU.

Ipratropium bromide has minimal systemic side effects because it is insoluble in lipids, and as such, is not absorbed systemically; this is particularly important in avoiding cardiac and central nervous system side effects [42]. Side effects include dry mouth, cough, pupillary changes, and rarely, paradoxical bronchoconstriction. Ipratropium bromide should not be administered as a solo first-line agent for severe exacerbations because of β-agonists' superiority in bronchodilation and rapid onset of action, but it can be mixed with albuterol in the nebulizer chamber for these children.

Corticosteroids

Corticosteroids play a vital anti-inflammatory role in the management of SA, and are recommended as part of the initial hospital management to expedite the resolution of the exacerbation [8]. Their mechanism of action includes suppression of certain immune functions (ie, reduction and decreased activation of lymphocytes, eosinophils, mast cells, and macrophages) and mediators of inflammation (ie, cytokines). These actions decrease airway hyperresponsiveness, edema, mucus secretion, and microvasculature leakage [6,18]. They also increase bronchodilation by augmenting the effects of catecholamines, and may be helpful in preventing down-regulation of β$_2$-adrenergic receptors in patients who are on chronic agonist therapy [6]. Furthermore, they restore damaged epithelium and a normal ciliated cell:goblet cell ratio which further decreases airway inflammation [18].

Corticosteroids can be administered enterally or parenterally—both are equally efficacious in acute asthma [43]. Despite the more rapid onset of action of parenterally administered corticosteroids, the time to peak effect is virtually the same with enterally administered steroids (8 hours versus 9 hours, respectively) [7]. The corticosteroid of choice in the management of acute asthma is a glucocorticoid (eg, prednisone, prednisolone, methylprednisolone). Because children in the PICU often are in respiratory distress, and as such, frequently NPO, management usually consists of a loading dose of IV methylprednisolone, 2 mg/kg, followed by 1 mg/kg every 6 hours. Furthermore, if the child is on chronic steroid therapy, additional stress dose glucocorticoid usually is indicated [8].

Corticosteroid therapy is administered routinely for at least 5 days and then is discontinued, at which time the child should be placed on inhalation steroids if indicated. If the child receives more than 5 days of systemic steroids, a taper may be indicated [27]. Steroid therapy is associated with a decrease in the rate of hospitalizations, improved recovery from an acute exacerbation—and with chronic inhalation—decreased rate of relapse [7]. Typically, side effects do not occur with short-term use, but may include hyperglycemia, hypertension, hypokalemia, nausea, vomiting, mood alterations, psychosis, and allergic reactions. In addition to these side effects, others that may occur with long-term use include adrenal suppression, Cushing's syndrome, fluid retention, gastric ulceration, and acne. Concomitant administration of a histamine-2 blocker often is recommended to prevent gastric ulcerations in the critically ill child who is receiving steroids.

Methylxanthines

The efficacy of methylxanthines (eg, aminophylline, theophylline)—once a standard in the management of acute and chronic asthma—recently has been questioned. Their mechanism of action is unclear with the following possibilities being purported: phosphodiesterase inhibitor, adenosine receptor antagonist, uncoupling of intracellular calcium, diuretic, stimulation of endogenous catecholamines, improvement of diaphragmatic contractility, increased binding of cyclic adenosine monophosphate, and prostaglandin antagonist [18,44]. They are believed to have anti-inflammatory, immunomodulary, bronchoprotective, and bronchodilatory effects [6,27]. Significant side effects include tachycardia, nausea, emesis, agitation, headache, tremor, seizures, encephalopathy, hyperthermia, hyperglycemia, hypokalemia, hypotension, and cardiac dysrhythmias [10,27]. Toxic side effects have been seen with a serum theophylline level of more than 15 μg/mL, although the therapeutic level ranges from 10 to 20 μg/mL [10,18]. The dosage is based on age and adjusted according to serum levels. Neonates and infants require smaller doses because of impaired clearance of theophylline.

Based on the narrow therapeutic window and potential for significant side effects, coupled with an unclear benefit to children who have SA, methylxanthines are not recommended in the management of children who have SA, specifically in the ED [10,27], but may be indicated for critically ill children. A recent randomized, controlled study supported the role of aminophylline in critically ill children and cited that children who received aminophylline (in addition to β-agonist, anticholinergic, and steroid therapy) were less likely to require mechanical ventilation and had greater improvement in pulmonary function and oxygen saturation, but increased adverse effects [45]. Another study of critically ill children found that for children who received mechanical ventilation, the addition of aminophylline hastened their recovery, as evidenced by improved clinical asthma score and more rapid meeting of discharge criteria; it was not associated with significant toxicity, other than an increase in emesis [44].

β-Agonist therapy is more effective in causing bronchodilation than methylxanthines [10]; however, methylxanthines may have a role in improving pulmonary function, and possibly avoiding mechanical ventilation in children who are affected most severely and are not responding to standard treatment.

Magnesium sulfate

The use of magnesium sulfate recently was re-examined; it was added to the armamentarium of alternative medications that are used in severe SA. It is believed to exert its effect by inhibiting calcium uptake and decreasing the release of acetylcholine at the neuromuscular junction. This results in smooth muscle relaxation, stabilization of mast cell membranes, and inhibition of histamine release, which decrease inflammation [46,47]. Magnesium also has sedating effects that may contribute to improvement in airway obstruction. Recent studies in pediatrics demonstrated that IV magnesium sulfate is a safe, effective adjunctive bronchodilator [12,47], that improved the PEFR as much as 80% [46,48] and decreased the rate of hospitalization [27,49] when administered in the ED. Doses as high as 100 mg/kg have been used safely in children [47], with a dosage range of 25 to 100 mg/kg [27,47]. Although the optimal serum magnesium level has not been established, most children tolerate magnesium therapy with serum magnesium levels of 3 to 5 mg/dL. They may experience side effects if the level exceeds 9 mg/dL [47]. Side effects associated with its use include nausea, flushing, vision changes, muscle weakness, and sedation [18,47]. Toxic effects to the respiratory, cardiac, and central nervous systems may occur if the serum magnesium level exceeds 12 mg/dL [18,47]. IV magnesium should be administered slowly to avoid hypotension and bradycardia. Nebulized magnesium sulfate also was shown to improve short-term pulmonary function when used in conjunction with albuterol for children who had mild to moderate asthma exacerbations [50].

Helium-oxygen mixture (heliox)

Heliox is the mixture of oxygen and helium which renders it less dense than air (nitrogen and oxygen). In children who have turbulent airflow, such as in airway obstruction disorders, the administration of heliox is effective in decreasing airway resistance and decreasing work of breathing. For children who have SA it may be beneficial in decreasing the work of breathing enough to stall respiratory muscle fatigue and allow β-agonist and corticosteroid therapy to take effect. Several studies demonstrated the benefits of heliox in patients who had acute asthma [51–53] at a concentration ranging from 60% to 80% helium, with the remainder being composed of oxygen (20% to 40%). One pediatric study did not appreciate any improvement in pulmonary function with short-term therapy (15 minutes) of 70% helium/30% oxygen mixture; however, although hospitalized children were analyzed, those who were unable to perform spirometry were excluded, which may be the population that could benefit most [54]. In two retrospective studies of mechanically ventilated children, heliox improved oxygenation as demonstrated by improved alveolar arterial (A-a) gradient [55], decreased peak inspiratory pressure (PIP), improved PaCO$_2$, and improved acidosis [56]. Furthermore, heliox is advantageous in enhancing the delivery of aerosol- ized medications to distal airways during mechanical ventilation, particularly at higher concentrations [57,58] as well as for spontaneously breathing asthmatics [59].

Although heliox does not have significant adverse effects and its administration may improve the status of the child who has SA, its delivery in a meaning- ful concentration (60% to 80% helium) may be lim- ited in the hypoxemic patient who requires increased fraction of inspired oxygen (FIO$_2$) concentrations. Furthermore, for intubated children who require in- creasing helium concentrations, the ventilator tidal volumes displayed may vary greatly from the pa- tient's actual tidal volume, and require close monitor- ing [56].

Ventilatory support

Noninvasive

In an effort to avoid the significant risks that are involved in intubating and mechanically ventilating the asthmatic patient, the use of noninvasive positive pressure ventilation by way of facemask or nasal prongs may be indicated. There are limited data to support its use; however, it was shown to decrease the work of breathing and dyspnea in children who had asthma exacerbations with no significant adverse ef- fects [60]. In adults, the application of bilevel positive pressure ventilation has improved pulmonary func- tion, hastened recovered, and decreased the rate of hospitalization when applied in the ED [61].

Invasive

All of the aforementioned therapies are insti- tuted in an attempt to avoid mechanical ventilation in the critically ill asthmatic child. Although the rate of children who have SA and require mechanical ventilation is low—1% reported in 1990 [7]—the rate of children who are admitted to the PICU and require mechanical ventilation ranges from 10% to 20% [5,62,63]. Air trapping, increased airway resis- tance, high end-expiratory lung volumes, prolonged time constants, and ventilator asynchrony complicate mechanical ventilation in the asthmatic [6]. Mechani- cal ventilation is associated with an increased risk of barotrauma, pneumothorax, pneumomediastinum, bronchospasm, and impaired venous return that results in hypotension and decreased cardiac output (Box 1). Hypotension may occur upon initiation of positive- pressure ventilation and should respond to a fluid bolus

---

Box 1. Complications of mechanical ventilation

Increased dynamic hyperinflation
Hypotension
Oxygen desaturation
Pneumothorax
Subcutaneous emphysema
Pneumomediastinum
Mucus plugging
Atelectasis
Nosocomial infections (ie, pneumo- nia, sinusitis)
Myopathy (with concurrent steroid use)
Arrhythmias

---

and alterations in manual bagging if appropriate (eg, decrease inspiratory tidal volume, decrease rate).

Indications for intubation and mechanical venti- lation include apnea, respiratory arrest, decreasing level of consciousness, severe hypoxemia, progres- sive exhaustion, or progressive hypercarbia despite maximized pharmacotherapy (Box 2). Arterial blood gas results should not be the sole criterion to intubate a child with SA. The results should be correlated with the patient's clinical status as well as the intensity of pharmacological management.

The asthmatic child who has severe respiratory distress that requires intubation will most likely be anxious, have severe bronchospasm, and possibly a full stomach which necessitates rapid sequence intu- bation. Medications commonly used include atro- pine, ketamine, benzodiazepine (eg, midazolam), and a short-acting nondepolarizing neuromuscular block- ing agent (eg, rocuronium, vecuronium). A cuffed endotracheal tube usually is necessary to minimize any air leak that may occur with the anticipated high inspiratory pressures. Goals of ventilation include: improving hypoxemia; resting of fatigued respiratory muscles; maintaining a PaCO$_2$ that is compatible with adequate alveolar ventilation, despite a possibly aci- dotic state; limiting inspiratory volumes and peak airway pressures; and allowing prolonged expiratory time [12]. The most optimal ventilation strategy for the child who has SA remains to be determined; vol- ume controlled and pressure controlled, as well as pressure support modes have been investigated. The goal is no longer to achieve normocarbia, which often resulted in increased dynamic hyperinflation that led to complications, such as airleak syn- dromes (eg, pneumothorax, subcutaneous emphysema, pneumomediastinum) and hypotension [12,18].

Box 2. Indications for intubation

Absolute

  Apnea
  Obtundation
  Bradycardia
  Respiratory arrest
  Cardiac arrest

Possible:

  Respiratory muscle fatigue
  Markedly diminished or absent breath
    sounds; absence of audible wheezing
  Pulsus paradoxus greater than 20–
    40 mm Hg; absent pulsus
    paradoxus indicates imminent
    respiratory arrest due to respiratory
    muscle fatigue [8]
  Deterioration in mental status
  Diaphoresis
  PaO_2 less than 70 mm Hg on 100% FIO_2
  Progressive hypercapnia despite max-
    imal pharmacologic therapy
  Metabolic or respiratory acidosis with
    pH less than 7.20
  Difficulty speaking
  Central cyanosis
  Inability to lie down

Volume control modes are applied with the goal of delivering a lower tidal volume (6–10 mL/kg) at a slow respiratory rate with prolonged expiratory time, no extrinsic PEEP, and a plateau pressure of less than 30 cm H_2O, thereby allowing hypercapnia in an effort to avoid overextension of the lungs [11,12]. This ventilation strategy, referred to as permissive hypercapnia or controlled hypoventilation, is an accepted approach to ventilating an asthmatic that is aimed at maintaining adequate oxygenation, while decreasing the risk of barotrauma by minimizing high airway pressures and allowing hypercarbia [64]. Often, a pH of at least 7.20 and $PaCO_2$ of less than 90 mm Hg will be accepted, with the administration of tromethamine or bicarbonate to improve the acidosis if necessary. The I:E ratio may be increased anywhere from 1:2 to 1:6 to allow for adequate exhalation and prevent air trapping. Risks of permissive hypercapnia include worsening of pre-existing increased intracranial pressure as a result of cerebral vasodilation, sub-

arachnoid hemorrhage, and myocardial depression if there is coexisting hypovolemia [65].

In volume control ventilation, it is hypothesized that the less obstructed airways will receive a greater amount of the tidal volume and result in uneven ventilation, a decrease in dynamic compliance, and higher peak inspiratory pressures [63]. Recently, pressure modes of ventilation have been promoted as more advantageous than volume control [63,66]. Pressure control, with its decelerating flow pattern, may be valuable by allowing more even distribution of inspired gas, improving dynamic compliance, and delivering more tidal volume at the same inflation pressures [63]. It allows for prevention of high PIP, yet can maintain adequate mean airway pressure. One of the disadvantages of pressure control is that abrupt changes in lung compliance could cause significant tidal volumes and result in barotrauma; therefore, the generated tidal volumes must be monitored closely.

Pressure support also has been reported as an effective mode of ventilation with the advantage of decreasing the inspiratory work of breathing but still allowing maintenance of the individual's own respiratory pattern and ability to maintain forced exhalation [66]. One study demonstrated an improvement in acidosis, hypercarbia, and respiratory rate for children who received pressure support ventilation [66]. Another method that may be advantageous, but has not yet been studied in the child who has SA, is pressure regulated volume control. This may be beneficial in that it allows for a high inspiratory gas flow with a set tidal volume, but it is pressure limited. Furthermore, this mode is now offered in synchronized intermittent mandatory ventilation mode; this may avoid the commitment to neuromuscular blocking agent administration, which is associated with myopathy when used in conjunction with steroids. In one case report, high frequency oscillatory ventilation successfully ventilated a child who had severe SA who failed conventional ventilation in the pressure-control mode [67].

The use of extrinsic PEEP is controversial in the intubated asthmatic; some investigators recommend no PEEP because of the concern for more air trapping, whereas others advocate for low PEEP (~3 cm H_2O) [18]. It is important to monitor and avoid auto-PEEP, and set extrinsically applied PEEP lower than auto-PEEP as determined by the end-expiratory airway occlusion method. Bear in mind that this method may underestimate auto-PEEP in certain patients and should be correlated with the plateau airway pressure [68].

In all conventional modes of ventilation, graphic monitoring of gas flow, volume, and pressure by way of the ventilator is helpful in children who have SA to assess changes in airway resistance and assure adequate expiration before the next inspiratory cycle. Assurance of adequate sedation and analgesia is indicated for these children, as well as the possibility of neuromuscular blocking agents to prevent ventilator asynchrony and tachypnea, particularly if permissive hypercapnia is instituted.

Anesthetic gases

The child who has refractory SA may benefit from inhalational anesthetics, such as halothane, isoflurane, or enflurane. The exact mechanism of action is unclear, but they have been used for many years to promote bronchodilation and improve severe bronchospasm. Their administration requires an anesthesiologist and may be associated with significant side effects, including hypotension, cardiac arrhythmias, and myocardial depression [12,18].

Antileukotriene agents

The use of antileukotriene agents or leukotriene receptor antagonists (eg, montelukast) in the management of asthma is a recent development. The role of leukotrienes in the pathogenesis of asthma led to the development and use of leukotriene receptor antagonists as a bronchoprotective therapy. They are effective in inhibiting the inflammation and bronchospasm that are mediated by leukotrienes in exercise and allergen-induced bronchoconstriction for patients who have mild to moderate asthma. There are limited data regarding their effectiveness in an acute asthma exacerbation, although they have demonstrated improved pulmonary functions in adults [69]. There are no data to support the use of antileukotriene agents in the critically ill child who has SA.

Other interventions

Ketamine is a dissociative anesthetic agent that is beneficial in asthmatics because of its bronchodilating effects. It is used often for children who require mechanical ventilation or as an agent for induction of anesthesia before intubation. It requires the coadministration of an anticholinergic agent (eg, atropine, glycopyrrolate) because of hypersalivation and increased bronchial secretions, as well as a benzodiazepine to prevent emergence reaction. It is contraindicated in children who have actual or the potential for increased intracranial pressure.

Bronchoscopy with bronchial lavage may be indicated if there is significant mucus plugging, severe atelectasis, or lobar collapse. Some asthmatics have massive bronchial casts that require bronchoscopy for removal.

Administration of nitric oxide is another adjunctive management approach for the child who has not responded to maximal conventional therapy. It was reported to dramatically improve ventilation by causing bronchodilation and possibly improve ventilation-perfusion mismatch through its direct pulmonary vasodilating effects [70].

In severe life-threatening asthma that has not responded to aggressive therapy, extracorporeal life support may be instituted. Although this is an experimental therapy for this population, children that have received extracorporeal life support for respiratory failure due to asthma had a surprisingly high survival rate of 88% [6].

Therapies that are not indicated in children who have SA include chest physiotherapy, administration of mucolytics, and antibiotics. Children who have SA may require antibiotics because of comorbid conditions, such as bacterial infections or sepsis; however, the routine administration of antibiotics is not indicated for SA.

Future therapies

Current management focuses on the reduction of inflammation, whereas future management may include therapies for preventing and managing the process of airway wall remodeling [15], as well as IV leukotriene-modifying agents [13]. In the future, disease severity and response to treatment may be monitored by measuring biologic markers of inflammation (eg, urinary leukotriene levels) [17]. Monitoring the response to treatment of the child who has asthma also may include noninvasive measurement of exhaled nitric oxide, because it is a marker of inflammation released from airway epithelium [12].

Management may be geared toward specific immune modulator therapy. Humanized monoclonal IgG anti-IgE antibodies are marketed for use on an outpatient basis for treatment of atopic asthma [4]. Antibodies for IL-5 and IL-4 receptors also have been developed and are being studied [4]. Another medication, tiotropium, a long-acting anticholinergic, is undergoing clinical trials to assess its effectiveness in patients who have asthma [11]. Further research is needed on the optimal management strategies for pediatric patients who have SA in the PICU. Therapies that were found to be ineffective in the ED may be beneficial in the child who has ongoing SA in the PICU and warrant further investigation.

Summary

SA in the PICU can progress to a life-threatening emergency. The goal of management is to improve hypoxemia and bronchoconstriction and decrease airway edema through the administration of continuous nebulized β_2-adrenergic agonists with intermittent anticholinergics, corticosteroids, and oxygen. Adjunctive therapies, such as magnesium, methylxanthines, IV β-agonists, heliox, and noninvasive ventilation, should be considered in the child who fails to respond to initial therapies. The restoration of adequate pulmonary functions, resolution of airway obstruction, and avoidance of mechanical ventilation should guide management. The child and family should be kept abreast of all changes in management and the ongoing plan of care. Children who have SA, if treated promptly and effectively, can return to their usual state of health, but require close management by their pediatrician, advanced practice nurse, or pulmonologist to prevent further severe recurrences.

References

[1] American Academy of Allergy, Asthma, and Immunology. Asthma statistics: media resources: media kit. Available at: http://www.aaaai.org/media/resources/media_kit/asthma_statistics.stm. Accessed January 3, 2005.

[2] Asthma in America - a landmark survey. Glaxo SmithKline. Available at: http://www.asthmainamerica.com/statistics.htm. Accessed January 2, 2005.

[3] National Institutes of Health - National Heart, Lung, and Blood Institute. Data fact sheet: asthma statistics. Available at: http://www.nhlbi.nih.gov. Accessed January 3, 2005.

[4] Guill M. Asthma update: epidemiology and pathophysiology. Pediatr Rev 2004;25(9):299–305.

[5] Roberts JS, Bratton SL, Brogan TV. Acute severe asthma: differences in therapies and outcomes among pediatric intensive care units. Crit Care Med 2002; 30(3):581–5.

[6] Isben LM, Bratton SL. Current therapies for severe asthma exacerbations in children. New Horizons 1999; 7(3):312–25.

[7] Qureshi F. Management of children with acute asthma in the emergency department. Pediatr Emerg Care 1999;15(3):206–14.

[8] National Asthma Education and Prevention Program. Practical guide for the diagnosis and management of asthma; 1997. Bethesda, US Department of Health and Human Services -National Institutes of Health National Heart, Lung, and Blood Institute, Publication #97–4053,1997.

[9] American Academy of Allergy, Asthma, and Immunology, Inc. Pediatric asthma: promoting best practice -

Guide for managing asthma in children. Available at: http://www.aaaai.org/media/resources/media_kit/asthma_statistics.htm. Accessed January 4, 2005.

[10] National Asthma Education and Prevention Program. Expert panel report: Guidelines for the diagnosis and management of asthma: update on selected topics 2002; 2003. Bethesda, MD: US Department of Health and Human Services; National Institutes of Health; National Heart, Lung, and Blood Institute. NIH Publication #02–5074.

[11] McFadden E. Acute severe asthma. Am J Respir Crit Care Med 2003;168:740–59.

[12] Bohn D, Kisson N. Acute asthma. Pediatr Crit Care Med 2001;2(2):151–63.

[13] Streetman DD, Bhatt-Mehta V, Johnson CE. Management of acute, severe asthma in children. Ann Phamacother 2002;36:1249–60.

[14] Kuster P, Pecenka-Johnson K. Nursing management of the child in status asthmaticus and impending respiratory failure. Crit Care Nurs Clin North Am 1999;11(4): 511–8.

[15] Bousquet J, Jeffery PK, Busse WW, et al. Asthma: from bronchoconstriction to airways inflammation and remodeling. Am J Respir Crit Care Med 2000;161(5): 1720–45.

[16] Barbato A, Turato G, Baraldo S, et al. Airway inflammation in childhood asthma. Am J Respir Crit Care Med 2003;168:798–803.

[17] Quinonez J. Asthma update. Medscape. Available at: http://www.medscape.com/viewarticle/495299. Accessed December 18, 2004.

[18] Werner H. Status asthmaticus in children: a review. Chest 2001;119(6):1913–29.

[19] Clark JA, Lieh-Lai M, Thomas R, et al. Comparison of traditional and plethysmographic methods for measuring pulsus paradoxus. Arch Pediatr Adolesc Med 2004;158(1):48–51.

[20] Wood DW, Downes JJ, Lecks HI. A clinical scoring system for the diagnosis of respiratory failure. Am J Dis Child 1972;123:227–8.

[21] Parkin PC, Macarthur C, Saunders NR, et al. Development of a clinical asthma score for use in hospitalized children between 1 and 5 years of age. J Clin Epidemiol 1996;49(8):821–5.

[22] Van Der Windt DA, Nagelkerke AD, Bouter LM, et al. Clinical scores for acute asthma in pre-school children. A review of the literature. J Clin Epidemiol 1994; 47(6):635–46.

[23] Angelilli ML, Thomas R. Inter-rater evaluation of a clinical scoring system in children with asthma. Ann Allergy Asthma Immunol 2002;88:209–14.

[24] Gorelick MH, Stevens MW, Schultz TR, et al. Performance of a novel clinical score, the Pediatric Asthma Severity Score (PASS), in the evaluation of acute asthma. Acad Emerg Med 2004;11(1):10–8.

[25] Kifle Y, Davenport PW. Magnitude estimation of inspiratory resistive loads in children with life-threatening asthma. Am J Respir Crit Care Med 1997;156: 1530–5.

[26] Guill M. Asthma update: clinical aspects and management. Pediatr Rev 2004;25(9):335–44.

[27] Warner JO, Naspitz CK. Third International Pediatric consensus statement on the management of childhood asthma. Pediatr Pulmonol 1998;25:1–17.

[28] McFadden E, Elsanadi N, Dixon L, et al. Protocol therapy for acute asthma: therapeutic benefits and cost savings. Am J Med 1995;99:651–61.

[29] Schuh S, Parkin P, Rajan A, et al. High-versus low-dose frequently administered, nebulized albuterol in children with severe, acute asthma. An Pediatr (Barc) 1989;83(4):513–8.

[30] Camargo CA, Spooner CH, Rowe BH. Continuous versus intermittent beta-agonists for acute asthma. Cochrane Database Syst Rev 2004;4.

[31] Katz RW, Kelly HW, Crowley MR, et al. Safety of continuous nebulized albuterol for bronchospasm in infants and children. Pediatrics 1993;92(5):666–9.

[32] Rodrigo GJ, Rodrigo C. Continuous vs. intermittent beta-agonists in the treatment of acute adult asthma: a systematic review with meta-analysis. Chest 2002; 122(1):160–5.

[33] Craig VL, Bigos D, Brilli RJ. Efficacy and safety of continuous albuterol nebulization in children with severe status asthmaticus. Pediatr Emerg Care 1996; 12(1):1–5.

[34] Carl JC, Myers TR, Kirchner HL, et al. Comparison of racemic albuterol and levalbuterol for treatment of acute asthma. J Pediatr 2003;143(6):731–6.

[35] Chiang VW, Burns JP, Rifai N, et al. Cardiac toxicity of intravenous terbutaline for the treatment of severe asthma in children: a prospective assessment. J Pediatr 2000;137(1):73–7.

[36] Stephanopoulos DE, Monge R, Schell KH, et al. Continuous intravenous terbutaline for pediatric status asthmaticus. Crit Care Med 1998;26(10):1744–8.

[37] Schuh S, Johnson DW, Callahan S, et al. Efficacy of frequent nebulized ipratropium bromide added to frequent high-dose albuterol therapy in severe childhood asthma. J Pediatr 1995;126(4):639–45.

[38] Plotnick LH, Ducharme FM. Combined inhaled anticholinergics and beta2-agonists for initial treatment of acute asthma in children. Cochrane Database Syst Rev 2004;4.

[39] Quershi F, Zaritsky A, Lakkis H. Efficacy of nebulized ipratropium in severely asthmatic children. Ann Emerg Med 1997;29(2):205–11.

[40] Goggin N, Macarthur C, Parkin P. Randomized trial of the addition of ipratropium bromide to albuterol and corticosteroid therapy in children hospitalized because of an acute asthma exacerbation. Arch Pediatr Adolesc Med 2001;155(12):1329–34.

[41] Craven D, Kercsmar CM, Myers T, et al. Ipratropium bromide plus nebulized albuterol for the treatment of hospitalized children with acute asthma. J Pediatr 2001;138(1):51–8.

[42] Satish B, McDonald N, Bara A. Anti-cholinergic therapy for acute asthma in children. Cochrane Database Syst Rev 2004;4.

[43] Barnett P, Caputo GL, Baskin M, et al. Intravenous versus oral corticosteroids in the management of acute asthma in children. Ann Emerg Med 1997;29(2):212–7.

[44] Ream RS, Loftis LL, Albers GM, et al. Efficacy of IV theophylline in children with severe status asthmaticus. Chest 2001;119(5):1480–8.

[45] Yung M, South M. Randomised controlled trial of aminophylline for severe acute asthma. Arch Dis Child 1998;79:405–10.

[46] Ciarallo L, Brousseau D, Reinert S. Higher-dose intravenous magnesium therapy for children with moderate to severe acute asthma. Arch Pediatr Adolesc Med 2000;154(10):979–83.

[47] Glover ML, Machado C, Totapally BR. Magnesium sulfate administered via continuous intravenous infusion in pediatric patient with refractory wheezing. J Crit Care 2002;17(4):255–8.

[48] Ciarallo L, Sauer AH, Shannon MW. Intravenous magnesium therapy for moderate to severe asthma: results of a randomized, placebo-controlled trial. J Pediatr 1996;129:809–14.

[49] Markovitz B. Does magnesium sulphate have a role in the management of paediatric status asthmaticus. Arch Dis Child 2002;86:381–2.

[50] Mahajan P, Haritos D, Rosenberg N, et al. Comparison of nebulized magnesium sulfate plus albuterol to nebulized albuterol plus saline in children with acute exacerbations of mild to moderate asthma. J Emerg Med 2004;27(1):21–5.

[51] Kudukis TM, Manthous CA, Schmidt GA, et al. Inhaled helium-oxygen revisited: effect of inhaled helium-oxygen during the treatment of status asthmaticus in children. J Pediatr 1997;130(2):217–24.

[52] Gluck EH, Onorato DJ, Castriotta R. Helium-oxygen mixtures in intubated patients with status asthmaticus and respiratory acidosis. Chest 1990;98:693–8.

[53] Manthous CA, Hall JB, Caputo MA, et al. Heliox improves pulsus paradoxus and peak expiratory flow in nonintubated patients with severe asthma. Am J Respir Crit Care Med 1995;151:310–4.

[54] Carter ER, Webb CR, Moffitt DR. Evaluation of heliox in children hospitalized with acute severe asthma. Chest 1996;109(5):1256–61.

[55] Schaeffer EM, Pohlman A, Morgan S, et al. Oxygenation in status asthmaticus improves during ventilation with helium-oxygen. Crit Care Med 1999;27(12): 2666–70.

[56] Abd-Allah SA, Rogers MS, Terry M, et al. Helium-oxygen therapy for pediatric acute severe asthma requiring mechanical ventilation. Pediatr Crit Care Med 2003;4(3):353–7.

[57] Goode ML, Fink JB, Dhand R, et al. Improvement in aerosol delivery with helium-oxygen mixtures during mechanical ventilation. Am J Respir Crit Care Med 2001;163:109–14.

[58] Habib DM, Garner SS, Brandeburg S. Effect of helium-oxygen on delivery of albuterol in a pediatric, volume-cycled, ventilated lung-model. Pharmacotherapy 1999;19:143–9.

[59] Anderson M, Svartengren M, Bylin G, et al. Deposition in asthmatics of particles inhaled in air or in helium-oxygen. Am Rev Respir Dis 1993;147: 524–8.

[60] Thill PJ, McGuire JK, Baden HP, et al. Noninvasive positive-pressure ventilation in children with lower airway obstruction. Pediatr Crit Care Med 2004;5(4): 337–42.

[61] Soroksky A, Stav D, Shpirer I. A pilot prospective, randomized, placebo-controlled trial of bilevel positive airway pressure in acute asthmatic attack. Chest 2003;123:1018–25.

[62] Malmstrom KM, Kaila M, Korhonen K, et al. Mechanical ventilation in children with severe asthma. Pediatr Pulmonol 2001;31:404–11.

[63] Sarnaik AP, Daphtary KM, Meert KL, et al. Pressure-controlled ventilation in children with severe status asthmaticus. Pediatr Crit Care Med 2004;5(2):133–8.

[64] Dworkin G, Kattan M. Mechanical ventilation for status asthmaticus in children. J Pediatr 1989;114(4 pt 1): 545–9.

[65] Mutlu GM, Factor P, Schwartz DE, et al. Severe status asthmaticus: management with permissive hypercapnia and inhalation anesthesia. Crit Care Med 2002;30(2): 477–80.

[66] Wetzel R. Pressure-support ventilation in children with severe asthma. Crit Care Med 1996;24(9):1603–5.

[67] Duval EL, van Vught AJ. Status asthmaticus treated by high-frequency oscillatory ventilation. Pediatr Pulmonol 2000;30:350–3.

[68] Leatherman JW, Ravenscraft SA. Low measured auto-positive end-expiratory pressure during mechanical ventilation of patients with severe asthma: hidden auto-positive end-expiratory pressure. Crit Care Med 1996; 24:541–6.

[69] Camargo CA, Spooner CH, Malice MP, et al. A randomized controlled trial of intravenous montelukast in acute asthma. Am J Respir Crit Care Med 2003;167: 528–33.

[70] Nakagawa TA, Johnston SJ, Falkos SA, et al. Life-threatening status asthmaticus treated with inhaled nitric oxide. J Pediatr 2000;137(1):119–22.

ELSEVIER
SAUNDERS

Crit Care Nurs Clin N Am 17 (2005) 481 – 494

CRITICAL CARE
NURSING CLINICS
OF NORTH AMERICA

Tsunami: Response to a Disaster

Dirk R.G. Danschutter, RN, CCRN, CP

Pediatric Intensive Care Unit, Free University Hospital, AZ-VU Brussels, Laarbeeklaan 101, Brussels B1090, Belgium

On December 26, 2004, 07:58:50 AM local time (02:58:50 PM Central European Time), an earthquake with a magnitude of 8.9–9.0 [1] on the Richter scale [2], occurred in the Indian Ocean at an unusually shallow depth and very near to Sumatra's coast (lat. 3,298° N; long. 95,779° E) [3]. The devastation caused by the powerful earthquake resulted in numerous casualties. Panic filled the streets and homes; people rushed out and laid down on the asphalt or walkways, others initialize rescue attempts in the collapsed buildings.

Earthquakes that are accompanied by vertical tectonic plate shift which occurs in the ocean floor, and that exceed 7.5 on the Richter scale, are capable of causing a "bump" in the global water volume located right above the epicenter [1,3,4]. The bump (in the case of December 26, 2004, a 1–3 meter shift) results in the formation of outward racing ocean waves known as Tsunami, which is Japanese for wave (nami) in harbour (tsu). These stealth waves travel at a very high speed and measure no more than 40 centimeters at open sea, but have enormous wavelengths (hundreds or thousands of km). When this mass energy of an ocean is moving with the speed of a jet airliner and reaches shallow water, velocity is reduced and the water mass starts to pile up. When the waves start to break at beach level, they have turned into walls of water that measure 10–15 meters high [5].

Because Sumatra's province Aceh was only 160 kilometers away from the epicenter, it took the ocean no more than 30 minutes to surprise the island residents with tons of debris, ships, cars, trucks, and

trees which were carried deeply into the land by the engulfing muddy water. Many people were trapped in the devastating whirling dirt yard, which hit their towns and beaches with every killer wave.

The same horror hit 10 countries over 7 hours and over 4500 kilometers of coast: Sri Lanka, Thailand, Malaysia, Myanmar, India, Somalia, the Maldives, Madagascar, Kenya, and Bangladesh. Many subsequent and powerful earthquakes (in Bangladesh, 7.4 on the Richter scale; in the Nicobar Islands, 7.3 on the Richter scale) followed minutes and hours later, which indicated that the tectonic plates had moved more than 15 meters laterally over a length of 1000 kilometers [1,4]. A 10-year-old girl (Tilly Smith from Oxshott, Surrey, UK) observed how the ocean drew back over an unusual distance of several hundred meters, a phenomenon that even surprised the fish. Many tourists were saved at Mai Khao beach (Thailand) by this little girl's intervention when she convinced her parents, in the little time left, about the things she learned at school [6,7]. Simuelue, an island in front of Sumatra and only 60 kilometers from the epicenter was first hit by waves of more than 10 meters high. In total, 7 of the 75,000 residents were killed. All had run uphill right after the earthquake and were shouting *"Semong! Semong!"* (Monster waves) because they remembered the stories their elders told about how thousands of people had been killed during the tsunami of 1907 [8]. In Sumatra however, these stories were forgotten and not enough time was left between local radio warnings and the rushing waves.

Aceh is a young province. Numerous babies and children died as did many young people who lived and worked in the towns. The area was severely hit and with every new wave engulfing the streets, Aceh

E-mail address: dirk.danschutter@az.vub.ac.be

DANSCHUTTER

lay down as a heavily wounded warrior, waiting for the final blow or waiting for mercy.

Earthquakes do often occur in this part of the world. About 150 kilometers west of Sumatra, the British naval vessel *HMS Scott* was on a mission of high-tech sonar readings to assess the stability of the region's tectonic plates, and on February 11, documented an impressive shift of earth's tectonic plates after the earthquake of December 26 [4,5,9]. The coral reefs show that tsunamis have seldom hit the Indian Ocean but when they did, it was with great force. Over the last decade researchers have urged government officials to establish tsunami warning systems. But among the many problems that trouble South Asia (such as civil wars, poverty, and diseases) rare, but deadly waves seemed to be a low priority [10,11]. When the earthquake struck, some experts around the world looked at graphs that were recorded on the world's most sophisticated monitoring equipment without realizing the larger threat. Others realized the danger but did not engage others for fear of being wrong or out of line. In India, air force officials received a mayday, possibly in time to save thousands of lives, but they never sent it out.

At the Hawaiian Pacific Tsunami Warning Center a researcher's attention was drawn to the signal coming from a seismic sensor far away on the Cocos Islands (southwest of Sumatra) which indicated the occurrence of a large earthquake in that area [10,11]. As the warning center's computer automatically sent a pager signal to a colleague, both men deliberated on the data. Initial readings indicated that the earthquake had a magnitude of 8.0 on the Richter scale and about the same reading as the Macquarie Sea earthquake of 3 days before, December 23 (located between New Zealand and Antarctica) [12]. This new earthquake was significant, and statistically speaking 8.0 earthquakes occur only once a year. It also happened outside the Pacific Ocean, which was their area of expertise and responsibility. At 03:14 PM (Hawaii time), the two men sent a bulletin on an automated e-mail and fax list to their colleagues around the Pacific Rim. The bulletin reported an earthquake located outside the Pacific and concluded: "No destructive tsunami threat exists based on historical earthquake and tsunami data" [10,11]. At that time the waves had rushed about 150 kilometers from the epicenter in ever-widening circles. In Sumatra, the first victims were about to die.

After the alarming earthquake that caused some buildings and houses to collapse, many of the people of Banda Aceh were outside inspecting their homes. It was a sunny, clear morning at the end of the monsoon season [11]. At about 08:30 AM (a half hour after the earthquake) the sound of an incoming train was heard. "Water! Big water!" they screamed, unable to find a name for this phenomenon.

The water swallowed up mothers and fathers, brothers and sisters, relatives and neighbors. It lifted fishing boats, trucks, and even an oil tanker, and dumped these in the middle of the city. Hundreds of bodies were dropped in the streets, trees, and stairways. The entire villages of Calang and Teunom disappeared, together with their 12,000 residents each, and left no trace as though they had never existed [13,14].

It was already much too late for the people of Aceh. A few hours earlier in Madras, the excursing needles of the local seismograph were documenting the 9.0 earthquake. Ten minutes later the New Delhi headquarters were informed by telephone. The air force base however was never called, and they in turn never called the Madras earthquake warning center. The wave was about an hour away from India [10,11].

At the US Geological Survey's National Earthquake Information Center, data from 350 monitoring stations around the globe came in on December 26. Comparing all the data, the earthquake's magnitude was thought to be 8.5 on the Richter scale, and a computer program to alert the White House, State Department, and other agencies was activated. The scientists at the Hawaii Tsunami Warning Center now started to realize that the earthquake was much larger than they previously estimated. A second bulletin was sent: "No destructive tsunami threat exists for the Pacific basin based on historical earthquake and tsunami data. There is the possibility of a tsunami near the epicenter." About an hour had elapsed between the quake and this bulletin. The wave was by now halfway across the Indian Ocean and had already killed most of the December 26 tsunami victims.

At the Hawaii center, the earthquake's magnitude was adjusted to 9.0 (10 times larger than the first estimate). The Hawaiian researchers now improvised a warning system as they started to phone consular officials across the Indian Ocean. This time the warning system proved effective. Many lives were saved in Kenya, Somalia, Madagascar, and Mauritius [11].

Response from Belgium

In Belgium, the Belgian Association for Pediatrics (BAP) decided, in the aftermath of the South Asia cataclysm, to join world solidarity. BAP is a small intellectual society for Flemish- and French-speaking pediatricians with no governmental support, and no real training to deal with catastrophe medicine. Within

24 hours, a medical team of 30 volunteers from 4 hospitals was rounded up. An Indonesian pediatrician who graduated in Brussels informed the society about the devastation at the Banda Aceh university hospital. The goal was to reach the Rumah Sakit Umum Dr. Zainoel Abidin General Hospital of Banda Aceh. The Belgian Medical Team (BMT) would leave as soon as possible to focus on the pediatric wards of this hospital. In the few days left before take-off, the BMT started to contact medical and pharmaceutical supply companies to collect medication, baby food, and medical equipment. From the hospitals they borrowed surgical, anesthesia, and nursing equipment. Sport and leisure companies donated solid metal transport cases, tents, mosquito nets, and protective products. With equipment from military stores the group tried to prepare themselves to face monsoon and the worst living conditions imaginable.

Two days before departure time, which was set for January 9, the local Indonesian pediatrician informed the BMT that the university hospital of Banda Aceh was not operational, and even worse, not accessible. The ocean had shifted several kilometers and water was still present in the hospital and in the wards. Officials estimated that nearly half of the personnel had died in the tsunami and the other half had disappeared. Many had probably escaped to the mountains or had joined other Banda residents to search for their missing relatives. Regardless, the hospital had a deficit of 600 nurses and 200 doctors (reported by hospital director M. Andalas, personal communication), and it remained unclear if there were many or any patients. It was presumed that most of the victims were carried away by the waves or were buried in the mud alongside the pavilions. Horrible stories were told about what happened in the hospital, but Indonesian soldiers and civilian volunteers had already started to clean the wards. As a result of this feedback, the BMT was split into three groups instead of going as one large group. Australian and German army forces had arrived at the hospital but had not reported on what kind of patients they were treating, so it was decided to first send a reconnaissance team. The equipment was reorganized when it became clear that the BMT was heading for what the military called ground zero. Also, because this group was much smaller, the number of transport cases was reduced and their contents were adapted to different scenarios. One transport case was for surgery and traumatology; another was for severe dehydration and infections. Plans had been made to send invasive intensive care inotropic support supplies to treat near drowning victims; however, those plans were dropped because BMT 1 would arrive on January 11 (Day 16 post-tsunami). No one could imagine that children would survive a near drowning incident in these conditions without therapeutic support because near drowning victims in more modern western practices often experience the complications of acute respiratory distress syndrome (ARDS) or severe infection within days.

Among the 30 BMT members, 11 people with previous experience in Africa, Bosnia, Bam, and Nicaragua were selected to form BMT 1. There were 5 nurses and 6 doctors. All nurses were senior nurses; 2 from Pediatric Intensive Care Units (PICU) and 3 from the Emergency Department (ER). The doctors included 2 surgeons, 1 anaesthesiologist, and 3 pediatric intensivists; 2 of them had additional ER certification. This group left Antwerp, Belgium, on January 9 at 04:00 AM with 250 kg of medical supplies and equipment in 8 large transport cases.

As we arrived at Banda Aceh, it struck us that we were facing a ghost town. The driver tried to explain to us with gestures where the capital was; however, we saw nothing but black. Nothing was visible for miles around. It was hard to believe that a town with 400,000 inhabitants was completely black and could only be found because someone was pointing us in that direction. A part of our small group, despite the curfew, went to inspect the hospital, which was about 10 minutes away by foot. They were not able to enter it because there was no light and debris was piled up everywhere so that no access to the building could be found. This was discouraging news. BMT 1 came to Sumatra to restart the pediatric wards of the university hospital. Now we had to look for another mission.

Refugee camps

The next morning BMT 1 headed for the United Nations (UN) headquarters which were located at the edge of ground zero. About 100 meters away, the streets stopped in muddy water. Our spokesman returned and told us there was no work for BMT 1 right now because many rescue workers had arrived at Banda Aceh and the coordination effort was very difficult. The UN headquarters asked us to return in the evening with the hope that there would be work for us.

We returned to our home base and realized that our closest European neighbors appeared to be the reporters of the British Broadcasting Corporation (BBC). They were staying in a house only a block away. We figured that journalists are likely to be informed and indeed they had heard of refugee camps where no one had received medical attention. On a map they had pinned on the wall, we were shown Lhoong and Meulaboh which seemed to be too far away, so we wrote down Sigli and we had ourselves a mission.

It was extremely hot at the refugee camp in Sigli. Our arrival was announced through the loudspeakers and many people hurried to meet us. The vans were unloaded and the improvised mosque served as the treatment place. About 50 of the 4000 children in the camp were presented at the consultation. All of them, in fact all camp refugees, had scurvy. We did a good job of treating scurvy, otitis, impetigo, and some small, infected wounds. On the other hand, we felt like we were losing precious time.

The next morning it was still raining heavily when we returned to the hospital (Fig. 1). We saw a few people dressed like officials with badges. We plodded our way through a thick black layer of slippery mud toward the seriously damaged building and what seemed like a main entrance. We used a small path that was made between a pile of beds, cupboards, bookcases, gas cylinders, and all kind of medical equipment. One of the officials understood English and we managed to explain that we were there to help. We came from far away to treat the sick anak (Anak is Indonesian for child). Ilmu Kesehatan ICU anak.

Our names were filed and we followed the guide through the black mud. We saw all kinds of equipment that gave us an idea of the potential of this hospital. It was a large hospital, with pavilions and two and three-story buildings. Large eels swam across the walkways, and large gas bubbles escaped from the mud, which later appeared to be the decomposing bodies of nurses, patients, and relatives as they tried to evacuate right after the earthquake.

Somewhere near the middle of the central corridor we reached the different pediatric wards: the Louser pavilion and next to it the Ilmu Kesehatan ward with the anak ICU and the rehidrasi unit (Fig. 2). The purpose of this last building was a very unfamiliar concept to us. This ward was for all children who had severe diarrhea. The unit had an open gutter all around. The feces splattered on the floor were then drained off by the nurses or relatives. All buildings had a brownish line at about 1,5 m which indicated the height of the mud before the water started to recede. Later and especially in the pavilions that were not cleared yet, some bodies were recovered between the furniture (Fig. 3). Of value were the white patient boards that hung on the walls of the pediatric wards. These boards had patients' names, ages, and reasons for admission (right before the tsunami). Many children suffered from dehydration. There was one case of leukemia. Some had tuberculosis and infectious diseases (measles, diphtheria and tetanus) which indicated a poor vaccination program. This was later confirmed when children who had tetanus were admitted. At the Ibu Anak maternity ward (Ibu means mother) we could read from the patient board that all babies had extremely poor weight. No baby weighed more than 2.5 kg and one baby weighted only 1.7 kg.

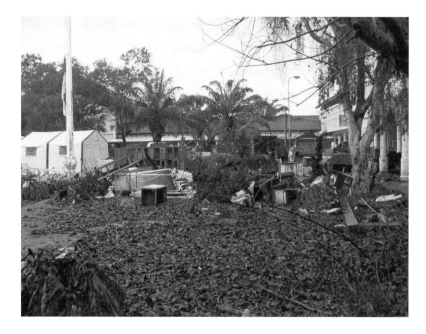

Fig. 1. Main entrance to Rumah Sakit Umum (RSU) Dr. Zainoel Abidin General Hospital of Banda Aceh.

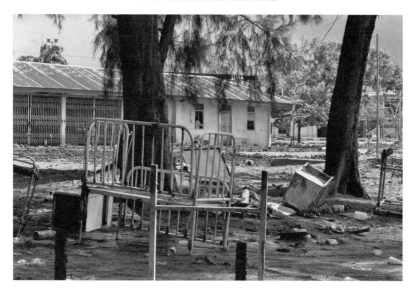

Fig. 2. The Ilmu Kesehatan Anak (Children's) Pavilion.

These babies were not hospitalized at the neonatal intensive care unit; this was considered normal weight. Another message board showed a giant mosquito and we all understood one word of the Bahasa Indonesian warning: Dengue.

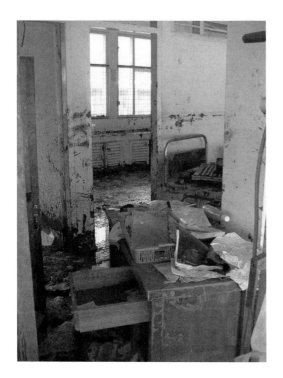

Fig. 3. RSU hospitalization ward.

Later it was explained to us that the first pavilion (Louser) was a unit for the richer Acehnese who paid for single patient rooms, air conditioning, and some fancy drawings on the walls. The second building was the building for the poor. The pavilion could be literally flooded by monsoon rainwater, so the patients were in about 10–20 cm of water once or twice a year. That is why some of the pavilions for the wealthier patients had floors that were about 50–100 cm higher. As we were guided through the building we first passed the pediatric ward that connected with the anak ICU. Between both wards a large crack crossed and bumped the floor; a remnant of the earthquake. Starving cats and dogs were freely entering the buildings in search of food. The anak ICU had been cleaned, but the cadavers of a snake and a dragon, and some feces still lay in the middle of it. The walls had oxygen, compressed air, and vacuum outlets (all out of use), with some oxygen masks still in place as plastic witnesses. All humidifiers were filled with green water. The toilets had not been cleaned yet and were covered with a thick layer of dry mud and excrement; they had been inundated by both the tsunami and a reverse flow. There was no water available from the taps and many of the electrical wall sockets had burned. There were no beds either and some children were lying down on beach chairs surrounded by their relatives and nurses who came from Langsa. They had not managed to insert intravenous (IV) lines in the acutely ill children and we immediately offered to help. There were no laboratory results available but some of the babies were obviously extremely dehydrated. We immediately split up into teams of doctors and nurses and started to insert central catheters (Fig. 4). The use of IV catheters was unfamiliar; the Langsa team had tried at several occasions to insert butterfly needles. We discussed the patients and suggested intravenous medication, then we heard that some very sick children were being observed in the ER. We went to the ER and indeed a few children who had survived a near-drowning insult were in severe respiratory distress. The Indonesian doctors kept repeating "tsunami pneumonia" and we tried to gain more specific information. These children were delegated to BMT 1.

The Belgian team deliberated briefly and decided not to install patients in the original anak ICU but to claim a multi-patient room on the Kesehatan pediatric ward. The Langsa team invited us to occupy "Tweety," a room where we could hospitalize six children. Because we had no beds for the young patients, no oxygen and no perfusion holders, we started to leave the building in search of this material, while a small group of the BMT stayed to examine and to treat the newcomers. Beds and cylinders were pulled out of the mud and cleaned using socks and muddy water. We also recovered alcohol from the mud so that the beds and mattresses could be disinfected. We were able to get a few rusty but cleaned hospital beds rather quickly and we dragged them to the Tweety unit.

We visited the German military camp of the Bundeswehr; 200 soldiers had arrived a few days before us. They were putting the white tents of their Lazarett in front of the hospital's main building. It would take them about a week to become operational with a two-bed intensive care station, an operating theater, and a pharmacy. In the meantime the German hospital ship *Berlin* was steaming for Aceh and was scheduled to arrive within a few days [15]. The command post of the Mobile Sanitätsrettungszentrum was located on the second floor and we literally had to slither our way to the stairs. What amazed us was that we could directly discuss our problems with Colonel Wachter, without protocol or intermediary steps. The result of our conference was even more surprising: the Germans would give us all that we needed as long as they had it somewhere in their tents or on the *Berlin*. For the hours and days after this meeting, the German soldiers were the ones that we could rely on, and they provided us with diesel power, water, oxygen, volume expanders, beds, and all that we asked. A few pavilions away, the Singaporeans were running an internal medicine ward and treating adult patients. Many of them suffered from tetanus. Two pavilions to the left of ours, the Sydney, Australia-based 1st Health Support Battalion with about 200 members (including 9 doctors), were mainly dealing with surgery patients [16]. They had installed an operating theater, a two-bed recovery room, and a hospital ward. They also had a few

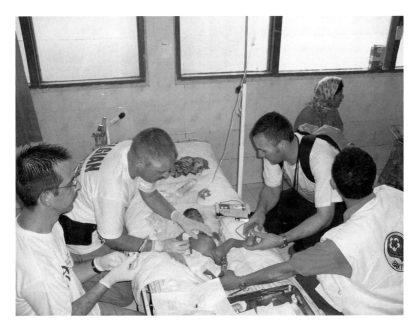

Fig. 4. The Belgian Medical Team (BMT) starts to insert intravenous lines.

surgery tents at the same location as the German Lazarett. We observed surgeons who were performing a necrotic bowel resection. So, there we were, between two armies and the Singaporeans on the other side of the corridor, installing our first little patients in the recovered beds. All of the Tweety children were near-drowning victims. They all survived the tsunami of Boxing Day. Mafouta had only his mother left. Maulida was a tsunami orphan and was accompanied by her aunt. Ikram lost his father, sister, and many other relatives. Niswa lost her father but her brother did not move an inch from her side as he constantly waved fresh air onto her little face. The father of Firda lost his wife and three daughters and was now caring for this little girl, the only precious thing that the tsunami left from his beautiful family.

Some members of the BMT were pediatric ICU nurses. From the beginning, even before we left Belgium, it was hard for us to hear the disaster coordinator explain that we were not going to treat severely ill children. What he meant was that there was no point to mechanically ventilating children, putting them on inotropic support, and then dragging them into multiple organ failure in an environment that is not equipped to handle the situation. According to the coordinator, we had to focus on surgery, infected wounds, dehydration and oral rehydration. It was hard to hear the officers and doctors of the 1st Health Support Battalion from Australia repeat exactly the same phrases. It was hard to hear Sidqi Anwar, the chief pediatrician of Zainoel Abidin's university hospital who survived the tsunami because he could swim, say that children had never been supported mechanically at the anak ICU before. If they required more than oxygen therapy and antibiotics, they were considered "lost cases." At Zainoel Abidin's hospital, 80% of the hospitalized children used to die. This was considered normal and acceptable.

Mafouta, a boy of 10 with "tsunami pneumonia," pneumopericardium and pleural effusions, would not live for many more hours (Fig. 5). His chest radiograph was a nightmare; everyone wondered how he still managed to have any gas exchange and cardiac output. He was completely exhausted, cachectic, dehydrated, with obstructive shock, and his scars reopened when we went to the Australians for treatment ideas, because we had no respirator. Probably because their recovery unit was unoccupied, the officer in charge decided to admit Mafouta and to offer the boy a 24-hour window. This offer was made on one condition: that the Belgians had to put in all of the lines and intubate the patient. This was done and Mafouta opened the door between the BMT and the Australians as both teams started to fight for his life.

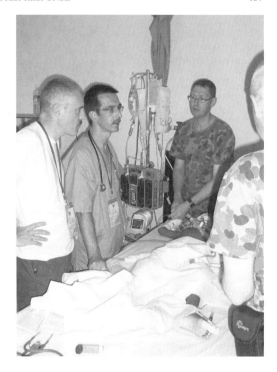

Fig. 5. Mafouta between the BMT and the Australian teams.

Despite their earlier statement, the Australians now inserted drains to evacuate pus and air and never deliberated on Mafouta's condition without us. But Mafouta needed inotropic support and that is where the story ended. Without dopamine as an option, both teams decided to continue treatment until Mafouta's heart stopped. His little heart stopped beating a few hours later.

Every day and night we felt new earthquakes, which later was described in the news bulletins as "if earth was ringing like a bell." The evening that Mafouta died, a strong earthquake (6.4) shook the roofs of the hospital buildings and we tried not to think too much about it.

Little orphan Maulida, a beautiful, tiny 9-year-old girl with radiographs similar to Mafouta's, could not be kept in her bed because she was panicking from severe hypoxia (Fig. 6). The two of us who had lost Mafouta decided to volunteer for the night shift back at the Kesehatan pavilion. The four children were critically ill with severe respiratory distress, uncontrollable temperature swings from hypothermia to high fever, dehydration, and exhaustion. The room temperature was intolerably high and the air was filled with hungry mosquitoes. Family members had spread their carpets around the beds to be at the sides of the sick children. Unfinished dinner plates and

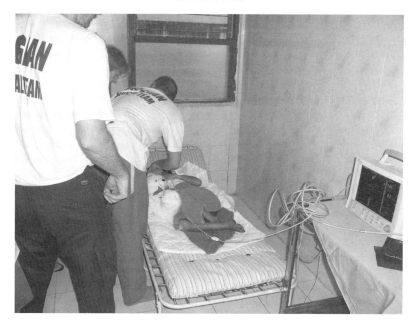

Fig. 6. Tsunami orphan, Maulida.

dishes sat on the floor where long colonies of ants feasted. Starving cats with oddly knotted tails passed by and jumped on empty beds.

Maulida died at 03:47 AM. For the rest of our lives the two of us will regret that we did not take her out of the bed to keep her in our arms as she was dying. Instead, we tried to keep her upright with a non-rebreather mask on her little face. She was literally asphyxiating in brownish pus that we tried to evacuate by suctioning her airway. She did not even gasp; she passed away very quickly with two desperate Belgians sitting on their knees.

Maulida's aunt was watching us from a little distance, sitting on the floor. Through a translator, we had been able to explain to her that her little niece would not make it through the night. It must have been hard for this courageous woman who saw her daughter, mother, and husband carried away by the black flood two weeks earlier. Several things began to happen simultaneously. Maulida's aunt tied the dead girl's legs and arms together and covered her with a blanket. The other residents reoriented their carpets in the direction toward Mecca (we also now saw the indicators on the ceiling of every room) as we started looking for some kind of local coordinator. A Langsa nurse came to the dead girl, knelt beside her, and with a long pair of scissors she cut off the uvula, opening the airway for the soul to raise to Allah without obstruction. We kept asking for a coordinator because we had learned that this word meant the same in

Indonesian. Then Ikram's mother faced Maulida's aunt and pronounced, loud and clear, the word "Inshallah" (the will of God). At last the coordinator came. He looked at our notes and the patient chart and went away without saying a word. Outside of the pavilion, however, he started to sing to Allah, and many others followed his example.

Maulida remained in the room until 10:00 AM. Then workers sent by the Indonesian coordinator took her away. Her aunt stayed for days because she was unable to return to her mountains. My partner of that night spent a whole day trying to arrange her return and finally he found an American army helicopter heading in that direction. He ignored the fact that she proposed to marry him, but we understood it well.

Every child of the Tweety room except from Ikram died from melioidosis (an infectious disease caused by the bacterium, *Burkholderia pseudomallei*). BMT 2 reported how Ikram recovered, after the microorganism that caused the "tsunami pneumonia" was identified by the Australian lab. Mascot Niswa, a 12-year-old girl with curly black hair, was also recovering, in spite of a paralytic ileus that did not result in bowel or stomach rupture, a catastrophic chest radiograph, and hypovolemic shock. This recovery took place without electrical power and with a gastric suctioning system adapted from feeding bottles. Someone had taught her to say "thank you and goodbye" the day we returned home (Fig. 7).

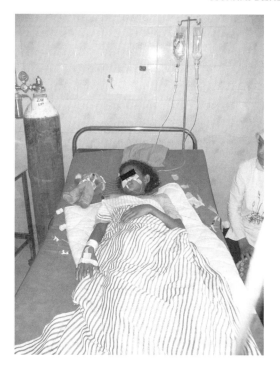

Fig. 7. Thank you and goodbye, Niswa.

This little phrase now has a very sad memory. BMT 3 sent us a cell-phone message that Niswa collapsed and died within a few hours of being admitted into an Indonesian army hospital.

Iqbal took Maulida's spot and was only one week old. He was dirty, had scurvy, and both the clinical signs and a radiograph similar to the other "tsunami pneumonias." He too was washed with drink water from our bottles. But then we realized that he was born after the tsunami. He had to be suffering from meconium aspiration and we were in very bad need of a respirator. Neither the Germans nor the Australians could help us this time, so we crossed the corridor and visited our Singaporean friends. They were in very bad need of morphine. And so we traded a brand new Viasys respirator for morphine. Iqbal got his own personal PICU: oxygen, an endotracheal tube, a resuscitation bag to recruit his alveoli, dial-flow controlled infusions, and diesel-powered prone ventilation, gastric suctioning, monitoring of ECG, blood pressure, and saturation. He recovered and was discharged like Ikram. A baby was saved for 10 ampoules of morphine (Fig. 8).

Belgian medical teams 2 and 3

BMT 2 created a pharmacy room and BMT 3 re-organized it into alphabetical order. The air con-

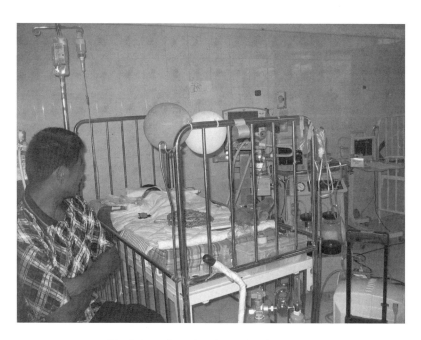

Fig. 8. A respirator for 10 ampules of morphine.

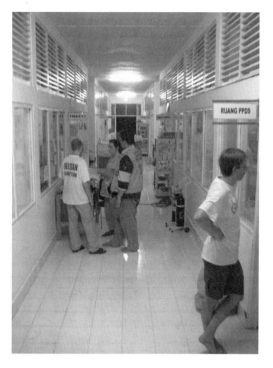

Fig. 9. the Ilmu Kesehatan repainted and fully operational.

ditioning was repaired and ventilators were whirling fresh air through the hallway of the Kesehatan unit. BMT 2 was the first to wash their hands with fresh water; the Germans from Katastrofenhilfe had assembled a 1000 liter water collector and a sanitary system on the ward. The windows were cleaned, doors, and sewage systems were repaired, and all of it, from ceiling to bottom, was repainted in white (Fig. 9). More and more patients were admitted and BMT 3 cared for about 25 children. Parents heard about foreigners who took care of the children and came to the hospital, even in the middle of the night. Some of them had traveled for 9 hours, leaving a wife or children behind.

In all, over the month that the BMT stayed at the Kesehatan ward, 50 children were admitted. Ten of them died; 5 of them shortly after admission, as the result of melioidosis. The others died from hypovolemic shock and two were born prematurely. The youngest one (27 weeks) stole a BMT 3 nurse's heart; she named him Tsunamo. In spite of her round-the-clock care, the improvised (gastric feeding tube) umbilical catheter, her warmth and space foil, he passed away after 4 days. Love surrounded him until the end.

Melioidosis

Melioidosis is a tropical disease [17], known for about 80 years [18], and is caused by *Burkholderia pseudomallei* [19]. This is a widespread environmental saprophyte most common in Southeast Asia but also in parts of Australia and South America [20,21]. Human and animal melioidosis arises through exposure to contaminated soil or muddy water. There was an unusual outbreak in France in the mid-1970s [18]. Bacteremia in melioidosis is associated with high mortality and most patients die early in the course of the disease [22]. Subacute and acute forms of the disease occur [23]. Eighty percent of the children living in Southeast Asia have antibodies by the age of four [19]. In most cases, the inoculation history is unclear or anecdotal, and ranges from near-drowning to insect bites, ingestion, inhalation, laboratory accidents, and person-to-person or animal-to-person spread [19]. The clinical features are varied, most patients present with pyrexia of unknown origin, pneumonia, abscesses or septic arthritis [24,25]. The microorganism can infect any organ system [26,27].

At least 10% of cases present with a chronic respiratory illness that mimics tuberculosis [25] (Fig. 10). Sixty percent of the patients present with septicemia or septic shock. Subacute disease can progress to cause severe systemic multi-organ involvement, which rapidly leads to death [21]. Predisposing conditions such as alcoholism, impaired cellular immunity, pre-existing renal failure, or diabetes mellitus enhance the severity of the disease [17,21,24]. Antibiotic therapy is initial intensive therapy with ceftazidime, meropenem, imepenem, or cotrimoxazole and

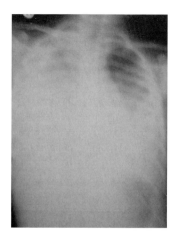

Fig. 10. Chest radiograph of Niswa with melioidosis.

later eradication therapy with doxycycline and chloramphenicol for three months [25].

What next?

Many children admitted by the BMT are still hospitalized; some are still suffering from "tsunami pneumonia," like Firdous or baby X, who is diagnosed with tetralogy of Fallot. As the ocean shifted to the front door of the university hospital, children attacked by venomous sea snakes were admitted to receive serum (Fig. 11). Some children suffered from head trauma because motorcycles are the main mode of transportation. Parents put their children between them while riding the motorcycle; sometimes they move a complete family of four at the same time. Traffic is hectic and the streets are in bad shape. Either the children fall from the vehicle or they are involved in a traffic accident.

The Spanish offered to help for about two weeks and they were incorporated into our working schedule. Once the *HMAS Kanimbla* had arrived, the Australians offered to help too. The helicopters from the *Berlin* and the *Kanimbla* provided us with oxygen, beds, and other medical equipment. Soldiers brought back the children that needed radiographs and the army laboratory technician came over to fetch the blood samples. We had never met such wonderful people. The Sumatran team from Langsa was friendly but seemed inhibited by our presence. After a week, Jakarta teams replaced them and the hospital started to recruit local nurses. The blending of cultures remained problematic, even though Indonesian coordinators had requested it. We had the impression that the Acehnese doctors and nurses did not fully trust our skills, but this was explained later when some anthropological differences were better understood. Historically, children were never examined at the Rumah Sakit Umum (RSU) and the consultation took place in the hospital hallway in the presence of the

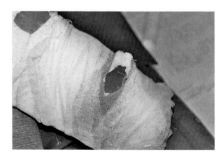

Fig. 11. Little boy admitted with venomous snake bite.

relatives. No blood or bacterial samples were collected. The Acehnese doctors fetched some medication from the pharmacy and the patient returned home. We understood later that physical examination and drawing blood was considered to be professional ignorance. Medical students need to examine and to collect samples. Fqihs or Hodjas do not. And according to the Koran, blood is a source of vitality. So, the Acehnese doctors and nurses believed that Belgium had sent its students or heathens instead of specialists. Maybe we insulted them right from the start.

At night it became clear that the local nursing level of care was different from what we were used to. The staff went away to sleep for six or seven hours and infusions were left unguarded. During the Idul Adha festivities, staff members were not in the area for four days, and left all patients behind in the care of the BMT. The staff did not measure patient temperatures, did not keep patient charts, had no idea of intake and outputs, had no signaling or alarm function, and started their morning shift by sweeping and cleaning the hospital floor. Cats and dogs were tolerated as they entered the pavilions and the patient rooms searching for food. No particular measures were taken to avoid errant animals; half empty dinner plates stayed on the floor and garbage was not discarded.

The Jakarta staff, however, was different. As they monitored our mortality rate, medical and nursing culture, they were convinced that teaching and education should be organized and continued in this area. Every morning at nine o'clock all teams gathered and briefed the hospital administrator and the coordinators from Jakarta. At the beginning there was no such organization, but after a few weeks the Indonesian, Belgian, Australian, German, American, Singaporean, Swiss, French, and Spanish doctors conferred. Different issues were discussed. First, there were too many patients and too many doctors but not enough nurses. The Belgian and French nurses were no longer able to fill in the night shifts, because they were completely exhausted. As a result, the continuity of care was jeopardized. Second, the mission of the hospital was discussed. It had a pediatric ward, an emergency room, two surgical units (Australian and German) and a general ward (Singapore). But it was in great need of an infectious diseases ward, a maternity ward, a pharmacy, a laboratory, a kitchen, and a radiology unit, especially when the Australians ran out of radiograph film. Third, the lack of coordination was discussed. The Sumatran and Indonesian teams (both the nurses and doctors) were replaced every week and this was unanimously considered to be a major problem. And finally, the need for teaching the Acehnese nurses was discussed. The Australian colleagues made one ex-cathedra teaching attempt, and the BMT tried to involve the local nurses and doctors in bedside training. It was clear that they were frightened by our presence, our techniques and how we adapted to unpredicted situations (power failure, absence of IV pumps and medical equipment, PICU charts). For example, a major difference in practice was that at night, they lit candles next to patients receiving oxygen therapy.

BMT 1, 2, and 3 have returned to Belgium. The French replaced them as they offered to take over the mission. Their team 5 has just returned from Banda Aceh with rather disappointing news: the Acehnese do not wish to continue working with them and the French government no longer wishes to support the Zainoel Abidin's mission. March 26 is "rehabilitation day" with subsequent closing of the Aceh borders, but the Indonesian government decided March 14 to agree to a visa extension of two months for those health care workers with unfinished projects. However, on March 26, the police begin to hunt down GAM rebels. In the meantime the home base of the Belgian team is brainstorming, reading, and searching for teaching programs or profiles that would possibly fit the Acehnese. The first priority is to get the teaching project outlined on paper and approved by the Banda Aceh hospital director. BMT 4 has already returned to Banda Aceh but needed to escape to higher ground because on March 28, 2005, a severe earthquake (8.7 on the Richter scale) hit Sumatra again. With an epicenter in the ocean very close to the island of Nias, the world's biggest threat was a rerun of Black Sunday. There were no deadly tsunamis this time, probably the tectonic plates did not buckle or heave. Nevertheless, many residents died under collapsing buildings. Nine of our Australian colleagues perished when their helicopter crashed during a humanitarian mission to Nias.

International pediatric intensive care disaster team

I was shocked to see and hear that children in the scope of a large disaster do not have the same value as an adult. I have never worked anywhere else but in a pediatric ICU in a western hospital, but I tried to understand this point of view. I believe I did. Disaster teams are often emergency or military units and are equipped mainly or solely to help with adult patients. The countries in which the most and recent disasters occurred are countries where many children are born and many die, even without a major disaster. Many times the children are not registered and sometimes they don't even have a name until they have survived measles. This could be a reason why people think and say that pediatric intensive care in such an environment is useless. Eventually the teams were split and equipment was removed. Now we are left with an unanswered question. What if? (Fig. 12).

What if we had enough respirators? What if we had used inotropic support? What if we had more antibiotics or immediate laboratory results? What if we had total parenteral nutrition components to mix, umbilical catheters, and volume expanders? What if we maintained pediatric intensive care until the patients could be transported to ships like the *Berlin* or the *US Mercy*? What if?

Our PICU mindset caused us to see the potential for much work in a disaster area where many caretakers were looking for a job and where even the UN could not provide us with one. There is no such thing as an International Pediatric Intensive Care Disaster Team (IPICDT): a team of specialists who head for every major event in the world to treat and care for

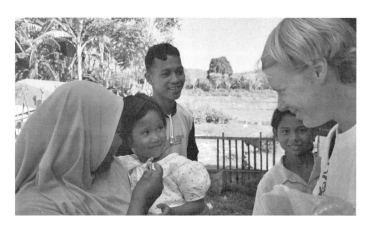

Fig. 12. BMT 3 on mission to Lhoong.

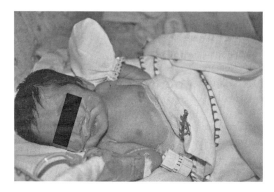

Fig. 13. Looking a dying baby in the eyes.

badly injured or very sick children; a team that could work in the conditions that we did; a team that would be able to provide care in a badly damaged hospital, a refugee camp, or a mobile hospital unit in a military or fire fighter camp.

Banda Aceh is slipping away now, out of the news, briefly browbeaten by Easter Monday's earthquake that targeted Nias. To teach Banda's nurses might be a good project. But other Banda Acehs will follow, some not that spectacular and others even larger.

The BMT is facing a 20% mortality rate in the aftermath of the tsunami, in a hospital where mortality was 80% prior to the tsunami. And yet this rate is unacceptably high, because the BMT arrived on day 16 and because tools were lacking. An earlier arrival and a different mindset might have resulted in a lower mortality rate. The arrival and departure time parameters are probably far more difficult to influence than the mindset. A small IPICDT that aims for a target (acutely ill) pediatric population and is equipped with the right tools should be able to buy time. In Banda Aceh buying time could have been enough to bridge the gap until the arrival of the hospital ships. This would not have saved Mafouta and perhaps not Maulida. But Firda, Niswa, Tsunamo and the others, they never had a real chance (Fig. 13). Disaster teams should focus on surgery, prevention and oral rehydration, even if it benefits only one child's life; that is what disaster managers say. But disaster managers did not look them in the eyes.

I did.

References

[1] http://www.earthquake.usgs.gov.
[2] http://www.neic.usgs.gov/neis/seismology/people/int_richter.html.
[3] http://www.neic.usgs.gov/neis.
[4] http://www.wikimedia.org/wiki/2004_indian_ocean_earthquake.
[5] http://www.en.wikipedia.org/wiki/tsunami.
[6] http://www.cbsnews.com.
[7] http://www.nationalgeographic.com.
[8] http://www.news.yahoo.com/asiadisaster.
[9] http://www.news.bbc.co.uk.
[10] Tsunami. Anatomy of a disaster. BBC March 28, 2005 documentary.
[11] Demick B. Catastrophe's warning signs went unheeded. The Los Angeles Times January 1, 2005.
[12] http://www.earthquake.usgs.gov/eqinthenews/2004/ussjal.
[13] Meek J. From one end to another, Leupung has vanished as if it never existed. The Guardian January 1, 2005.
[14] Sipress A. Not a living soul seen on long trek home. The Washington Post January 1, 2005.
[15] Ein lazarett für Banda Aceh, die Bundeswehr hilft beim Wiederafbau. Reuter archiv 07.01.2005.
[16] Murdoch L. Tent wards go up outside smashed hospital. The Australian January 9, 2005.
[17] Schwarzmaier A, Riezinger-Geppert F, Schober G, et al. Fulminant septic melioidosis after a vacation in Thailand. Wien Klin Wochenschr 2000;112(20):892–5.
[18] Dance DA. Melioidosis: the tip of the iceberg? Clin Microbiol Rev 1991;4(1):52–60.
[19] Dance DA. Ecology of Burholderia pseudomallei and the interactions between environmental Burkholderia spp. and human-animal hosts. Acta Trop 2000;74(2–3):159–68.
[20] Loveleena, Chaudhry R, Dhawan B. Melioidosis; the remarkable imitator: recent perspectives. J Assoc Physicians India 2004;52:417–20.
[21] Tran D, Tan HH. Cutaneous melioidosis. Clin Exp Dermatol 2002;27(4):280–2.
[22] Mukhopadhyay A, Lee KH, Tambyah PA. Bacteraemic melioidosis pneumonia: impact on outcome, clinical and radiological features. J Infect 2004;48(4):334–8.
[23] O'Carroll MR, Kidd TJ, Coulter C, et al. Burholderia pseudomallei: another emerging pathogen in cystic fibrosis. Thorax 2003;58(12):1087–91.
[24] Jesudason MV, Anbarasu A, John TJ. Septicemic melioidosis in a tertiary care hospital in south India. Indian J Med Res 2003;117:119–21.
[25] Currie BJ. Melioidosis: an important cause of pneumonia in residents of and travellers returned from endemic regions. Eur Respir J 2003;22(3):542–50.
[26] Ip M, Osterberg LG, Chau PY, et al. Pulmonary melioidosis. Chest 1995;108(5):1420–4.
[27] http://www.edvos.demon.nl/bahasa-indonesia.

Further readings

Ban lifted, foreign aid workers arrive. The Jakarta Post, December 30, 2004.

http://www.acehnews.com.

http://www.acheh-eye.org.

http://www.asnlf.net.

http://www.encarta.msn.com/encyclopedia.

http://www.en.wikipedia.org/wiki/aceh.

http://www.en.wikipedia.org/wiki/infrasound.

http://www.en.wikipedia.org/wiki/pacinian_corpuscle.

http://www.en.wikipedia.org/wiki/rayleigh_waves.

http://www.gimonca.com.

http://www.heute.de/ZDFheute/inhalt.

http://www.hosted.ap.org.

http://www.hrw.org.

http://www.indonesiaforum.org.

http://www.indonesia-ottawa.org.

http://www.let.leidenuniv.nl.

http://www.members.chello.nl.

http://www.nedindie.nl.

http://www.pro-regenwald.de/new_tsu3.

http://www.singapore.com.

http://www.story.news.yahoo.com.

http://www.tapol.org.

http://www.timesonline.co.uk.

http://www.unesco.bbk.org.

http://www.wrm.org.uy.

Sanders E. (1990) Eponiemen woordenboek. Amsterdam: Nijgh en van Ditmar.

ELSEVIER
SAUNDERS

Crit Care Nurs Clin N Am 17 (2005) 495–510

CRITICAL CARE
NURSING CLINICS
OF NORTH AMERICA

Cumulative Index 2005

Note: Page numbers of article titles are in **boldface** type.

0899-5885/05/$ – see front matter © 2005 Elsevier Inc. All rights reserved.
doi:10.1016/S0899-5885(05)00112-7

ccnursing.theclinics.com

United States Postal Service
Statement of Ownership, Management, and Circulation

1. Publication Title	2. Publication Number	3. Filing Date
Critical Care Nursing Clinics of North America	0 8 9 9 - 5 8 8 5	9/15/05

4. Issue Frequency	5. Number of Issues Published Annually	6. Annual Subscription Price
Mar, Jun, Sep, Dec	4	$100.00

7. Complete Mailing Address of Known Office of Publication (Not printer) (Street, city, county, state, and ZIP+4)

Elsevier Inc.
6277 Sea Harbor Drive
Orlando, FL 32887-4800

Contact Person
Gwen C. Campbell

Telephone
215-239-3685

8. Complete Mailing Address of Headquarters or General Business Office of Publisher (Not printer)

Elsevier Inc., 360 Park Avenue South, New York, NY 10010-1710

9. Full Names and Complete Mailing Addresses of Publisher, Editor, and Managing Editor (Do not leave blank)

Publisher (Name and complete mailing address)

Tim Griswold, Elsevier Inc., 1600 John F. Kennedy Blvd. Suite 1800, Philadelphia, PA 19103-2899

Editor (Name and complete mailing address)

Maria Lorusso, Elsevier Inc., 1600 John F. Kennedy Blvd. Suite 1800, Philadelphia, PA 19103-2899

Managing Editor (Name and complete mailing address)

Heather Cullen, Elsevier Inc., 1600 John F. Kennedy Blvd. Suite 1800, Philadelphia, PA 19103-2899

10. Owner (Do not leave blank. If the publication is owned by a corporation, give the name and address of the corporation immediately followed by the names and addresses of all stockholders owning or holding 1 percent or more of the total amount of stock. If not owned by a corporation, give the names and addresses of the individual owners. If owned by a partnership or other unincorporated firm, give its name and address as well as those of each individual owner. If the publication is published by a nonprofit organization, give its name and address.)

Full Name	Complete Mailing Address
Wholly owned subsidiary of	4520 East-West Highway
Reed/Elsevier Inc., US holdings	Bethesda, MD 20814

11. Known Bondholders, Mortgagees, and Other Security Holders Owning or Holding 1 Percent or More of Total Amount of Bonds, Mortgages, or Other Securities. If none, check box → ☐ None

Full Name	Complete Mailing Address
N/A	

12. Tax Status (For completion by nonprofit organizations authorized to mail at nonprofit rates) (Check one)
The purpose, function, and nonprofit status of this organization and the exempt status for federal income tax purposes:
☐ Has Not Changed During Preceding 12 Months
☐ Has Changed During Preceding 12 Months (Publisher must submit explanation of change with this statement)

(See Instructions on Reverse)

PS Form **3526**, October 1999

13. Publication Title		14. Issue Date for Circulation Data Below
Critical Care Nursing Clinics of North America		June 2005

15.	Extent and Nature of Circulation		Average No. Copies Each Issue During Preceding 12 Months	No. Copies of Single Issue Published Nearest to Filing Date
a.	Total Number of Copies (Net press run)		1850	1800
b. Paid and/or Requested Circulation	(1)	Paid/Requested Outside-County Mail Subscriptions Stated on Form 3541. (Include advertiser's proof and exchange copies)	1273	979
	(2)	Paid In-County Subscriptions Stated on Form 3541 (Include advertiser's proof and exchange copies)		
	(3)	Sales Through Dealers and Carriers, Street Vendors, Counter Sales, and Other Non-USPS Paid Distribution	123	114
	(4)	Other Classes Mailed Through the USPS		
c.	Total Paid and/or Requested Circulation [Sum of 15b. (1), (2), (3), and (4)] ▲		1396	1093
d. Free Distribution by Mail (Samples, complimentary, and other free)	(1)	Outside-County as Stated on Form 3541	62	82
	(2)	In-County as Stated on Form 3541		
	(3)	Other Classes Mailed Through the USPS		
e.	Free Distribution Outside the Mail (Carriers or other means)			
f.	Total Free Distribution (Sum of 15d. and 15e.) ▲		62	82
g.	Total Distribution (Sum of 15c. and 15f) ▲		1458	1175
h.	Copies not Distributed		392	625
i.	Total (Sum of 15g. and h.) ▲		1850	1800
j.	Percent Paid and/or Requested Circulation (15c. divided by 15g. times 100)		96%	93%

16. Publication of Statement of Ownership
☐ Publication required. Will be printed in the **December 2005** issue of this publication.   ☐ Publication not required

17. Signature and Title of Editor, Publisher, Business Manager, or Owner

[signature]   Date 9/15/05
Tim Palucci - Executive Director of Subscription Services

I certify that all information furnished on this form is true and complete. I understand that anyone who furnishes false or misleading information on this form or who omits material or information requested on the form may be subject to criminal sanctions (including fines and imprisonment) and/or civil sanctions (including civil penalties).

Instructions to Publishers

1. Complete and file one copy of this form with your postmaster annually on or before October 1. Keep a copy of the completed form for your records.
2. In cases where the stockholder or security holder is a trustee, include in items 10 and 11 the name of the person or corporation for whom the trustee is acting. Also include the names and addresses of individuals who are stockholders who own or hold 1 percent or more of the total amount of bonds, mortgages, or other securities of the publishing corporation. In item 11, if none, check the box. Use blank sheets if more space is required.
3. Be sure to furnish all circulation information called for in item 15. Free circulation must be shown in items 15d, e, and f.
4. Item 15h., Copies not Distributed, must include (1) newsstand copies originally stated on Form 3541, and returned to the publisher, (2) estimated returns from news agents, and (3), copies for office use, leftovers, spoiled, and all other copies not distributed.
5. If the publication had Periodicals authorization as a general or requester publication, this Statement of Ownership, Management, and Circulation must be published; it must be printed in any issue in October or, if the publication is not published during October, the first issue printed after October.
6. In item 16, indicate the date of the issue in which this Statement of Ownership will be published.
7. Item 17 must be signed.

Failure to file or publish a statement of ownership may lead to suspension of Periodicals authorization.

PS Form **3526**, October 1999 (Reverse)

Changing Your Address?

Make sure your subscription changes too! When you notify us of your new address, you can help make our job easier by including an exact copy of your Clinics label number with your old address (see illustration below.) This number identifies you to our computer system and will speed the processing of your address change. Please be sure this label number accompanies your old address and your corrected address—you can send an old Clinics label with your number on it or just copy it exactly and send it to the address listed below.

We appreciate your help in our attempt to give you continuous coverage. Thank you.

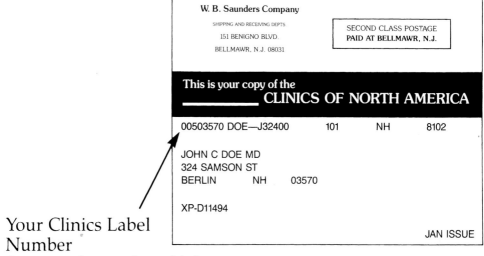

Your Clinics Label Number
Copy it exactly or send your label along with your address to:
W.B. Saunders Company, Customer Service
Orlando, FL 32887-4800
Call Toll Free 1-800-654-2452

Please allow four to six weeks for delivery of new subscriptions and for processing address changes.